The First Miracle Drugs

THE FIRST MIRACLE DRUGS

How the Sulfa Drugs
Transformed Medicine

JOHN E. LESCH

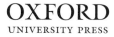
OXFORD
UNIVERSITY PRESS

2007

OXFORD
UNIVERSITY PRESS

Oxford University Press, Inc., publishes works that further
Oxford University's objective of excellence
in research, scholarship, and education.

Oxford   New York
Auckland   Cape Town   Dar es Salaam   Hong Kong   Karachi
Kuala Lumpur   Madrid   Melbourne   Mexico City   Nairobi
New Delhi   Shanghai   Taipei   Toronto

With offices in
Argentina   Austria   Brazil   Chile   Czech Republic   France   Greece
Guatemala   Hungary   Italy   Japan   Poland   Portugal   Singapore
South Korea   Switzerland   Thailand   Turkey   Ukraine   Vietnam

Copyright © 2007 by John E. Lesch

Published by Oxford University Press, Inc.
198 Madison Avenue, New York, New York 10016

www.oup.com

Oxford is a registered trademark of Oxford University Press

Library of Congress Cataloging-in-Publication Data
Lesch, John E. [date]
The first miracle drugs : how the sulfa drugs transformed medicine /
John E. Lesch.
p. ; cm.
Includes bibliographical references and index.
ISBN-13 978-0-19-518775-5
ISBN 0-19-518775-X
1. Sulphonamides—Therapeutic use—History.   2. Antibacterial agents—History.
I. Title.
[DNLM: 1. Sulfonamides—history.   2. Bacterial Infections—drug
therapy.   3. History, 20th Century.   4. Sulfonamides—therapeutic use.
QV 265 L625f 2006]
RM666.S88L47 2006
615'.32938—dc22   2005036136

9   8   7   6   5   4   3   2   1

Printed in the United States of America
on acid-free paper

For Paula

Preface

We live in an age of powerful medicinal drugs. Antibiotics cure or prevent bacterial infections, diuretics and other medicines help to control hypertension, antiretrovirals add years to the lives of those infected with HIV. The list of substances that cure or palliate our ills is very long and getting longer every year. This book is one historian's attempt to understand how we arrived at such a place, which is unprecedented in the long history of medicine and humanity before the twentieth century. I have concluded that the answer lies in the industrialization of science and medicine, and that within this historical process the introduction of the sulfa drugs in the 1930s was the event that did most to set us on our present course.

My path to this conclusion was not a direct one. This book had its origins in reflections on the relationships of industrialization and science that began in graduate school with my reading of Jerome R. Ravetz's *Scientific Knowledge and Its Social Problems*. What did it mean to say that science became industrialized, I wondered, and what were the ramifications and limitations of such a line of analysis? Joined to my prior interest in the relationships of the laboratory sciences and medicine, such questions drew me eventually to the history of medicinal drugs and the pharmaceutical industry. I chose to work on the sulfa drugs because their study promised to allow exploration of issues surrounding industrialization of science and medicine, because their importance seemed out of all proportion to the slight attention they had received in the historical literature, and because it was clear from the very beginning of the project that the crucial role played by research in several national settings would permit, indeed would require, comparative analysis and study of transnational connections in medicine and science. As I moved further into the research and writing, the pivotal role of the sulfa drugs in initiating the modern era of medicinal drugs emerged with increasing clarity.

Little did I know what I was getting into. I am an admirer and sometime reader of Charles Dickens, but never thought of myself as a Dickensian character until I read *David Copperfield* and discovered Dr. Strong. Headmaster of a school that David attends, Dr. Strong works at compiling a dictionary of roots—not, as David at first thinks, of the botanical kind, but rather of the etymological variety. What caught my eye was not the nature of the project, but the pace at which it was prosecuted. Taking note of this, one of Dr. Strong's students does a simple calculation and finds that his dictionary will likely be completed in one thousand six hundred and forty-nine years. While I suspect that, from time to time colleagues, family and friends have performed similar calculations on my book, I am glad to report that it has come in substantially ahead of the figure projected for Dr. Strong.

In the course of this work, I have accumulated many debts (another Dickensian motif?) that I can only begin to acknowledge here. Funding for research, and for the invaluable leaves from teaching that make it possible, has come at different times from the National Science Foundation (SES 81-11985 and SES-8409848), the National Institutes of Health (NIH-R01 LM04231), the John Simon Guggenheim Memorial Foundation, and, on two occasions, University of California–Berkeley Humanities Research Fellowships. I have also benefited from research assistantship support from the Center for German and European Studies at UC Berkeley and from numerous small grants from the UC Berkeley Academic Senate's Committee on Research.

Parts of this book have been published in different form. I am glad to have this occasion to thank the editors Seymour H. Mauskopf, *Chemical Sciences in the Modern World* (University of Pennsylvania Press, 1993), and Gregory J. Higby and Elaine C. Stroud, *The Inside Story of Medicines: A Symposium* (American Institute of the History of Pharmacy, 1997), for invitations to the conferences that gave rise to these books and for their help in bringing my contributions to publication.

This book would not exist without the resources of numerous archives and libraries and the skills and generosity of their staffs. These include, more or less in order of their appearance in the notes, the Alan Mason Chesney Medical Archives of the Johns Hopkins Medical Institutions, with special thanks to Nancy McCall; the Bayer Archive in Leverkusen, Germany, where I was assisted during my visit by Peter Göb, and subsequently by Michael Pohlenz; the Nobel Archives in Stockholm; the Hoover Institution Library in Stanford; and the Archives of the Institut Pasteur, Paris. In London, Malcolm Goodson and Robert J. Moore facilitated my research at the Medical Research Council Archives. At the Royal Society Archives, I was helped by Mary Sampson and Sandra Cumming; at the Wellcome Institute for the History of Medicine, by William F. Bynum; and at the Contemporary Scientific Archives Centres in London and Oxford, by J.G.A. Sheppard and by Margaret Gowing and J.B. Alton, respectively.

My visit to the May & Baker Archives at Rhône-Poulenc-Rorer (now Sanofi-aventis) in Dagenham, United Kingdom, was greatly facilitated by Peter J.T. Morris, who first made me aware of its collections, and by John Salmon (then of Rhône-Poulenc-Rorer), who also helped to put me in touch with individuals who had been involved in research and development on M&B 693. Jeffrey Sturchio helped to arrange my visit to the Merck Archives in Whitehouse Station, New Jersey, where Joe Ciccone and Amber Olterzewski responded readily to my various requests for information and documents. Many people assisted my research at the National Archives in Washington, DC, among them notably John Taylor and George Wagner at the Modern Military Branch. Thanks are due also to Michael G. Rhode at the National Museum of Health and Medicine, Armed Forces Institute of Pathology, Washington, DC, for location of a photograph used in chapter 10. Finally, I am grateful to the staff of the Bodleian Library, Oxford, for their help with the Donald Devereux Woods papers.

I have depended heavily on other libraries, not for archival materials but for their rich collections of published sources and skilled and responsive staffs. Especially important for this project have been the libraries of the University of California–Berkeley, the Lane Medical Library of Stanford University, the Kalmanovitz Library of the University of California–San Francisco, and the National Library of Medicine in Bethesda, Maryland.

The Department of History of the University of California–Berkeley has been a wonderful intellectual environment in which to work, and I am grateful to a succession of chairs of the department for their steady support of this project. No less important has been the intellectual community and material support provided by UC Berkeley's Office for History of Science and Technology. I am especially grateful to its directors, John Heilbron, Roger Hahn, and Cathryn Carson, and its excellent administrator, Diana Wear, for their assistance in a myriad of ways over the years.

Margaret Anderson, John Parascandola, John Swann, and Paula Fass read the whole manuscript of this book in its penultimate version and offered detailed and valuable comments that have made the final version better than it might have been. I have not been able to incorporate all of their suggestions, but I am grateful for their insights and, in several instances, for their corrections of errors. The faults that remain are, of course, entirely my responsibility.

Many others have had a hand in this book, by reading and commenting on parts, by helping to locate sources, or in other ways. Among them are Matthew Bailey, Marcel H. Bickel, Gert Brieger, Glenn Bugos, Adele Clarke, Gerald D. Feldman, Tore Frängsmyr, Robert Frank, Jordan Goodman, Mirko D. Grmek, J.F. Hodgson, Ernest Hook, Thomas P. Hughes, Jeffrey Alan Johnson, Jonathan Liebenau, Patrick Malloy, Maria Mavroudi, Michael Miers, Harry M. Marks, E.W. Parnell, Scott Podolsky, Karen Reeds, Wolfgang Sadee, Arlene Shaner, Judy Slinn, Doreen Strang, Molly Sutphen, Andrew Taylor, R.F.B. Welford, and Christine Woollett.

My thinking on the problems and themes of this book has been developed and sharpened in countless classroom presentations and discussions, and for that I am glad to thank my students. It is something of a cliché in academia that teaching and research should benefit one another. In this case there is no doubt of the fact.

Students have contributed to this project in a more direct way, as research assistants or by helping to enter my longhand drafts on the computer. My thanks go to Jesse Berrett, Renee Coury, Ki Won Han, Marianne Miller, Julia Rechter, Jonna Van Zanten, and Alex Wellerstein. For typing and other crucial tasks, I am also indebted to Department of History staff at different stages of the project, especially Nadine Ghammache and Sherrill Young.

Going from a manuscript to a book is in itself a process of many stages, and I am indebted to the people at Oxford University Press who have made it happen. Special thanks go to Jeffrey House, who first welcomed the manuscript; to my editor, Carrie Pedersen, who managed its progress with diplomacy, skill, and good feeling; to Regan Hofmann, who with energy and tact kept me focused on the task at hand; to my copyeditor, Trish Watson; and to Keith Faivre, who managed the book's production.

More important than anything else has been the support of my family. My daughter Bibi and my son Charlie literally grew up with this project, and their presence has made the journey a wonderful one at every stage. In numerous conversations around the dinner table, Charlie urged me to find ways to make the book more accessible, and Bibi has inspired me with her own enthusiasm for science and medical research. Paula Fass has been there from the beginning, encouraging, admonishing, reading, and criticizing drafts and accommodating my work in many other ways in the midst of our family life and her own very busy career. We have made this trip together, and I gladly dedicate this book to her.

Contents

The First Miracle Drugs

Introduction

On Christmas Day 1932, the German chemical combine I.G. Farbenindustrie filed a patent application on behalf of a red dye that its medical researchers and chemists had found to have a remarkable ability to cure certain kinds of bacterial infections in mice. By the time the patent was awarded just over two years later, the dye, now called by the trade name Prontosil, had been found to have the same curative powers in humans. Announced in a brief publication in a German medical journal in February 1935 by Gerhard Domagk, the medical researcher responsible for the work, Prontosil went on the market and became available to doctors in April 1935.

In retrospect, it is clear that the introduction of Prontosil marked a turning point in the history of medicine. As the first of the compounds called sulfonamides or, more familiarly, sulfa drugs, Prontosil initiated a revolution in the therapeutics and management of bacterial infections. Within a few years, feared diseases such as streptococcal infections (including childbed fever and septicemia), pneumonia, meningitis, dysentery, gonorrhea, and urinary tract infections, were brought under a substantial measure of control by chemotherapy. The medical success of the sulfa drugs gave a powerful impetus to the expansion of the international pharmaceutical industry and of the research and development enterprise within it. The same success contributed heavily to the opening of what was widely referred to as an era of miracle drugs, with its attendant optimism and raised expectations of medicine, accelerated appearance of new medicines as a result of increased levels of research, regulatory dilemmas, and unanticipated therapeutic problems. Finally, the sulfa drugs proved extraordinarily fruitful as starting points for molecular modifications that led to new drugs or classes of drugs not only for bacterial infections (eventually including tuberculosis) but also for leprosy

3

(Hansen's disease), diabetes, hyperthyroidism, gout, heart disease, and hypertension. The reach of research based on the sulfa drugs extended beyond human into veterinary medicine and even to the discovery of new herbicides.

Other writers have used the phrase "therapeutic revolution" to refer to the discontinuity in the history of medicine initiated by the introduction of the sulfa drugs. In this usage, the therapeutic revolution is a compact denotation of an aggregate of events, including rapid expansion of pharmaceutical research, development, and production, that issued a steady and, in quantitative terms, unprecedented flow of new medicines onto the market and into medical practice, a flow that has continued from the late 1930s to our own day and that has transformed the practice of medicine.[1]

If the sulfa drugs were the first act of the therapeutic revolution, they were also a culminating event in a larger historical process stretching back to the 1880s, which may be called the industrialization of pharmaceutical innovation. Behind this process was the rise of a fine chemicals industry (that is, one that manufactures products such as dyes, pharmaceuticals, and photographic products) based on synthetic coal tar chemistry beginning in the 1860s, especially in Germany, and the industrialization of invention within this industry between 1880 and 1914.

For all human history until the 1880s, medicines had been derived almost exclusively from natural products, plant, animal, or mineral. Among these sources, plant extracts were by far the most important. The first great medical achievement of analytical organic chemistry in the nineteenth century was the isolation of active principles of plants, including morphine from opium and quinine from cinchona bark, and their characterization as members of a new chemical class, the alkaloids.[2]

With rapid development of analytical, synthetic, and structural organic chemistry in the middle decades of the nineteenth century, chemists moved beyond isolation of natural products to their synthesis. More important, they began to recognize the potential medical usefulness of organic compounds prepared in the laboratory. A crucial turning point came in the 1880s, with the realization by German chemists that certain coal tar derivatives have powerful fever- and pain-reducing properties. One of these compounds, phenacetin, introduced in 1887, was manufactured by the German fine chemicals company Bayer and found widespread use in medicine. Recognition of the pharmaceutical potential of coal tar derivatives, joined with increasing industrial connections to academic organic chemistry and legal and economic incentives for diversification, propelled companies such as Bayer, which were already in possession of extensive knowledge of coal tar chemistry through work on synthetic dyes, into pharmaceutical research. One of the important early products of the Bayer pharmaceutical laboratories, established in the 1890s, was acetylsalicylic acid, marketed in 1899 under the trade name Aspirin.[3]

The same decades that saw the establishment of research within the German fine chemicals industry also witnessed spectacular developments in bacteriology and the germ theory of disease. By the early 1900s, microbial parasites had been associated with more than a score of serious human and animal diseases. Synthetic organic chemistry and the germ theory were joined in Paul Ehrlich's program for chemotherapy, which aimed to identify compounds that would destroy infectious organisms without harming the host, and in the 1910s the German chemical industry took another major step by incorporating Ehrlich's research program into its own pharmaceutical research effort. From 1900 through the 1920s, a variety of new medicines came out of German industrial pharmaceutical research, including barbiturates, local anesthetics such as Novocain, the sleeping sickness medicine Bayer 205 (Germanin), and the antimalarial Atabrine.[4]

Meanwhile, France, Britain, and the United States lagged behind in building up industrial research and development in pharmaceuticals. The 1914–1918 war shocked other countries into recognition of their dependence on Germany for imports of fine chemicals, including drugs. In the 1920s and 1930s, efforts were made in France, Britain, and the United States to develop synthetic organic chemicals manufacturing and industrial, or industry-linked, pharmaceutical research. In areas of drug innovation that were not so dependent on medicinal chemistry in the sense of molecular synthesis and molecular modification, but rather on the isolation, purification, and chemical and physiological characterization of naturally occurring compounds such as hormones and vitamins, much important work was done outside of Germany between 1900 and 1935. In many cases, the development of such research for medical and commercial purposes entailed academic–industrial cooperation and stimulated expansion of industrial–pharmaceutical research. By the late 1930s, when the sulfa drugs arrived on the scene, the beginnings of industrial pharmaceutical research and the links of such research to academic science were in place in France, Britain, and the United States, although none of the these countries could yet challenge German leadership in medicinal chemistry.[5]

This situation was transformed first by the response of French, British, and U.S. industry to Prontosil and its effective component, sulfanilamide, and then by a new World War. The sulfa drugs helped to spark an expansion of pharmaceutical production and research and development that began before World War II and that was accelerated by it. The war removed German pharmaceutical manufacturing and research from serious competition, at least until postwar recovery began. The result was the emergence after the war of a larger and more truly international pharmaceutical industry in which the United States had replaced Germany in a leading position.[6]

The sulfa drugs therefore stand at a pivotal moment in the history of twentieth-century medicine. They are at once the culminating event of the first major phase of the industrialization of pharmaceutical innovation, and the initial event of the second great phase of that process, the therapeutic revolution that continues in our time.

Those who witnessed the introduction of the sulfa drugs into medicine recognized that a major break with the past was under way. One of the earliest attempts at an appraisal was made by F. Sherwood Taylor, whose book *The Conquest of Bacteria: From Salvarsan to Sulphapyridine* appeared during the war in 1942. Writing for a lay audience, Taylor presented the sulfa drugs as the triumphal outcome of long research based on Ehrlich's program and ultimately on the bacteriology and synthetic organic chemistry of the late nineteenth century. Looking to the future,

he called for more substantial public support of research in chemotherapy. Also
written for a general audience, although in this case by a physician, Iago Galdston's *Behind the Sulfa Drugs: A Short History of Chemotherapy* (1943) presented the sulfa drugs as the "crowning achievement" of curative medicine, with
antecedents much like those described by Taylor.[7]

Neither Taylor nor Galdston mentioned penicillin, which was the object of a
crash wartime Anglo-American development project when their books appeared.
By the time that American medical researcher Boris Sokoloff published *The Miracle Drugs* in 1949, again for a general audience, the sense of dramatic change
persisted, but its content had been reshaped to take into account penicillin and
other antibiotics, substances with powerful antibacterial action that, unlike the
sulfa drugs, were derived in the first instance from living organisms. Sulfa drugs
still counted as miracle drugs in Sokoloff's account, but his book allotted them a
relatively small proportion of its pages and included information on toxicity and
bacterial resistance.[8]

For the most part, those who wrote on the sulfa drugs in the 1930s and 1940s,
including Taylor, Galdston, and Sokoloff, focused on their importance as antibacterial agents and their role in reviving interest in chemotherapy. As penicillin and
other antibiotics displaced sulfa drugs from news headlines and medical practice,
popular awareness of the historical role of the sulfa drugs in initiating a new era in
medicine receded. Nevertheless, by the late 1950s and 1960s, it was clear to some
observers more intimately familiar with pharmaceutical research that the importance of the sulfa drugs extended well beyond the chemotherapy of bacterial infections. By the 1960s, chemists and medical researchers, often working in
industrial laboratories enlarged or created in part because of the earlier success of
the sulfa drugs and exploiting knowledge or insights gained in research on the
sulfa drugs, had employed molecular modification to develop new drugs or
classes of drugs for a variety of diseases and conditions most of which were not
infectious. Among the most articulate commentators on these developments was
Max Tishler, who served as director of the Merck, Sharp & Dohme Laboratories
from 1957 to 1969 and president of the American Chemical Society in 1972, and
who reflected on the recent history of medicinal chemistry in a series of papers
and talks in the late 1950s and 1960s.[9]

By the 1980s, perceptive writers on the history of medicinal drugs began to
describe the sulfa drugs as the leading edge of what was increasingly seen as a
wider therapeutic revolution embracing bacterial chemotherapy, antibiotics, and
the many other new kinds of drugs that followed, but also rapid expansion of
pharmaceutical production and research, new precision manufacturing methods,
and new drug evaluation and regulatory problems.[10]

In 1988, Daniel Bovet, a Nobel laureate in Physiology or Medicine for work
on synthetic curares and antiallergy medicines, and himself a participant in a crucial early episode in the development of the sulfa drugs, published *Une chimie qui
guérit: histoire de la découverte des sulfamides (A Healing Chemistry: History of
the Discovery of the Sulfonamides)*. This wide-ranging, informative, and often
engaging study did justice to the international character of the sulfa drugs story,
with discussions of developments in France, Germany, Britain, the United States,

and Switzerland and of cross-national influences. On a number of points, Bovet departed from conventional accounts, for example, in his emphasis on the role of the chemists in comparison to the medical researchers in the collaborative work that resulted in the early sulfa drugs, and in his revision of usual descriptions of research at the Pasteur Institute in Paris based on his own participation in events. Above all, Bovet called for recognition of the historical and medical importance of the sulfa drugs and greater public appreciation of the complex and difficult research behind the achievements of modern therapeutics.[11]

In the same year that Bovet's book appeared, Marcel H. Bickel, a pharmacologist and medical historian, published a concise overview of the history of the sulfa drugs that emphasized both their role in effecting "a true revolution of chemotherapy" and some of their principal consequences for drug research and pharmacology. He subsequently explored the latter topic in more detail in the context of his study of Johns Hopkins pharmacologist Eli Kennerly Marshall, Jr.[12]

Since Bovet's and Bickel's overviews, other historians have examined facets of the sulfa drugs story. Several of these studies have brought out the ways in which the introduction of the sulfa drugs directly or indirectly played a role in the passage, content, and implementation of the landmark U.S. Food, Drug, and Cosmetic Act of 1938. Other work has examined the reception of the sulfa drugs in the United States prior to U.S. entry into World War II, emphasizing changes in the chemical and pharmaceutical industries and in the attitudes of physicians and patients.[13]

In spite of these valuable efforts, the pivotal role of the sulfa drugs in the history of twentieth-century medicine is not yet sufficiently appreciated by historians or by the wider circles of those interested in medicinal drugs, including the vast majority of the public who make use of them. My aim in this study is to build upon existing scholarship, to extend and revise it with new research and interpretation, and above all, to show how the development of the sulfa drugs resulted from the long process of the industrialization of pharmaceutical innovation and at the same time effected a significant change in the direction of medicine.

My perspective is primarily that of a historian of science and medicine interested in the process of innovation in medicinal drugs. I emphasize the development and study of sulfa drugs by researchers and physicians and the crucial role of industrial research. My perspective is also international. The story of the sulfa drugs cannot be confined within national boundaries, and one of its advantages as a historical subject is the opportunity it presents for national comparisons and for study of the cross-national traffic of ideas, research programs, and people.

I have selected for detailed examination some of the more important episodes in the history of the sulfa drugs, but I am aware that the path I have taken is not the only way to approach the sulfa drugs story. Scholarship in the history of medicine has emphasized the need to examine medical innovations at the level of day-to-day therapeutic practice or from what John Harley Warner has called the therapeutic perspective. The sulfa drugs offer a wide field for such investigations, but one that I have not entered except incidentally in this book. Other aspects of the story, including the technology and engineering dimensions of manufacturing processes; the business and commercial problems of finance, marketing, and distribution; and the economic impact of the new drugs, also invite closer scrutiny by historians. I hope that the present study, by underlining the importance of the sulfa drugs for twentieth-century medicine, will encourage historians to take up these and other problems.[14]

This book has three parts. Part I, "The Industrial Origins of Prontosil," shows that an industrial research setting was crucial to the success of chemotherapy. It examines the background of the first sulfa drug in Paul Ehrlich's program for chemotherapy and in the embedding of chemotherapeutic research in an industrial research organization, that of Bayer and I.G. Farbenindustrie. Efforts to enact Ehrlich's program in nonindustrial institutional settings often met with limited success or failure. This is illustrated by the vogue for mercurachrome, an antiseptic developed at Hugh Hampton Young's Brady Urological Institute at Johns Hopkins and touted by Young as a chemotherapy for bacterial infections. The failure of mercurachrome suggests the limitations of U.S. institutional arrangements for chemotherapeutic research in the 1920s and places in relief the strengths of the I.G. Farben organization. Prominent among these strengths was the institutionalization of an interdisciplinary approach to research that associated medical researchers and chemists in long-term collaborative work, supported by the vision of research managers who were not averse to risk. Prontosil emerged from such an industrial research program.

Part II, "The Making of the First Miracle Drugs," shows how differences in national political and institutional circumstances shaped the reception of the first sulfa drugs and the ways in which the initial discoveries were extended in new research. It traces the reception of Prontosil, the recognition of sulfanilamide as its effective component, and the beginnings of the development of other sulfa drugs in the late 1930s. The break with the past effected by the introduction of the sulfa drugs was not immediate but was spread out over several years. The transition also occurred differently in different countries.

In the case of Germany, the coincidence of the introduction of Prontosil and the further development of the sulfa drugs with the Third Reich and World War II means that the stories of the sulfa drugs and their makers provide one window on the fate of science and medicine under National Socialism. At the same time as it continued its research and development efforts, the I.G. Farben establishment came under multiple pressures from the National Socialist regime and related organizations.

One of the first challenges came from the German antivivisectionist movement, which made a determined effort to end the use of animals in I.G. Farben pharmaceutical research by harnessing antisemitic and ultranationalist ideologies in harsh attacks on the chemical combine. The regime's programs of autarky and rearmament were felt in the I.G. Farben pharmaceutical research establishment in the form of secrecy rules imposed on research results and compulsory participation in weapons development. Hitler's decree forbidding Germans to accept Nobel Prizes resulted in jail time and subsequent Gestapo surveillance for Gerhard Domagk, I.G. Farben's leading medical researcher on the sulfa drugs. Finally, the war brought attrition of staff, materials shortages, and subordination of research to war production. These challenges were met by Heinrich Hörlein, leader of I.G. Farben's pharmaceutical research, with a mixture of combativeness and accommodation that aimed to preserve the organization he had built.

Through all of this, and despite a significant measure of hostility to scientific medicine within the National Socialist movement, the sulfa drugs were widely accepted by German doctors, and their production and use on a substantial scale continued through World War II.

Outside of Germany, in France, Britain, and the United States, medical researchers, physicians, and the public recognized the importance of the new medicines by the middle of 1937, but the path to recognition was markedly different in each case. Comparison of these three national settings reveals important differences in the closeness with which pharmaceutical developments in Germany were followed, the degree of skepticism greeting claims for new drugs in general and those from Germany in particular, procedures for evaluating new drugs, relations between the medical community and the pharmaceutical industry, the status of foreign (in this case, German) patent law, and the roles of professional and popular media in publicizing and creating demand for new medicines.

General recognition of the medical and commercial value of Prontosil and sulfanilamide touched off an international competition in the pharmaceutical industry to discover and market derivatives of sulfanilamide that would be effective in treatment of infections not influenced by the first two sulfa drugs, or that would carry less risk to the patient. By the mid-1940s, some 5,000 sulfonamide derivatives had been synthesized, and a small fraction of these had made their way onto the market and into medical practice. Much of this work was done in industrial laboratories.

The first major success of this effort came with the introduction of sulfapyridine (or M&B 693) in 1938 by the British company May & Baker. Of outstanding medical importance as the first effective chemotherapy for pneumonia, sulfapyridine also merits closer study as a product of industrial innovation typical of the generation of sulfa drugs that followed Prontosil and sulfanilamide. Although initially received with reservations by some medical researchers, especially in the United States, sulfapyridine found a strong positive response among physicians, stimulated in part by enthusiastic coverage in newspapers and other media. In the United States, sulfapyridine was the first important new drug to be reviewed under the U.S. Food, Drug, and Cosmetic Act of 1938. Its medical and commercial success encouraged British and American pharmaceutical manufacturers to expand their research and development establishments, an undertaking that began well before U.S. entry into World War II.

By the early 1940s, the sulfa drugs were in wide use, but researchers were just beginning to understand how they worked. Part III, "Practice and Theory," documents the substantial impact of the sulfa drugs on the American war effort. It also shows how researchers finally arrived at a successful theory of their mechanism of action and how that theory in turn became a basis for discovery of new medicinal drugs in the 1940s and 1950s.

Sulfa drugs were used extensively in treatment of casualties at Pearl Harbor, and physicians credited them with the minimal morbidity and mortality from infection among the wounded in that attack. U.S. preparation for wartime production and use of the sulfa drugs began long before Pearl Harbor, however, and that circumstance enabled a rapid deployment of the medicines in the months that followed American entry into the war. In parallel with preparations for production and use came large-scale U.S. government–sponsored organization of medical research, including research on the sulfa drugs, that continued for the duration of the war.

During the war, the U.S. military used sulfa drugs in treatment or prophylaxis of a variety of diseases and conditions, including pneumonia, gonorrhea, meningitis, bacillary dysentery, hemolytic streptococcal infections, and wounds and burns. In addition to control of bacterial infections in the wounded, sulfa drugs also contributed to the saving of millions of man-hours of active service that would otherwise have been lost to gonorrheal infections, to the prevention of epidemics that might otherwise have disrupted large-scale mobilization by the U.S. Navy in the middle of the war, and to control of dysentery in field conditions where good sanitation was difficult or impossible.

It was in the context of extensive use of sulfa drugs by the U.S. military during the war that bacterial resistance to chemotherapeutic agents first emerged as a serious problem. U.S. government–sponsored wartime research on the sulfa drugs eventually led to changes in the ways the medicines were used by doctors, although for the most part these changes took effect only after the war. Finally, this study shows that penicillin, introduced into military medicine relatively late in the war, entered a field of practice already occupied by the sulfa drugs and tended to supplement rather than to replace the older medicines.

The sulfa drugs were in widespread use in medicine for years before any consensus emerged in the medical and scientific community as to how they worked, that is, their mechanism of action. By the mid-1940s, such a consensus did develop around a theory proposed in 1940 by British bacteriologist Paul Fildes and British biochemist Donald D. Woods. Joining to the work of other investigators elements from their own training and research backgrounds, Woods and Fildes concluded that sulfanilamide and, by extension, other sulfa drugs acted by competing with and displacing a compound utilized by a bacterial enzyme to produce a needed nutrient. Unable to grow or reproduce, pathogenic bacteria were then destroyed by the defenses of the human or animal host. Fildes generalized this result by suggesting that other antibacterial agents could be found by identifying compounds similar in structure to substances needed by the bacterial cell and that would therefore competitively inhibit the cell's use of the needed substance.

By the mid-1940s, other investigators had further generalized Fildes's formulation beyond the realm of bacteria in the concept of antimetabolite, defined as a substance that interfered with the action of an essential metabolite in a living cell. The antimetabolite concept inspired a number of efforts at rational drug design from the 1940s to the 1960s. None of these resulted in medicines of stature comparable to that of the sulfa drugs, but notable successes with drugs for treatment of leukemia and of tuberculosis and other bacterial infections demonstrated the long-term value of the approach.

Even after they had been relegated to secondary status in the therapeutics of bacterial infections by penicillin and other antibiotics, the sulfa drugs continued to give impetus to pharmaceutical innovation not only through application of the antimetabolite concept but also through the direct or indirect roles that they played in the development of other new drugs and classes of drugs.

By the 1950s, the therapeutic revolution that the introduction of the sulfa drugs had done so much to initiate was in full swing. With the flow of new medicines, and in part precisely because of their number and power, came also a rising awareness of their costs and limitations. Criticisms and reassessments of the more extravagant hopes and expectations of the age of miracle drugs began to emerge. An early cloud on the horizon was the appearance of bacterial resistance to sulfa drugs, then to antibiotics, a problem accentuated by overuse and indiscriminate use of the medicines. Close behind followed recognition of widespread iatrogenic illness associated with recently introduced drugs, or what American physician Robert H. Moser pointedly described as "diseases of medical progress." Most fundamental, perhaps, was Rene Dubos's critique of medical utopias associated with recent successes of scientific medicine. Dubos, a prominent microbiologist at the Rockefeller Institute in New York, rejected the notion that medicine would ever be able to eliminate all disease, or even necessarily reduce the overall burden of disease carried by human societies.[15]

By 1981, when physicians began to puzzle over the first cases of what would later be termed AIDS, even strong partisans of the therapeutic revolution had come to recognize that it had problems and limitations. The unfolding of the AIDS pandemic in the decades since has driven home that recognition, as has increasing public awareness of problems such as bacterial resistance to antibiotics and the sometimes fatal consequences of medical error, including misuse of powerful medicinal drugs.

In the enormity of its impact, its complexity, and its human costs, the AIDS pandemic is unmatched in its challenge to late twentieth- and early twenty-first-century medicine. Despite the best efforts of the world's biomedical researchers, as of this writing there is no cure and no vaccine. Nothing has been more revealing of the insufficiency of a narrowly biomedical model of disease, that is, one that focuses exclusively on the identification of specific therapies for specific biologically defined pathologies. As a disease, AIDS has been incomprehensible except as an entity with demographic, political, cultural, and economic dimensions as well as biological ones. Attempts to come to grips with it have reinforced increasingly holistic understandings of disease and underlined the need for multifaceted preventive efforts.[16]

All of this said, it cannot be denied that the AIDS pandemic has also thrown into relief the continuing strength of the premises that have driven the therapeutic revolution. Underlying the AIDS activist movement of the 1980s and 1990s was the conviction that the disease is caused by a specific virus and that a specific therapy could and would be found if only the right resources (scientific, clinical, organizational, financial) were marshaled in the right way. Sustained by this view, AIDS activists effected important changes in the U.S. system for developing and approving new drugs.[17] The ongoing search for more effective drugs and vaccines and efforts to improve the delivery of existing drugs to affected populations at manageable costs remain prominent components of the worldwide struggle with AIDS.

The therapeutic revolution started by the sulfa drugs continues. The idea that one important task of medicine is to find specific therapies for specific diseases is alive and well and is periodically reinforced by the perceived promise of new lines of investigation, such as those opened by the human genome project and stem cell research. Medicinal drugs comprise a significant fraction of the American health care system and are likely to do so in the future. The pharmaceutical industry continues to lead innovation, even as it is challenged for its contribution to the financial burden of health care. We need to come to terms with this ongoing revolution in all its promise, complexity, limitations, and costs. Part of the insight we need will surely come from historical understanding of the medicines that first set us on this path.

PART I

The Industrial Origins of Prontosil

CHAPTER 1

Beginnings

In 1913, Paul Ehrlich stood before an audience of the Seventeenth International Medical Congress in London and predicted substantial progress in the chemotherapy of bacterial diseases within the next five years. His optimism was based in part on confidence that the combined efforts of many researchers would be bent to the task. The principle of *viribus unitis* (with united forces) was happily borne out, he said, by the international congress where thousands, gathered "from all countries of the world, have come to bear witness that in science all boundaries between nations have fallen."[1]

In the short run, at least, neither form of optimism proved justified. Within months of Ehrlich's speech, the nations of Europe had embarked on a long and terrible war that would weaken or efface the internationalism of science. Achievement of an effective bacterial chemotherapy was to require not five years but more than two decades. Yet Ehrlich's talk gave voice to a burst of optimism and activity in chemotherapy in the years before and after World War I that his own work both exemplified and had a powerful role in creating. In another speech seven years earlier, at the inauguration of his Institute for Experimental Therapy in Frankfurt, Ehrlich had introduced the term "chemotherapy" to stand for the destruction of disease-causing microorganisms in the human or animal host by means of chemical compounds introduced into the host organism. Ehrlich's persuasive formulation of the theoretical basis of chemotherapy, derived in part from earlier work in biological staining and immunology (for the latter he received the Nobel Prize in Physiology or Medicine for 1908), and still more his striking practical success with the introduction of Salvarsan and Neosalvarsan against syphilis in 1910 and after, played a major role in the initiation of other research in the next two decades. Early successes were scored with the finding of chemotherapies for diseases caused by spirochetes, such as syphilis, and for others caused by protozoans, such as leishmaniasis (kala-azar) and trypanosomiasis (sleeping sickness).[2]

The chemotherapy that Ehrlich held up as the promise of the future was born of the confluence of two great historical movements of the half century before the first World War. One of these, the bacteriological revolution in medicine, transformed scientific understanding of the causation of many diseases by associating them with specific microbial parasites, including certain species of bacteria or protozoa and the vectors (e.g., insects) that carried them to their human hosts. The other, the rise of a hugely successful fine chemicals industry based on synthetic organic chemistry, brought with it not only vast numbers of new chemicals not found in nature, with multiplying uses as dyestuffs, pharmaceuticals, and other products, but also, and more important, the appearance of some of the first industrial research laboratories.

By the early 1900s, the newly defined field of infectious diseases loomed as a major challenge facing Western societies and their colonies. In the three decades between 1875 and 1906 alone, investigations including and following on the pioneering work of Louis Pasteur in France and Robert Koch in Germany identified causative agents for more than a score of diseases. Among these were such major scourges as typhoid fever, malaria, tuberculosis, cholera, diphtheria, pneumonia, plague, bacillary dysentery, sleeping sickness, and syphilis.[3]

Despite public health measures and rapidly advancing knowledge in bacteriology and related fields, bacterial infections still took a heavy toll in lives and health. The ten most significant causes of death in the United States in 1900 included pneumonia, tuberculosis, infections of the gastrointestinal tract, and diphtheria, all of them caused by bacteria, which together accounted for more than a third of all deaths in the American population.[4]

Pneumonia, to take only one example, was described by Johns Hopkins professor William Osler in the 1899 edition of his authoritative *The Principles and Practice of Medicine* as "the most widespread and the most fatal of all acute diseases" and second only to tuberculosis as a cause of death in the United States. Hospital statistics indicated a mortality for pneumonia of between twenty and forty percent. In patients sixty or more years of age, mortality ranged from sixty to eighty percent, leading Osler to remark that "in this country at least . . . one may say that to die of pneumonia is the natural end of old people." Possible complications of pneumonia, especially meningitis (an infection of the membranes enclosing the brain and spinal cord) and endocarditis (an infection of the membrane lining the heart), increased the danger still further.[5]

In the face of these threats, there was little that physicians could do for patients beyond provision of good nursing care and appropriate diet. As Osler put it, "pneumonia is a self-limited disease, which can neither be aborted nor cut short by any known means at our command." He gave his readers a skeptical survey of various measures then in use in treatment of pneumonia patients, including bleeding, drugs, serum ("still in the trial stage"), and methods for symptomatic relief. But he warned that "the young practitioner may bear in mind that patients are more often damaged than helped by the promiscuous drugging, which is still only too prevalent."[6]

Knowledge of microbial agents did not in itself affect these facts. It did bring sharply into focus the paths that practical measures might take. In the domain of prevention, public health could look beyond filth, miasmas, and bad water to more precise targets, microbial pathogens and their vectors. Vaccines could be developed to maximize resistance to specific infective agents. In therapeutics, surgeons could apply antisepsis and asepsis, opening up new fields for surgical practice. Medical researchers could develop serums or antitoxins based on immune reactions of animals and humans to specific microbes. Finally, researchers could imagine the creation of a chemotherapy in which molecules prepared in the laboratory could attack infecting microbes without serious harm to their human hosts.[7]

For the emergence of chemotherapy, the prior development of synthetic organic chemistry and of the industry based on it was decisive. Rapid growth of organic chemical analysis early in the nineteenth century made possible the appearance of structural and synthetic organic chemistry after the mid-nineteenth century. After William Perkin's introduction of the first synthetic dye, aniline purple (mauve) in 1856, strong worldwide demand drove the expansion of synthetic dyestuff synthesis and manufacture, especially in Germany, from the 1860s to 1914. By the beginning of the twentieth century, thousands of dyes, and extensive expertise in dye chemistry, were available to researchers.[8]

Connections between the new synthetic dye chemistry and medical research began early. By the 1870s, microscopists were using dyes to develop improved techniques for staining tissues and cells. In the 1880s, researchers in the chemical industry realized that some synthetic dyes, or the intermediate compounds used to prepare them, had medicinal qualities. Interest in chemical therapies for microbial infections spurred research at the founding centers of bacteriology, the Pasteur Institute in Paris and Robert Koch's Institute for Infectious Diseases in Berlin.

Ehrlich and Chemotherapy

It was Paul Ehrlich who, in this context, most clearly grasped the historical opportunity and who most clearly defined a program for chemotherapy. Born in comfortable circumstances in Upper Silesia in 1854, Ehrlich followed his Gymnasium education with study of medicine at several universities, finally taking his medical degree at Leipzig in 1878. After nearly a decade of service as physician at the Charité Hospital in Berlin, and two years in Egypt recovering from a bout of tuberculosis, Ehrlich returned to Berlin and accepted a position at Koch's Institute. There he helped Emil von Behring develop effective therapeutic serums, especially the new diphtheria antitoxin.[9] Serums, or antitoxins, were prepared by extracting the liquid part of the blood, or serum, from animals inoculated with a specific bacterium. This serum contained antibodies produced by the animal in response to the infection and could be used to treat humans infected with the same type of bacterium, a kind of therapy called passive immunization.

In 1896, recognizing Ehrlich's skill in devising methods to test serums, the Prussian government made him director of its new Institute for the Investigation

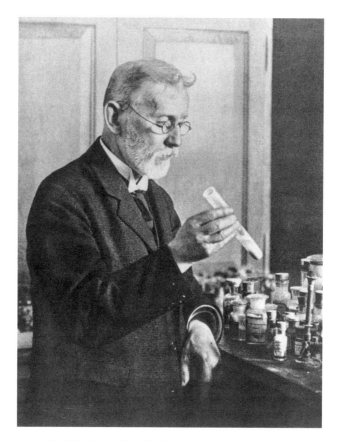

Figure 1.1. Paul Ehrlich (1854–1915) in his laboratory (© Bettman/Corbis).

and Control of Sera. In 1899 this institute, with Ehrlich still in charge, was transferred to Frankfurt-am-Main. Finally, in 1906, Ehrlich became director of a second institute, set up beside the Serum Institute with private funds and devoted to research in chemotherapy.[10]

From the time that he completed his M.D. thesis on the theory and practice of histological staining in 1878 to the end of his career, Ehrlich's research was closely bound up with the new synthetic dyes and their selective affinities for living tissues. Taken in one direction, this interest led him to develop new staining techniques such as those he applied to a definitive classification of white blood cells. Taken in another direction, the same interest led him to reflect on the therapeutic potential of dyes. He had shown, for example, that methylene blue selectively stained cells of the peripheral nervous system. Would it also alleviate pain associated with those nerves? Therapeutic experience confirmed that it did have such an effect, although a temporary one.[11]

Ehrlich further reasoned that, just as with dye compounds, where part of the molecule attaches to the substance to be dyed while another part is responsible for the color, so too with therapeutic compounds: one part will attach to a specific tissue while another part is responsible for the therapeutic effect. Applying this concept to the problem of parasitic infection, Ehrlich reasoned that the goal should be to identify a compound with a selective affinity for the parasite but not for the cells of the host. To this compound should then be attached a toxic component that would kill or disable the parasite. Such a compound, *prepared in the laboratory* and administered in the right way, should *disinfect* the host organism by eliminating the parasites. In Ehrlich's memorable phrase, it would be a "magic bullet" in the same sense as those substances (antibodies) produced by the natural process of immunization, that is, compounds that selectively seek out and destroy the parasites.[12]

Ehrlich's first major effort along these lines focused on diseases caused by trypanosomes. Among these was sleeping sickness, which devastated large areas of central Africa. Alphonse Laveran in France had opened the way to chemotherapeutic research by showing how to create and maintain experimental trypanosome infections in mice. Now, Ehrlich and his collaborator, Japanese physician Kiyoshi Shiga, vied with Pasteur Institute researchers in Paris to find effective compounds to treat such infections. Both research teams tested hundreds of synthetic dyes, with Ehrlich relying heavily on help from dye chemist Arthur Weinberg, and the Pasteur Institute investigators drawing on the resources of the Bayer chemical company. Beginning in 1904, both teams reported promising results, with trypan red the best compound from Ehrlich's laboratory. Although neither group produced a cure for sleeping sickness, Ehrlich judged that even the limited successes achieved by 1906 "should encourage us to continue, without deviation, along this path."[13]

As it happened, Ehrlich was prompted to deviate from his path by a report from the Liverpool School of Tropical Medicine that atoxyl, an organic arsenic compound, was more effective than inorganic arsenic in the treatment of trypanosomal infections. Ehrlich set his chemists to synthesis of organic arsenicals, and they soon produced hundreds. Two of these, numbered 418 and 606, seemed especially promising.[14]

Meanwhile, Ehrlich's attention had been drawn to syphilis, for which the causative organism, a spirochete, had been discovered in 1905 by German zoologist Fritz Schaudinn. Schaudinn's opinion that the spirochete was related not to bacteria but to trypanosomes led Ehrlich to test his organic arsenical compounds against syphilis. Fortunately for this endeavor, an animal experimental model for syphilis had already been developed by Sahachiro Hata, a Japanese bacteriologist who joined Ehrlich's laboratory in 1909. Subjecting Ehrlich's compounds to tests on experimental infections in rabbits, Hata found that compound 606 was highly active.[15]

Ehrlich devoted the next few years, until his death in 1915, to the development of compound 606 into an effective chemotherapy for syphilis. Marketed in 1910 by the German chemical company Höchst under the trade name Salvarsan, compound 606 (also known as arsphenamine), transformed the treatment of syphilis. Although plagued by problems of toxicity and difficult to administer, Salvarsan and the related compound Neosalvarsan represented the first clear practical triumph of chemotherapy.[16]

Behind the fervent optimism of Ehrlich's 1913 speech, therefore, lay a theoretical formulation of the rational basis of chemotherapy and a practical research program that had already achieved notable successes. To these Ehrlich added a broad historical appreciation of changes in medicine since the 1860s that highlighted the potential role and opportunities of chemotherapy.

Looking at the sweep of medical history since the 1860s, Ehrlich easily discerned a broad pattern of advance. Isolation of pathogenic bacteria; study of protozoa; discovery of filterable viruses; recognition of insects as intermediate hosts and transmitters of disease; study of immunity, antitoxins, immunology, and sera; and the development of new diagnostic tests all contributed to an increasingly effective prevention, control, and therapy of infectious diseases. The place of chemotherapy was, wherever possible, to "fill gaps in the lines of attack, particularly, by curing diseases in which the natural powers of the body are inadequate." Since, to Ehrlich's mind, the scientific foundations of chemotherapy were in place, he felt confident in asserting that "the way lies in full view before us, a way which will not at all times be easy to follow, but which, nevertheless, it will be possible to follow."[17]

The chemotherapy of bacterial infections proved even more difficult and elusive than Ehrlich had predicted. By the end of the war, the five-year mark set in Ehrlich's optimistic 1913 prediction had come and gone without a major breakthrough in bacterial chemotherapy. If Ehrlich's hopes had not yet been realized, the urgency of the problem and belief in the possibility of a solution persisted, and the 1920s opened with ample evidence of international response to his program and example. In the minds of many leaders in relevant fields of biomedical science, the question was not whether there would be a chemotherapy of bacterial disease, but when and through what mix of research organization, theory, models, and methods it would be accomplished.

The Vogue for Mercurachrome

The felt need, the optimism, and equally, the limitations of chemotherapeutic investigation in the 1920s are well exemplified by the vogue for mercurachrome that rose, peaked, and fell within the space of a decade. Its initiator was Hugh Hampton Young, a surgeon who had joined the faculty of the Johns Hopkins University Medical School in 1898, after coming to Johns Hopkins for postgraduate work in 1895. Young was an innovator in the surgery of the genitourinary system, and in the 1910s was in the early stage of a career that would bring him fame as a founder of urology as a medical specialty. In that career, chemotherapy played a small but noteworthy part.

Young was in the audience when Ehrlich spoke on chemotherapy to the International Medical Congress in London in 1913. He later remarked, "I returned to America greatly impressed by the magnitude of Ehrlich's researches, and the remarkable character of his results inspired me to add to the Brady Urological Institute, then in the course of construction, a laboratory for chemical investigation."[18]

Creation of the Brady Institute, to which Young added facilities for chemotherapeutic research, was an episode in the flow of private wealth into scientific medicine in the United States in the decades around 1900. In 1912, Young had operated on James Buchanan (Diamond Jim) Brady for a urinary obstruction caused by a chronically enlarged prostate. The flamboyant Brady had been turned away by other doctors because of complications: he had, among other things, diabetes, Bright's disease (nephritis), infection of both kidneys, inflammation of the bladder, and severe heart disease, from which he later died. Surgeons in New York and Boston had told him that an operation would kill him. Young successfully removed the obstruction with a new instrument he had invented, without need for the general anesthesia that concerned others he had consulted. Brady was enormously relieved and grateful, though he continued to suffer from his other conditions and remained a patient of Young's until his death in April 1917.[19]

Reflecting on the vast sums Brady had spent—and in Young's view squandered—backing plays, actors, and actresses and on lavish entertainments, it occurred to Young that the fortune of the Standard Steel Car Company's head of sales might more profitably be employed elsewhere. Since soon after his arrival at Johns Hopkins in 1895, Young had been developing the field of urological surgery, initially at the prompting and with the support of William Halsted. By 1911, Young had become convinced of the need for special research facilities in urology, not only to extend urological surgery but also to devise new diagnostic methods and laboratory tests. In that year, he had drawn up plans "with the firm conviction that someone could be persuaded to erect a building for this purpose." That someone was now before him in the person of Brady. Young's pitch proved persuasive, and the James Buchanan Brady Urological Institute was dedicated on the grounds of the Johns Hopkins Hospital on May 4, 1915.[20]

Young's firm intention to integrate research and practice in urology was embodied in the design of the building. The institute's eight floors formed a sandwich, with research facilities at top and bottom enclosing clinics and patient rooms in between.[21]

The dual mission of the institute was reflected in its bifurcation of staff into clinical and research divisions. A good part of what made the institute special in Young's eyes was its nature as a "complete unit for a special subject," namely, urology. In this sense, it was an institutional embodiment of this new field of medicine. Henry Wade, a visiting English surgeon, agreed, calling Young's creation "undoubtedly . . . the most complete Institute of Urology that exists in any part of the world."[22]

Even before the institute was built, Young, moved by Ehrlich's ideas and example, had begun his own search for effective urinary tract antiseptics, and this work had brought him into a cooperative relationship with the Baltimore-based pharmaceutical company of Hynson, Westcott, and Dunning.[23]

A strong supporter of American entry into the war, Young quickly volunteered his services. In May 1917, General John Pershing commissioned him as a major in the American Expeditionary Force Medical Corps, and Young sailed with Pershing to France. In July, Young was put in charge of all urological and venereal disease work in the expeditionary force, with the official title of Director of the Division of Urology. He played a leading role in organizing the force's programs for control and treatment of venereal disease. In 1918 he was promoted to colonel, and in

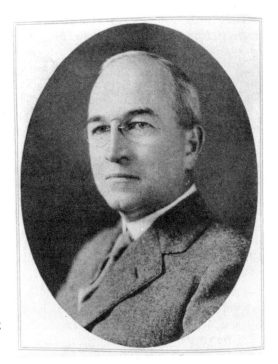

Figure 1.2. Hugh Hampton Young (1870–1945) c. 1918 (*Munsey's Magazine*).

1919 he received the Distinguished Service Medal. Along the way, he co-authored *The Manual of Military Urology*. For the duration of the war, Young set aside a yearly civilian income that ranged from $100,000 to $250,000.[24]

The war gave fresh urgency to the problem of urinary tract antisepsis as the incidence of venereal disease rose and with it the need for prophylactic and therapeutic measures. Young later recalled that his wartime experience reinforced his conviction of the value of antiseptic therapy and of the search for new compounds. After the war, Young's institute continued to focus on preparation and testing of compounds as possible new urinary tract antiseptics.[25]

In notes for a 1920 report on Brady Institute research activities, Young highlighted the institute's development of a new compound called mercurachrome-220, "for use in gonorrhea, chancroid, and other infections of the urinary tract and elsewhere." The steps leading to mercurachrome-220 provide a window on the nature of chemotherapeutic research at the Brady Urological Institute.[26]

Young and his collaborators laid down six criteria to be met by a compound destined for local use as a urinary antiseptic. It should readily penetrate the tissues in which the infection existed, be nonirritating to the tissues, have high germicidal activity, be readily soluble in water, not precipitate in urine, and be of sufficiently low toxicity to be harmless if absorbed into the system.[27]

To satisfy the first criterion, the researchers decided to seek a penetrating dye. The substance did not need to be a germicide itself, but merely to serve "as a carrier in which a germicidal group could be substituted." Citing both clinical experience and chemical reasoning indicating that basic dyes were more irritating to tissues than acid ones, Young and associates narrowed their search to acid dyes. Among these, eosin was attractive because of its use as a cytoplasmic stain. Chemical scrutiny, however, revealed that the sites on the molecule where substitution might occur were already occupied by bromine. The researchers found that the same was not true of the closely related compound dibromofluorescein, which "could undergo substitution by the germicidal group we chose" while retaining much of the staining power of eosin.[28]

As the "active germicidal principle to be substituted in the dye molecule," Young and his collaborators chose mercury. If the long history of mercury as a specific agent against syphilis played any role in this choice, it was not revealed here. Instead, the researchers referred exclusively to general antiseptics. They viewed the inorganic salts of mercury as highly irritating, toxic, and probably of low ability to penetrate tissues. Substituted in an organic compound, however, the metal generally lost much of its irritating quality and toxicity while preserving the greater part of its germicidal power. The collaborators thought that these traits, together with the great variety of possible combinations, made organic mercury compounds promising candidates in the search for local antiseptics of the genitourinary tract.[29]

Edwin C. White, who had joined the Brady Institute in 1916 as full-time chemist, prepared some 265 compounds. Of these, only three (nos. 205, 220, and 253) were considered by Young, White, and Swartz to merit further testing. One of these, number 220, stood out in test-tube, animal, and, eventually, clinical trials. It was a deep red dye obtained by substituting one atom of mercury in the molecule of dibromofluorescein. For the benefit of clinicians, the Brady Institute team set aside the unwieldy chemical name, dibromooxymercuryfluorescein, replacing it with the generic term mercurachrome-220, reflecting the series number of the compound. Eventually the number was also dropped, and the trade name became mercurachrome.[30]

In early clinical use, Young and his associates found mercurachrome to be an effective antiseptic for local use in the genitourinary tract. They did not seek to use it in systemic bacterial infections. By Young's later account, it was the failed experiment of a Philadelphia physician that provoked the Brady Institute team to try intravenous use of mercurachrome. Dr. Edmund D. Piper had tried to save the life of a woman suffering from puerperal septicemia (childbed fever) with intravenous injections of one percent mercurachrome. He had failed in this and four other cases. Hoping for greater success with increased dosages, he had visited Young in Baltimore.[31]

On December 30, 1922, a man was admitted to Young's clinic complaining of pain in the kidney. Young introduced a catheter into the ureters, finding pus on both sides. The man developed a chill and fever, his temperature rising to 103.4°F. On January 2, he was irrational, with continued high temperature, and a blood culture showed a high concentration of colon bacilli. Consultations confirmed the diagnosis of general septicemia, and Young and his colleagues estimated that the man had four hours to live. In this desperate circumstance, Young decided to try intravenous mercurachrome. After the patient received 34 cc of a one percent solution in an arm vein, his temperature first rose to 104 degrees, but then fell to normal within six hours. By the following morning, Young reported, the man's condition was "completely transformed," and he said that he felt quite well. Blood and urine cultures were found to be sterile and remained so, and the patient was well and discharged six days later. "In this case," Young remarked, "which was the first positive demonstration of the value of mercurachrome as an intravenous germicide against septicemia and urinary infection, the research, which had been commenced six years before, in an effort to produce a new urinary germicide, was concluded."[32]

A number of other successful cases followed, and in October 1923 Young made his first public report on the intravenous use of mercurachrome at a meeting of the New York Medical Society in Buffalo. The following year, Young and a colleague, the bacteriologist Justina H. Hill, published a paper in the *Journal of the American Medical Association* (*JAMA*) recommending use of intravenous mercurachrome in both local infections and general septicemias. In October 1924, Young spoke to the Academy of Medicine of Cleveland, Ohio, summarizing 255 clinical cases in which mercurachrome had been used intravenously. The examples were collected from the Brady clinic, personal communications from other physicians, and a handful of published cases.[33]

Surveying the array of clinical cases, Young seemed to waver between slightly abashed recognition that there was still little he could say with certainty about the therapeutic value of mercurachrome, and a barely restrained enthusiasm. He admitted that all intravenous medication required great care, that mercurachrome could produce violent reactions, that mercurachrome could not be effective without help from the body's defenses, that mercurachrome therapy frankly failed in many cases, and that in many others it could not positively be credited with the recovery. "In therapeutics," he conceded, "it is so easy to confound propter hoc with post hoc and also so easy, in the enthusiasm of a new idea, to view facts in a biased way that the exact truth is difficult to get." Nevertheless, by his most cautious reading of the evidence, he believed that mercurachrome had "cured or contributed largely to the cure" of an astonishing variety of conditions, including twenty-five cases of septicemia, two of meningitis, two of epidemic encephalitis, twelve of pneumonia, one of general peritonitis, one of retroperitoneal and one of perinephritic abscess, four of erysipelas (a skin infection), and one of furunculosis (boils). He thought its use in venereal infections to be "most promising." "Making every allowance," he concluded, "I believe I can safely say that [mercurachrome] has already saved many lives, and has assisted the body's defences in throwing off grave local and general infections. Intravenous therapy does not supplant surgery, but it may be of vast assistance and turn the tide for the patient."[34]

The tone of Young's speeches and publications on mercurachrome is expansive and leaves the impression that in the mid-1920s many physicians were using, or at least trying, the compound in a variety of conditions. Young himself later called the work with mercurachrome "the first important effort to apply Ehrlich's principles of chemotherapy." Such a statement reveals an ignorance of the chemotherapy literature of the 1910s and early 1920s, and perhaps also a misapprehension of Ehrlich's principles. By 1913 Ehrlich was moving away from the general antiseptic model and was emphasizing the search for specific therapies. Young's whole program, in contrast, was emphatically an embodiment and extension of the general antiseptic model. He referred to the general antiseptics mercuric chloride and mercuric cyanide in describing his decision to use mercury as the toxic element in the organic compounds he had synthesized. He called mercurachrome a "germicide" (i.e., a topical or local antiseptic) even after it was being used to treat systemic infections. Most important, in his presentation of the many different pathological conditions for which mercurachrome treatment might be effective, there was no trace of a recognition that chemotherapeutic agents were typically, or even occasionally, specific in their action.[35]

Young and his team did not rely on correlation between *in vitro* (test-tube) tests and therapeutic effectiveness. They carried out test-tube and animal tests—the latter mostly to assess toxicity—but gave these little weight in the assessment of new compounds. Instead, they tried out mercurachrome in a more-or-less hit-and-miss way in clinical practice. They did not do controlled studies, either did not report failures or discounted them, and drew freely on the testimonials of other physicians. On this basis, Young was willing to draw tentative but sweeping conclusions. "In many cases it is difficult to interpret the clinical results," he noted, "and the skeptical will decide that nature cured them while enthusiasts, like myself, may attribute it to mercurachrome." Even later, when evidence accumulated against the effectiveness of mercurachrome, Young persisted. He was still using it in 1942, seven years after the introduction of the sulfa drugs. Led on by his enthusiasm, Young established an early commanding lead over his evidence, and never lost it.[36]

The emphasis Young placed on clinical case reports, versus *in vitro* and especially animal trials, was in part a consequence of the aims and structure of the Brady Institute. Young's overriding purpose, perhaps best expressed in the first issue of the *Journal of Urology*, was to build a new medical specialty. The work of the journal and the institute was to bring together contributions of whatever sort to urology as a specialized field. Chemotherapeutic research was a part, but only one part, of the larger project. The Brady Institute seems to have embodied in microcosm the Johns Hopkins ideal, combining medical teaching, clinical practice, and research, in close proximity and interaction. Of the three, clinical practice and, to a lesser extent, clinical research dominated both architectural space and action. The same aims and distribution of resources explain the institute's nearly exclusive concentration of effort on organic mercury compounds against urological and related general infections. The institute's goal was to find an efficient antiseptic for the genitourinary tract. Mercurachrome appeared to be such a compound. In addition, it seemed to have the unexpected virtue of working against many systemic infections. Young and his colleagues did not envision or put into practice a long-term research effort to examine other groups of compounds in other kinds of infections. They established no system of innovation in chemotherapy. With mercurachrome in hand, and within the framework of goals they had set, they felt no need for one.[37]

Concentration on mercurachrome was also reinforced by the institute's perennial shortage of research funds. Small and uncertain budgets prevented the expansion of chemotherapeutic research much beyond the handful of mercurial compounds from which mercurachrome emerged. At the same time, the need to show dramatic results to attract and retain private support led Young and his staff into inflated hopes for mercurachrome and its promotion beyond what could reasonably be justified by laboratory and clinical results.

In 1934, Young wrote to a correspondent that, despite the institute's excellent design and facilities, it had "never had sufficient funds for research, and for maintenance of the laboratories." The problem was there from the beginning. James Buchanan Brady's annual contribution during his lifetime fell far short of expenses, and a promised increase in the endowment that would solve the problem was never written into his will. Young struggled to make up the difference by contributions from his private income and by soliciting donations from grateful patients and philanthropic sources. Young put it candidly when he wrote that "we have faced yearly the necessity of begging and borrowing and going into our own pockets to continue the active work in our laboratories and clinical departments. Being poor—as compared with richly endowed institutions—has made us work harder to produce more in order to impress philanthropic men with the value of our work."[38]

One of the men whom Young struggled to impress was Francis P. Garvan. A millionaire and Yale graduate, described by one source as "a positive, intense, short stocky man, a resolute, aggressive fighter," Garvan had worked in the office of the Alien Property Custodian during the war. There he had become acutely aware of the strategic importance of the synthetic dye industry and of previous U.S. dependence on German industry for its products, which could include high explosives and poison gases as well as dyes. The death of one of his children from rheumatic fever brought home to him in addition the connection between synthetic dyes and medicines. In a statement prepared in defense of U.S. protective tariffs on coal tar chemicals, Garvan later wrote that "the American coal tar chemical industry is indispensable to the health, the prosperity and the national defense of the American people. Coal tar dyes are indispensable also in research into the cause, prevention, and cure of human diseases." Garvan concluded his statement by quoting Julius Stieglitz, a University of Chicago chemistry professor who had chaired the National Research Council's Committee on Synthetic Drugs during the war. "The pitiful calls from our hospitals for anesthetics to alleviate suffering on the operating table, the frantic appeals for the hypnotic that soothes the epileptic and staves off seizure, the almost furious demands for remedy after remedy, that came in the early years of the war, are still ringing in the ears of many of us," Stieglitz had written.[39]

At the end of the war, Garvan set up the Chemical Foundation, a semipublic organization, with himself as president and stockholder. Acting as Alien Property Custodian, he arranged for some 4,500 German chemical patents to be sold to the Chemical Foundation for the low price of $250,000. Personal gain was not a motive, for Garvan and his associates drew no salary and received no dividends from their stock, which conferred only voting privileges. Their aim was to prevent both the return of the patents to Germany and their direct acquisition by American private interests that might create a monopoly. Instead, the Chemical Foundation leased patent rights to any American chemical manufacturer, in the hope that a thriving and competitive American chemical industry would emerge. Royalties

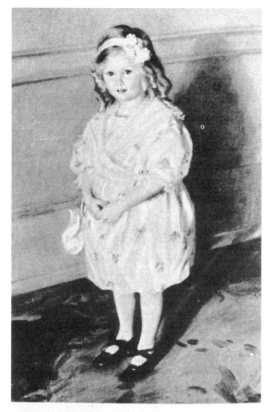

MAY THE MEMORY OF LOST CHILDREN URGE US ON

Figure 1.3. Portrait of Patricia Garvan. Her death from rheumatic fever helped motivate her father, Francis P. Garvan, to found the Chemical Foundation to promote the expansion of the American chemical industry. Frontispiece to *Chemistry in Medicine: A Cooperative Treatise Intended to Give Examples of Progress Made in Medicine with the Aid of Chemistry* (New York: Chemical Foundation, 1928).

from lease of the patents were directed by the foundation into chemical and medical research.[40]

By early 1925, Hugh Young had met with Garvan on several occasions, describing the Brady Institute's work on antiseptics and warmly praising the Chemical Foundation's efforts on behalf of American chemistry and pharmacology. Contacts continued through the spring and summer. In June, Young submitted a report on the institute's current research and, on the basis of this, received in October the first quarterly installment of an annual subvention of $10,000 from the foundation. Acknowledging the check, Young wrote to William Buffum, the foundation secretary, that "it lifts a load of anxiety which was bearing us down and will enable us to continue work which I hope will be even more successful in the immediate future than in the past."[41]

Chemical Foundation support, though welcome, placed Brady Institute research under a spotlight and lent new urgency to the push for tangible results. The foundation required occasional reports, which Young supplied. When, in 1928, his report was delayed because of his wife's and his own illnesses, foundation funding was temporarily suspended. On at least two occasions, foundation contacts brought invitations for Young to speak to chemical industry and professional chemical groups. Young's rising reputation as American representative of chemotherapy is reflected in Charles H. Herty's letter inviting Young to speak to the Synthetic Organic Chemical Manufacturers Association of the United States in 1926. Herty was "very anxious that at this meeting which brings together so many representatives of this industry there should be presented the all-important subject of the contribution that chemistry can make in the further advancement of medicine." Young seemed the obvious choice. "We all feel," Herty continued, "that you better than any other man in the country can speak on this subject with authority and in a manner which will not only inspire those who hear you but will reach a wider field through the press and thus serve to concentrate public thought on this subject which is so intimately bound up with the good of the nation."[42] Between 1925 and 1930, the year when Chemical Foundation support ceased, a firm association existed, at least in Young's mind, between the success of mercurachrome and the continuing flow of checks from the foundation. Also keenly interested in mercurachrome's fortunes was the Baltimore pharmaceuticals firm of Hynson, Westcott, and Dunning, which manufactured the drug and with which Young had a close cooperative relationship based on mutual interest.

From 1925, Young became aggressive in his advocacy of mercurachrome in both local and intravenous treatment of a variety of bacterial infections. He chafed at criticism and impatiently awaited general recognition of the drug's value by the medical profession. Acknowledging receipt of a Chemical Foundation check, Young wrote to William Buffum in 1927 that,

> as you know, we have had great difficulty in getting this work across to the medical profession, which is very skeptical, and requires a continuous stream of papers, and hundreds of experimental and clinical cases before they will admit new and fundamental truths of great value, but our day of justification is rapidly approaching, and I think we will undoubtedly get the recognition which this work deserves.

In case Buffum had missed the point, Young made it explicit: "In the meantime," he concluded, "the continued assistance of the Chemical Foundation is of the greatest value; in fact without it we would have to greatly curtail our work."[43]

At least through the end of 1930, Young worked closely with Hynson, Westcott, and Dunning to supply samples of mercurachrome, and literature on its use, to interested practitioners. To Young, each letter, reprint, or sample sent out was a shot fired on behalf of wider recognition of mercurachrome.[44]

Hostile fire was not lacking. In December 1927, for example, Young wrote to H.A.B. Dunning complaining of an item in *JAMA*. In reply to a doctor's inquiry, a member of the journal's editorial staff had advised against intravenous use of mercurachrome in gonorrhea because of risk of kidney damage. "What in the devil is the matter with these people?" Young exploded. "Why do they take this attitude when all of us know it is absolutely untrue and has proved to be many times?" Young urged Dunning in reply to take a full page in the journal to present "all the facts in the literature of intravenous therapy with mercurachrome." In 1928, Young worked closely with Hynson, Westcott, and Dunning and with an independent investigator favorable to mercurachrome, W. Dandridge Reddish, to confront criticisms of the drug that again appeared in *JAMA*. This time the critic was a Major Simmons. Reddish, urged on and advised by the company and by Young, arranged with the *JAMA* editor, Morris Fishbein, to publish a reply to Simmons alongside the latter's article.[45]

At least through the end of 1929, Young's hopes for mercurachrome and efforts on its behalf continued unabated. He wrote to William duPont about the latter's use of intravenous mercurachrome in veterinary cases and, perhaps with visions of financial support in mind, invited duPont to visit the institute. He tried to persuade his former student John W. Churchman, now a professor of experimental therapeutics at Cornell University Medical College, to come to Baltimore to inspect the institute's records on mercurachrome and to include the information in a book Churchman was writing on synthetic dyes. When phenolsulfonphthalein and mercurachrome were used to treat the King of England, Young discreetly but eagerly sought to get all details of the case. For all that, there is a plaintive note in Young's remark to H.A.B. Dunning about the same time: " '*per aspera ad astra.*' Sometime we will get our work recognized by all the medical profession."[46]

The general recognition that Young sought for mercurachrome never came. By the early 1930s, his efforts in this direction had been defeated by the dual blows of a precipitous decline in institute research funds brought on by the Depression and accumulating criticism of mercurachrome from medical and scientific sources. Chemical Foundation support ceased in 1930.

After 1930, the Brady Urological Institute continued to use mercurachrome both as a topical antiseptic and in intravenous treatment of bacterial infections. The institute's scarce research money ceased to flow into chemotherapy, however, and little new work was done. In a list of sixty-nine publications by Young and other institute staff that appeared between 1934 and 1939, only one included mercurachrome in the title, and that referred to its use as topical antiseptic. No new compounds were synthesized and tried. By 1937, institute staff were experimenting with sulfanilamide in the treatment of gonorrhea, but that, like other sulfa drugs soon to follow, came to the institute from other sources. The days of the Brady Urological Institute as a site for the development of new chemotherapeutic agents had passed.[47]

Mercurachrome in Decline

How many physicians made use of mercurachrome in their practices is not known. What is certain is that already by the mid-1920s Young's work was being criticized, at least implicitly, by researchers whose aims were to develop rigorous methods for the evaluation of new chemotherapeutic agents and, if possible, to establish a rational basis for chemotherapy. These investigators shared Young's optimism and sense of urgency regarding bacterial chemotherapy, his appeal to Ehrlich as an inspiration and model, and his focus on mercury dyestuffs, including, but not exclusively, mercurachrome. Where they differed from Young and his associates was in the priority they gave to methods of evaluation and fundamental principles over clinical applications, the emphasis they placed on controlled animal experiments and attention to biomedical variables, and their embrace of concepts of specific or semispecific action.

In April 1925, George W. Raiziss, M. Severac, and John C. Moetsch discussed their work on bacterial chemotherapy using mercury dyestuffs before the American Chemical Society's Section on Chemistry of Medicinal Products. The speakers held positions at the Dermatological Research Laboratories in Philadelphia, which was part of the pharmaceuticals company Abbott Laboratories. Raiziss and his associates noted the intense interest of chemists and physicians in bacterial chemotherapy. They pointed out that a decade of effort by chemists, pharmacologists, and physicians had produced hundreds of new compounds, some of which "gave rise to great hopes and were used extensively in medicine only to be abandoned because of their toxic effects upon the patient or disappointing curative results." Yet the need was, if anything, more urgent, since, as the speakers pointed out, serum therapy appeared to have "exhausted its efforts in an attempt to combat such diseases as tuberculosis, pneumonia, and various types of septicemia." The speakers saw a basis for optimism in the successes of trypanosomal and spirochetal chemotherapy but viewed bacterial infections as more difficult targets, perhaps because they were "in most cases acute, causing greater amount of damage to the vital functions of the body."[48]

Raiziss and his associates were convinced that the path out of the uncertainty and failure that had prevailed so far lay in controlled animal trials. They gave close attention to choice of type of bacteria, its virulence, the quantity of the bacteria to be injected, and timing of administration of the compound. Partly with the Brady Institute work in mind, they selected four compounds for comparison: mercurachrome, metaphen (synthesized by the authors), benzurin (benzuchrome), and a compound called simply preparation number 565. They established experimental infections of *Staphylococcus aureus* in white rats and rabbits. A key variable in their tests turned out to be the timing of administration of the compound. At first they treated rabbits one, two, or three hours after infection. The result was that treated animals died even earlier than controls. Puzzled, Raiziss and his colleagues delayed administration until forty-eight or seventy-two hours after infection. Although at a loss to explain the much more favorable results obtained through the delay, they welcomed the finding because the greater interval between infection and treatment seemed to better approximate clinical conditions. They speculated that the delay occurred because the drugs acted not directly on the microorganisms, but indirectly through "mobilization of immune bodies."[49]

Summarizing their results in a table, Raiziss and his colleagues concluded that organic mercury compounds did increase the chances of survival of experimentally infected animals. Of the four tested, they said, benzurin appeared the most promising in therapeutic efficacy and to have lower toxicity than mercurachrome.

Since mercurachrome had "sometimes been employed in the treatment of patients suffering from streptococcic and staphylococcic septicemia," they recommended extended clinical trials for benzurin.[50]

More directly critical of Young's claims were Ernest Linwood Walker and Marion A. Sweeney, collaborators in chemotherapeutic research at the University of California Medical School in San Francisco. In work published in 1926 and 1927, Walker and Sweeney lamented the uncertainty surrounding recent therapeutic claims for mercurachrome and other compounds. Noting that "the indiscriminate intravenous use of these substances has become prevalent in clinical medicine," they pointed out that little weight could be given to the "favorable and even enthusiastic" reports so far made of them. They allowed that "single patients or small groups of patients, suffering from local or general infections with staphylococci, streptococci, gonococci, colon bacilli, or what not, have been treated and recovered," but pointed out that whether these recoveries were "in consequence or in spite of the treatment, it is impossible to say in absence of controls or larger series of cases."[51]

Walker and Sweeney saw two ways out of the impasse. The first was to make a fresh evaluation of the main chemotherapeutic agents currently in use against bacterial infections. To do so, they needed to establish standard methods of testing compounds against experimental bacterial infections, methods that could then be applied to any future compound. In their view, components of such a standard testing procedure would have to include choice of experimental animal, choice of pathogenic bacteria, standardization of the virulence of the bacteria, characterization of chemical compounds used and their sources (e.g., pharmaceutical companies), and methods of infecting experimental animals. In this case, the compounds they tested were ones that had come into clinical use during or just after the war: acriflavine, gentian violet, and mercurachrome. Walker and Sweeney chose the mouse as their experimental animal, and among the pathogenic bacteria they used was *Streptococcus pyogenes hemolyticus*. They specified as their source of mercurachrome the Baltimore firm of Hynson, Westcott, and Dunning, which also supplied the Brady Institute. Walker and Sweeney emphasized the gulf that separated *in vitro* tests and animal trials, pointing out that many compounds found to be germicidal in the test tube failed entirely in infected animals. At the same time, while they acknowledged the difference between mice and men, they held that tests on mice did bear comparison with intravenous treatment of human infections and, in any case, provided the best available methods for comparing the chemotherapeutic action of different compounds.[52]

On the basis of their controlled experiments, Walker and Sweeney were willing to give qualified endorsement to therapeutic use of acriflavine, gentian violet, and mercurachrome. The qualifications, however, were substantial. Chief among these was that each substance was "more or less specific in its chemotherapeutic action." Gentian violet acted only against staphylococcal infections. Mercurachrome was more effective in streptococcal than in staphylococcal infections. Acriflavine was more effective in staphylococcal than in streptococcal infections. Also telling against claims made for the three compounds was that none appeared to act more than feebly unless brought into direct contact with the pathogenic bacteria.

That is, the substance had to be introduced into the body at or near the site of infection. Walker and Sweeney allowed only a weak action of mercurachrome against streptococcal infections when the compound was introduced intravenously, as suggested by Young and his associates.[53]

Evaluation of mercurachrome and other compounds was, for Walker and Sweeney, a means to an end. Part of their purpose was, as mentioned above, to establish rigorous methods of evaluation for new chemotherapeutic agents. Even more was at stake. Chemotherapy had been empirical. It needed to become rational, to be based on fundamental principles. Thus, the second path they offered out of the impasse of bacterial chemotherapy was "to establish so far as possible the relation between chemical constitution and therapeutic action, in order that research might proceed in a scientific manner."[54]

The problem, they thought, could be approached analytically or synthetically. That is, investigators could start with compounds already in use in chemotherapy and try to determine what it was about their chemical makeup that made them work. Or researchers could begin with a relatively simple molecule and study the therapeutic consequences of variations in its constituents or structure. Walker and Sweeney chose the latter course, laying down the requirement that the simple compound chosen "be capable of extensive chemical modification without destruction of its fundamental structure and that it contain a definite bactericidal group." As their starting molecule, Walker and Sweeney chose the benzene ring, with an atom of mercury substituted for one of the carbons. They produced variations on this mercurated benzene by substituting other elements or radicals for other carbons on the ring or by joining other elements or radicals to the mercury. They held the mercury content constant in the various derivatives, with the mercury present in preparations given to experimental animals measured by reference to mercuric chloride as unity. They made their tests on mice infected with a standardized fatal dose of *Staphylococcus aureus* following the procedures developed in their evaluation of mercurachrome and other compounds.[55]

Walker and Sweeney gauged the effectiveness of each compound they tested by percentages of animals saved. In a first series of trials, they brought the compound being tested into direct contact with the bacteria by injecting a single dose into the peritoneum of the mouse immediately after intraperitoneal infection. From these trials, they concluded that chemotherapeutic activity depended "not only upon the chemical groups introduced into the ring, but also upon the relative positions of these groups to one another and to the mercury in the ring." They realized that the value of these conclusions was limited, however, by the lack of correspondence between experimental conditions and the conditions of practical chemotherapy. In clinical conditions, the action of a compound was often blocked by organotrophism, which Walker and Sweeney defined as "any action or condition in the animal body that tends to divert the chemotherapeutical from the invading microorganisms." Such conditions might include, for example, "slow absorption of the chemical, failure to penetrate the foci of infection, fixation of the tissues, decomposition into inactive substances, or rapid excretion from the body." A second set of trials of the same compounds began to address this problem by following intraperitoneal infection of the mice by subcutaneous administration of each compound, so that contact between bacteria and chemical agent could be achieved only via the bloodstream. As they had expected, these trials showed a dramatic drop in therapeutic action for the compounds tested, compared with the first series.[56]

Recognizing that development of effective chemotherapeutic agents required a combination of low toxicity with therapeutic action, Walker and Sweeney conducted a separate set of trials in which healthy mice received intraperitoneal injections of the same mercuribenzene derivatives. Their findings pointed to a complex relationship between toxicity and chemical constitution.[57]

Walker and Sweeney concluded that two chemical factors were principally involved in the action of organic mercurial compounds on staphylococcal infections. One of these was the bactericidal mercury group, or toxophore; the other, the therapeutic-action–enhancing or chemophore groups in other positions in the benzene ring. Referring to similar studies of other kinds of infections that they intended to publish later, Walker and Sweeney ventured that while a toxophore group, like mercury, might be effective against all bacterial infections, the chemophore groups appeared to be more or less specific for each type of infection. This conclusion, if true, would be of fundamental importance, for it "would render any attempt to prepare a panchemotherapeutical for bacterial infections futile." It meant that "a chemotherapeutic treatment for the various bacterial infections, if such be possible, must be developed for each independently." It also told against the view, prevalent in the 1920s, that chemotherapeutic agents acted indirectly by stimulation of the body's defenses rather than directly on specific kinds of bacteria.[58]

Raiziss and colleagues and Walker and Sweeney were not alone in their reservations about mercurachrome or in their call for more rigorous standards of research in chemotherapy. The spectrum of expert opinion on both sides of the Atlantic in the late 1920s and early 1930s ran from cautious endorsement of mercurachrome as a local or topical antiseptic, through suspended judgment pending further investigation, to outright dismissal. Possibly with the vogue for mercurachrome in mind, the author of a major American textbook on chemotherapy complained in 1926 that,

> unfortunately, many investigators, probably the majority, have not systematized their work or stuck long enough to any one group of compounds to permit them to study these fundamental relations, a feverish desire to evolve remedies of striking properties quite generally preventing the less spectacular, but nevertheless highly desirable, systematic studies devoted to a painstaking and persistent study of chemical constitution in relation to toxicity and parasiticidal activity and employing the simplest biological methods in order to render all tests strictly comparative with the minimum of experimental error, which will permit the influence of minor alterations in chemical constitution to be properly evaluated.[59]

In an article published in the Chemical Foundation's volume *Chemistry and Medicine* (1928), and intended to paint a bright future for chemotherapy, Carl Voegtlin included a carefully worded statement allowing that mercurachrome appeared to be of value in treatment of urinary tract infections and might also be useful as a prophylactic in preparing patients for genitourinary operations. He passed over in silence claims made for mercurachrome as an agent against systemic infections.[60]

The best shots of its critics failed to kill mercurachrome. Instead, it appears to have entered a slow decline. The more extravagant claims were abandoned, the more modest ones were hedged with qualifications, and some clinical use continued. In the seventh edition of their well-known textbook of bacteriology, published in 1934, Hans Zinsser and Stanhope Bayne-Jones mentioned the great research and therapeutic activity surrounding organic mercury compounds since 1920 and, in particular, the extensive use made of mercurachrome both as topical antiseptic and as chemotherapeutic agent in many infections. They took note of, but kept at arm's length, the many reports of favorable results from use of mercurachrome. "In our opinion," they remarked, "the claims for it have not been extensively substantiated. . . . We would place it just below tincture of iodine as a surface antiseptic."[61] Evidence of decline is more marked in an important British textbook published five years later, the second edition of G.M. Findlay's *Recent Advances in Chemotherapy*. Findlay stated flatly that "mercurachrome has unfortunately failed to fulfill the hopes which were at first entertained of it as an antidote to septicemia." Citing studies indicating that the bactericidal properties of organic mercury compounds were neutralized by their binding with serum protein, Findlay pointed out that sterilization of the bloodstream with mercurachrome would require administration of many times the fatal dose. Although he mentioned reports that questioned the value of mercurachrome even as a germicide, Findlay was willing to allow that "as antiseptics for such purposes as cleansing the skin before operations [mercurachrome and other organic mercurials] possibly possess some value."[62]

The Prospects of Chemotherapy

Looking back in 1955 at what he called "the immense vogue" for mercurachrome in the 1920s, British physician Lawrence P. Garrod marveled that so many people seriously believed the compound to be an efficient intravenous antiseptic. His own explanation, that the episode was a case of therapeutic fraud, is surely mistaken. The vogue for mercurachrome emerged from, and placed in sharp relief, several features of the medical world of the 1920s. It expressed the intense desire of researchers, physicians, and patients alike for some defense against the relentless suffering and death associated with bacterial infections. It expressed even more clearly an optimism, motivated in part by Ehrlich's program, in part by other successes of chemotherapy, and in part perhaps by the spectacular impact of insulin against a very different kind of disease, that such a thing as bacterial chemotherapy was even possible. And it expressed, or was made possible by, a lack of settled consensus on principles, methods, and standards of evaluation in chemotherapy. Mercurachrome rose on a wave of need and expectation. When it declined, the need remained, but expectations inevitably cooled as well. For some, by the early 1930s, the failure of mercurachrome and countless other compounds warranted an increasing pessimism where bacterial chemotherapy was concerned. For most of those engaged in research, it meant not so much pessimism as a new sobriety, a concentration on methods and standards of investigation, and a sense that bacterial chemotherapy would emerge not from a quick victory but from long, steady, and determined effort.[63]

The pre-sulfa drugs decade of the late 1920s and early 1930s has sometimes been portrayed as a time of increasing gloom over the prospects for bacterial chemotherapy.[64] A survey of leaders of the scientific and medical communities in Europe and America, however, found little evidence of genuine pessimism. More evident are varied assessments of the achievements of chemotherapy so far, a proliferation of diagnoses of its shortcomings, and prescriptions for its future success.

At the Toronto meeting of the British Association for the Advancement of Science in 1924, the president of the association's section of physiology, Henry H. Dale, spoke on the "progress and prospects in chemotherapy." Dale was both critical of the current state of chemotherapeutic theory and expansive on the practical achievements and future prospects of the field. On the theoretical side, he questioned Ehrlich's views on the mode of action of chemical agents on microbes as ad hoc and insufficiently precise in a biochemical sense and called for greater attention to the interactions of synthetic compounds with host organisms. He pointed to the need for such knowledge, and of knowledge of microbial physiology, if chemotherapy was to be put on a rational basis. At the same time, just because of the limits of theory to date, he expressed

> wonder and admiration that so much of practical value has already been achieved—the treatment of spirochetal infections, syphilis, yaws and relapsing fever, revolutionized; leishmania infections, kala-azar and Baghdad boil and bilharzia infections which crippled the health of whole populations in countries such as Egypt, now made definitely curable; trypanosome infections, such as the deadly African sleeping sickness, after years of alternating promise and disappointments, brought now at last within the range of effective treatment.

And the end was nowhere in sight, he continued, for "if such results have already been attained, in a period during which practice has inevitably and often outrun theory, we may well be hopeful for a future in which fuller understanding should make for more orderly progress."[65]

Although Dale nowhere mentioned bacterial chemotherapy, his optimism seemed to embrace prospects for treatment of all infectious disease. The author of the foremost American textbook of chemotherapy, John A. Kolmer, was much more explicit in his hopes for bacterial chemotherapy. Kolmer, a professor of pathology and bacteriology at the University of Pennsylvania medical school, devoted most of his *Principles and Practice of Chemotherapy* (1926) to syphilis. Not only had chemotherapy's greatest successes been scored against syphilis, he argued, but the treatment of syphilis provided a model for laboratory and clinical investigations of the chemical therapy of other infectious diseases. Among these, he gave bacterial infections a prominent place. Some 140 pages of the 1,000-page text were devoted to chemotherapy of bacterial diseases, a figure that reflected both the relative lack of progress of the subfield and Kolmer's close attention to what had been done.[66]

Kolmer was aware of the difficulties. He referred to "the skepticism so frequently expressed in regards to the future of the chemotherapy of bacterial diseases." He noted that while the bacteria, because of their relative simplicity and greater distance from mammalian organisms, might have been considered easier targets for chemotherapy than protozoa or metazoa, exactly the opposite had been the case. He even suggested that the discovery of spirochetes and trypanosomes and of the means of conducting large numbers of inexpensive experimental infections with them "was a wonderfully fortunate circumstance, for had the early experiments in chemotherapy been conducted with the bacteria, disappointments would probably have extinguished enthusiasm by a lack of sufficient success and encouragement as subsequent events have amply indicated."[67]

Whatever the problems, Kolmer thought that grounds for optimism could be found in recent work in bacterial chemotherapy that had produced drugs of practical value. Among the latter, he included the work of Young and his associates on mercurachrome and that of himself, J. F. Schamberg, and Raiziss on synthesis of other mercurial compounds, including mercuraphen. Kolmer brightened the picture of recent work and future prospects considerably by loosening his definition of bacterial chemotherapy to include local as well as systemic treatment.[68]

Kolmer's broad-ranging optimism was echoed two years later by Voegtlin, a pharmacologist with the U.S. Public Health Service's Hygienic Laboratory, in his chapter for the Chemical Foundation's *Chemistry and Medicine*. Voegtlin's tone, as befitted the volume as a whole, was forward-looking, militant, and upbeat. He pointed to the real triumphs of chemotherapy against protozoal diseases and to promising beginnings in bacterial chemotherapy. Although Voegtlin regarded these successes as "a sufficient demonstration of the practical value of this new science," he, like Dale, lamented the contemporary lack of knowledge of mechanism of action of drugs and of microbial physiology. Such ignorance, he thought, blocked establishment of a scientific foundation for chemotherapy and slowed discovery of useful drugs.[69]

A cooler view of the state of the field, and especially of bacterial chemotherapy, was taken by Findlay in the first edition (1930) of his major British textbook. Findlay was acutely aware of the tendency for hope to triumph over experience in a field with potentially enormous impact on medical practice. "In perhaps no other department of science," he remarked, "is there psychologically so great a will to success as in chemotherapy."[70] In Findlay's view, bacterial chemotherapy had so far proved a failure in both local and systemic infections. He regarded all chemical antiseptics then in use as general protoplasmic poisons. As such, they killed bacteria but at the same time weakened the body's defenses by inhibiting phagocytosis by leukocytes and weakening the leukocytes' bactericidal action. Only their rapid elimination from the body, he thought, prevented them from seriously compromising the body's defenses. He pointed out that, even when applied locally, as in infected wounds, known antiseptics quickly lost effective concentrations and, while present, interfered with the action of leukocytes. Findlay's strictures applied to mercurachrome as well as to many other compounds. From them, he also drew the conclusion that *in vitro* tests of an antiseptic's action could throw little or no light on its effectiveness *in vivo*.[71]

Failure so far did not preclude future success, however, and Findlay had no hesitation in listing the properties of an ideal compound for use in bacterial infections. It should have

> a well-marked bactericidal action when brought into contact with bacteria in the presence of tissue fluids; it should be non-toxic to tissue cells; it should stimulate the bactericidal powers of the leucocytes; it should retain its bactericidal powers for a prolonged period when present in blood or tissue fluids; and it should readily diffuse from the blood into serous cavities and tissue spaces.

Such a compound had not yet been found, but the very act of defining its ideal properties affirmed the possibility.[72]

Findlay's prescription for cure of chemotherapy's troubled state emphasized more rigorous research methods. At the base had to be experimental infections in appropriate laboratory animals. *In vitro* tests alone were unreliable, Findlay held, and the chemotherapeutic activity of powerful compounds such as the arsphenamines in syphilis, Bayer 205 (Germanin) in sleeping sickness, or Plasmoquine (chloroquine) in malaria "could hardly have been determined" without trials on infected animals. Chemotherapeutic action in animals did not guarantee chemotherapeutic action in humans, he admitted, but "broadly speaking, it may be said that any drug which is devoid of action in experimental animals will also be devoid of action in man." Passing through the sieve of animal trials was therefore a necessary, but not sufficient, condition for the success of a compound as chemotherapeutic agent. Clinical trials were also required. To ensure the value of animal trials, Findlay specified six criteria to be satisfied regarding kinds and numbers of animals used and the experimental conditions. He offered the clinician a parallel list of eight measures to be taken to establish credible results in tests of chemotherapeutic agents on humans.[73]

The most novel aspect of Findlay's exhortation was his call for application of statistical methods to chemotherapy. Findlay urged laboratory researchers and clinicians to familiarize themselves with simple statistical concepts. Not only could use of such methods save considerable time and energy, he argued, but "little solid progress can be made in chemotherapeutic research until both the laboratory worker and the clinician realise the errors into which lack of elementary statistical knowledge may lead them." With statistical thinking would come "a healthy skepticism," to be applied to a researcher's own work as well as that of others.[74]

A cautious and critical reserve was also the keynote of the 1934 edition of Zinsser and Bayne-Jones' *Textbook of Bacteriology*. The authors devoted a chapter to "the effects of chemical agents on bacteria" but restricted its coverage almost entirely to antiseptics or disinfectants. They did not formulate a program for research, did not mention Ehrlich's program, did not issue a call for more effort in bacterial chemotherapy, and thought that any results claimed to be achieved so far against systemic bacterial infections were at best unproven, at worst unsuccessful. All of this added up to a relatively passive and expectant optimism. Not pessimism, surely, but equally not a posture that was likely to drive innovation.[75]

Finally, more than a decade after Dale's optimistic remarks, a note of frustration and resignation was struck by Max Gundel in his German textbook on infectious diseases. Gundel, a physician and medical researcher at the Robert Koch Institute in Berlin, aimed the multiauthored anthology at practitioners. Following brief introductory sections, the first, longest, and most elaborately subdivided portion of the text covered bacterial infections. Gundel himself contributed the first subsection, on streptococcal infections. He regarded most chemotherapeutic agents as having failed in streptococcal infections. He looked grimly ahead to a long struggle in which chemotherapy did not play an explicit, let alone a prominent, role. "If one looks over the whole field of the streptococcal infections of humans," he reflected, "then one comes in every respect to an ever more resigned attitude." Neither the biology of streptococci nor the specific therapy of streptococcal diseases had made any essential advance in recent decades, Gundel believed, and "only the most intensive common work of all disciplines will perhaps bring progress, which is all the more urgent and to be desired, as with the streptococcal infections it is a matter of diseases of the greatest significance for public health."[76]

Gundel's emphasis on sera and vaccines at the expense of chemotherapy, an emphasis evident elsewhere in his text, reminds us that more was involved in the status of chemotherapy than the record of its own past achievements or lack of them. Other approaches to infectious disease competed for the attention and energy of investigators and the institutions that funded them. By the mid-1930s, vast effort had been expended on the development of sera alone. Major successes had been scored in serum treatment of diphtheria and pneumococcal pneumonia, and pharmaceutical companies and clinicians continued to test sera against other bacterial infections. Serum therapy of streptococcal infections was frustrated in part by the large number of varieties of the target organism, *Streptococcus pyogenes*. It would be a presentist fallacy, however, to see something inevitable in the triumph of chemotherapy and to fault investigators of the early 1930s for failure to anticipate it. In the struggle with bacterial infections, it was by no means obvious in what direction success might be found.[77]

Whatever their views on the most promising path to be taken, several investigators of the pre-1935 decade called for major new efforts in the search for treatments of bacterial disease. A common theme in these appeals was a perception that previous efforts had been inadequate in both quantity and quality. Gundel thought that only research "of an entirely other extent" from that of the present, "put in motion from the most various directions and focuses," would improve the prognosis for streptococcal infections. Kolmer made his optimism on the prospects for bacterial chemotherapy conditional on a tremendous expenditure of brains and money not yet thrown into the struggle. To these would have to be joined "hard, conscientious, and unremitting, but systematized toil coupled with the ever alluring chance of making a 'lucky strike.' "[78]

The most emphatic, and the most carefully thought out, call to action came from Voegtlin. Commenting on the treatment of tuberculosis, he remarked rue-fully that "it is very likely that if but half of the energy and money which has been spent in the search for a serum, had been devoted to chemotherapeutic investiga-tion, greater progress might have been recorded." In this context, he ascribed the disproportionate emphasis on sera and vaccines to physicians' lack of chemical training: "There are few Paul Ehrlichs in medicine."[79]

In mentioning Ehrlich, Voegtlin had in mind not only the need for chemically trained doctors. More fundamental were the commitment of resources and the or-ganization of research exemplified by Ehrlich's institute. Voegtlin conceded that valuable discoveries had been made in laboratories not organized specifically for chemotherapeutic research. He pointed out, however, that work in such locales was often hindered by inappropriate use of personnel and equipment, by lack of financial resources, or by unwillingness of laboratory directors to wait the years often necessary for practical results. Ehrlich's institute embodied a formula for success that should be adopted in the United States, Voegtlin argued. The essen-tial ingredients included mobilization of substantial financial resources and their long-term commitment to chemotherapeutic research. With these resources labo-ratories should be organized that embodied cooperative associations of chemists, pharmacologists, bacteriologists, and other specialists, all working full time on problems of chemotherapy. Equally important, in Voegtlin's view, was the close association of such a laboratory with the fine chemicals industry. "The secret of the success of the immense organic chemical industry in Germany," he remarked, "is to a great extent due to their policy of establishing within the works true re-search laboratories which, as far as personnel and equipment is concerned, are not surpassed by the chemical departments of German universities." The same in-dustrial laboratories also maintained consulting arrangements with leading aca-demic chemists. Voegtlin lamented that, despite its growth since the war, the U.S. organic chemicals industry did not yet encourage fundamental research, still pre-ferring to exploit existing knowledge.[80]

That Voegtlin's blueprint for chemotherapeutic research was not yet realized in the United States despite the availability of its separate ingredients points to the limitations of American optimism about the field. The venture into chemotherapy that resulted in mercurachrome embodied the optimism, but also the constraints of funding, focus, and organization that characterized many efforts in the field in the 1910s and 1920s. What Voegtlin did not take note of was that in Germany the fine chemicals industry not only cooperated with institutes like Ehrlich's but also had long ago incorporated Ehrlich's program into its own research organizations. By the time Voegtlin's comments were published in 1928, the pharmaceutical re-search division of one such company was already embarked on work that would produce a major breakthrough in the chemotherapy of bacterial infections.

CHAPTER 2

A System of Invention

In 1939, the Nobel Prize in Physiology or Medicine was awarded to Gerhard Domagk, a medical researcher employed by the German fine chemicals company I.G. Farbenindustrie. Domagk was cited for his "recognition of the antibacterial activity of Prontosil," by that time recognized as the first of a new class of antibacterial agents, the sulfa drugs. Domagk's first findings related to Prontosil were dated 1932, and the first publication, 1935. In fact, the research program from which Prontosil emerged had been initiated in 1926. And the successful result of that program depended heavily on Domagk's close collaboration with two of the company's chemists, Fritz Mietzsch and Joseph Klarer, whose roles the Nobel award passed over in silence.

Indeed, contrary to the impression conveyed to the world by Domagk's Nobel Prize, the research that produced the first sulfa drugs was a collaborative effort in which biomedical researchers and chemists played distinct and complementary roles. Behind their association were the vision and experience of a company research manager, Heinrich Hörlein. Hörlein approached the problem of bacterial chemotherapy with an expansive view of the potential uses of chemistry in medicine and a systemic approach to innovation, and as director of a research organization with a record of recent successes in work on closely related problems. Behind Hörlein was I.G. Farben, for which the venture into antibacterial chemotherapy was among the latest in a series of steps in a diversification that led from synthetic dyestuffs through pharmaceuticals to chemotherapy.

Involvement of the German fine chemicals industry with pharmaceuticals stretched back to the 1880s, long antedating even Ehrlich's early work in chemotherapy. The industry's attention to pharmaceuticals increased at the same time that it was expanding its commitments to research. As Georg Meyer-Thurow has shown for Bayer, one of the major component companies of I.G. Farben, the establishment of research and its contribution to Bayer's success were the results of an evolutionary process in which legal and economic as well as scientific developments played important roles. Major components of this process included the opening of a main scientific laboratory in 1891; the building up of a research infrastructure to support the main laboratory, including a library, a literary department, a patent bureau, a control laboratory, a training laboratory, and an experimental dye house; and the increasing focus of management on the organization of research and on the introduction of related managerial techniques, including labor contract regulations, financial incentives, conferences, regular progress reports, and creation of the role of research administrator. Research became increasingly differentiated, specialized, and decentralized with the setting up of new laboratories, including, by 1902, a pharmaceutical and a bacteriological laboratory. Largely in place by the beginning of World War I, the establishment of research within Bayer had as one major consequence the industrialization of invention, as technical innovation at Bayer became a bureaucratically managed, routinized process carried out by teams of cooperating specialists.[1]

It was within such an industrial research setting that the first compounds effective against bacterial infections in humans were developed. Their story is therefore more than that of the two or three individuals most directly engaged in the research and most visible in the historical record. It is also the story of a particular kind of organization and of the ways in which it shaped the careers, research programs, and working relationships of investigators who were part of it.

An internal company report of 1930, prepared for the information of higher management, is revealing of the aims, organization, and system of innovation of I.G. Farben's pharmaceutical division. The report was strictly confidential and distributed in numbered copies to a small group of high executives. It was intended to familiarize its readers, especially those in the other divisions of the company, with the inner workings of the pharmaceutical division. The occasion for the report was completion of the fusion of the pharmaceutical parts of I.G. Farben's component companies into a single organization, a process begun in 1925 with the formation of I.G. Farben. The most important components of the new entity so far as pharmaceuticals were concerned were Bayer and Höchst, and the leaders of their pharmaceutical divisions, Rudolf Mann and Alfred Ammelburg, respectively, were singled out for special thanks. The report was also meant to be a critical stock-taking, for its authors conceded that in spite of the overall success of the merger, there was still room for improvement.[2]

All five component companies of the unified division—Bayer, Höchst, Kalle & Co. of Biebrich, Leopold Casella & Co. of Frankfurt am Main, and Agfa (Aktiengesellschaft für Anilinfabrikation) of Berlin—had begun as producers of synthetic dyes and had later expanded into pharmaceuticals. The continuing pressure for diversification in this direction is visible in a section of the report on the "significance and use of our bacteriological dyes in medicine." The authors reviewed current uses of dyes in diagnosis (including pathology), in therapy (including chemotherapy), in surgery as markers of lines of incision, as indicators of acidity and alkalinity, in botany, and in nutritional chemistry. They saw a wide field of

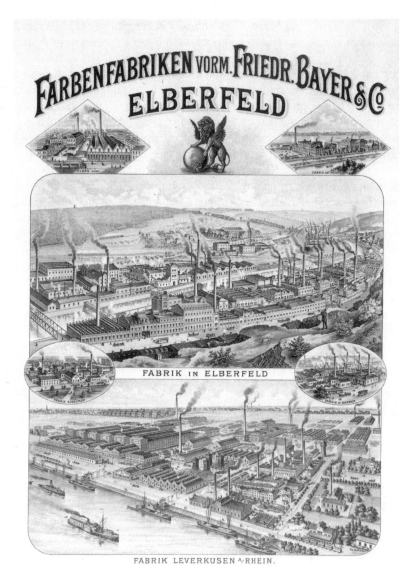

Figure 2.1. A 1900 Bayer advertisement showing factories at Elberfeld and Leverkusen (reprinted courtesy of the Bayer Archive).

use for dyes in medicine, but one that was so far more impressive in its potential than in its realization. They conceded that "surprises are always possible in the field of dye therapy." The keynote of the relationship of dyes to medicines was therefore unpredictability, but an unpredictability that the authors chose to read in an optimistic way.[3]

One of the more striking features of the report was its effort to convey to its executive readers the typical cycle of development of a new pharmaceutical product within I.G. Farben. Drawing upon the component companies' nearly half-century of experience with pharmaceuticals, the authors were able both to take a long view and to abstract from particulars. They recognized a periodicity in the development of pharmaceuticals in which times of relatively quiet stability alternated with periods of rapid or revolutionary change. They noted that new scientific ideas usually did not have an immediate payoff in the manufacture of new products, but that it was precisely in the lag time between new ideas and new products that purely scientific work became most important. Steady scientific research was necessary, they argued, in order to meet practical needs with new products that would replace existing ones. The relatively rapid turnover of pharmaceutical products required a permanent source of innovation, and this source was scientific research.[4]

At the same time, the report conceded, the company's scientific laboratories needed to keep in touch with the needs and desires of medical practice. One source for such contact was the medical literature. Another was reports by scientific or medical people in external service, who made regular personal visits to clinics. From these sources came ideas and stimuli that helped to shape guidelines for research within the company.[5]

The authors pointed out that rational drug design, that is, the deliberate search for medicinal drugs of definite effect, was possible only in a very limited way because of lack of knowledge of the relation between chemical constitution and pharmacological action. Thus, the route from chemical laboratory to new product was not direct or predictable. An elaborate series of steps intervened, at any one of which a promising compound might be eliminated. A compound was first subjected to pharmacological scrutiny in the form of "wide-ranging animal tests" in company laboratories at Elberfeld, Höchst, or Mainkur. If these tests gave reason to believe that the compound might have some definite therapeutic action, it was sent on to Leverkusen and referred to the central testing site. Here, pharmacological data were gathered to arrive at a statement of indications, dosage, and standards to be set for the preparation. At this stage, the substance would be subjected to preliminary clinical testing on a restricted basis, presumably either within the company or under its close supervision. The immediate goal of the preliminary clinical tests was to establish tolerance. If the substance appeared to be well tolerated by human subjects, dosages were increased to establish optimal dosage levels. Only after these steps had been completed would the compound be released for further clinical tests by qualified individuals outside the company, who were supplied with scientific information on the preparation and adequate quantities of samples.[6]

The testing period for new preparations averaged one year. Within this time, the pharmaceutical division had to gather, compare, and judge results from its various sources. Typically, problems or complications arose, due, for example, to failure to follow guidelines, overdosing, or intolerances in individual cases. Such difficulties were treated with special care, since an understanding of them often improved knowledge of the compound. Evaluation involved ongoing exchanges of information and ideas with the research laboratories, including regular discussions in Elberfeld and Höchst and larger conferences that brought in scientific people in external service. The whole process might have one of three outcomes:

introduction of the preparation into commerce and medicine, its discontinuance, or further testing. A decision taken by a major conference to introduce a compound triggered a number of technical preparations, including manufacture in quantity and creation of packaging, prospectuses, and advertising, all in cooperation with the appropriate parts of the company. In all of this, a central coordinating role was played by Leverkusen.[7]

The report also assessed costs and profits of the pharmaceutical division in recent years. It identified major problems facing the division and came to a judgment on its future prospects. Not surprisingly, the authors gave pride of place to the need to maintain profitability. This could be achieved in the first instance, they argued, by increasing volume of business. Business volume, in turn, could result either from an increase in numbers of "truly promising products" or through participation in companies whose activities were closely related to those of the division. As to the first goal, the authors noted that "our gaze is confidently directed to our research laboratories." In general, the authors insisted, costs had to be lowered through "the closest contact between factory, laboratory, and marketing, which we fortunately may affirm is already long established."[8]

The report concluded that, all things considered, the future looked bright. Conceding that the critical situation of the world economy had created uncertainty, they still admitted to "a healthy optimism" and looked forward to "a constant development with increasing improvement of profits." The key to this success, the authors affirmed, would be leadership: "As everywhere, so also here, the choice of the right leading personalities will be decisive."[9]

Of the leading personalities referred to in the 1930 report, perhaps the most important was Hörlein, who was principal architect of that part of I.G. Farben's pharmaceutical research organization contributed by the former Bayer company. Like the German fine chemicals industry itself, his early career had moved between dyestuffs and pharmaceuticals. Born in 1882, the son of a vineyard owner in Wendelsheim, Rheinhessen, Hörlein was educated at *Realschulen*. He studied chemistry first at the *Technische Hochschule* in Darmstadt, and then at the University of Jena, where he took his doctorate in 1903 under Ludwig Knorr, an organic chemist and the discoverer of antipyrine. At Jena, Hörlein studied physics and political economy as well as chemistry, and his doctoral examination was awarded *summa cum laude* in all three subjects. From 1904 to 1908, Hörlein was assistant and collaborator to Knorr and concentrated on the chemical structure of morphine. In 1908, Carl Duisberg, himself a chemist and by then director of Bayer, was looking for a new chemist for Bayer's pharmaceutical division. At that year's Jena meeting of the Society of German Chemists, over which he presided, Duisberg put the question to Knorr, whom he knew from earlier days in Munich. Knorr pointed out Hörlein and subsequently wrote to Duisberg that "Hörlein has a very intelligent, clear head, and is an outstanding, skillful chemist. He possesses extensive knowledge of chemistry and political economy, is a swift and reliable worker, and has the most important characteristic for a technologist [*Techniker*], a tenacious, systematic energy." Hörlein got the job.[10]

After joining Bayer in 1909, Hörlein worked for several months in dyestuffs chemistry with the aim of deepening his knowledge of its methods. He then returned to pharmaceutical chemistry and in 1910 was instrumental in introducing Luminal (phenobarbital), a sedative that came to play an important role in the treatment of epilepsy.[11]

By this time, Duisberg had ample evidence to confirm Knorr's judgment of Hörlein's energy and talents. In 1910, he placed him in charge of Bayer's pharmaceutical-scientific laboratories, and Hörlein thereby joined the governing body of the pharmaceutical research division in Elberfeld. Under Hörlein, and with Duisberg's support, the pharmaceutical research division at Elberfeld began a long-term expansion. To the existing chemical, pharmaceutical, and bacteriological laboratories, a new chemotherapeutic laboratory was added in 1910, with a student of Ehrlich's, Wilhelm Roehl, as first director. Through the 1910s and 1920s, Hörlein expanded the existing laboratories and added others. When I.G. Farben was formed in 1925, the company controlled not only the Bayer laboratories at Elberfeld and Leverkusen but also others at Höchst and Mainkur. Of these, the Elberfeld establishment was the largest and had the most subdivisions.

As of 1927, Hörlein presided over seven laboratories, with a total staff, including assistants, numbering eighty-two. There were two chemical laboratories, one of which included among its staff Domagk's collaborators Klarer and Mietzsch. There was one special laboratory, one chemical trials room, one physiological and biochemical laboratory, and one chemotherapeutic laboratory. Domagk's laboratory of experimental pathology, which became the eighth unit under Hörlein's direction, was inserted into a carefully constructed, large-scale, ongoing co-

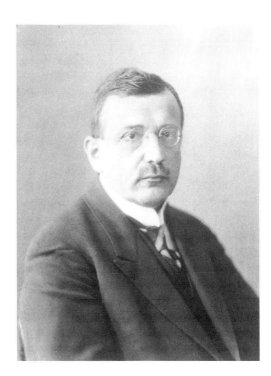

Figure 2.2. Heinrich Hörlein (1882–1954) c. 1920 (reprinted courtesy of the Bayer Archive).

operative research effort. Duisberg in 1934 described the Elberfeld research establishment as a "rounded whole" that comprised "the collected theoretical fields of a medical faculty."[12]

Hörlein's rise in the company paralleled his building up of its pharmaceutical research division. In 1914 he was named *Prokurist*, in 1919 deputy director, and in 1921 deputy member of the executive board of Bayer. In 1931, he became a regular member of the executive board (*Vorstand*) of I.G. Farben, member of the technical committee (TEA, *technische Ausschuss*) of I.G. Farben, and director of the pharmaceutical and plant-protection divisions in Elberfeld. Hörlein took over direction of the Elberfeld works in 1933 and in 1935 became chairman of the pharmaceutical major conference of I.G. Farben, in which the directors of all pharmaceutical units, including those for research, manufacture, advertising, and marketing from Leverkusen, Höchst, and Elberfeld, took part. Without exaggeration, Hörlein may be called the leading figure in the management of pharmaceutical research and development at Bayer and I.G. Farben between the world wars.[13]

His position is reflected in an admiring bit of doggerel penned by Walther Wolff, who visited the company in March 1930:

> The car brings me quickly
> To the I.G.'s entrance
> First the announcement, then up we go
> To the I.G. Farben main office,
> Therein Bonhoeffer and Hörlein preside,
> In order to make dividends.
>
> —
>
> Long ago, in narrow ways,
> I earlier saw the work bestir itself,
> Small buildings, the air was filled
> With the scent of chemicals,
> The ground green, violet, blue
> The whole building wrapped in steam.
>
> Yet today the ways are broad,
> The huts defy time,
> And newly arisen, where once the dye
> House earned fame for Friedrich Bayer
> Is many a structure of pharmacy
> As an ornament of chemistry.
>
> —
>
> On the other side of the Wupper
> A new edifice grows out of nothing,
> Erected by pure science:
> Concentrated pharmacology!
>
> Shall I praise the building
> That unveils the philosopher's stone?

Whose bright windows give
Light to the strivings of young researchers?
—

Here is fought the curse of the tropics.
Malaria in microscopes,
Anopheles and Tsetse flies.
To conquer the devil's effects
Is Heinrich Hörlein's great deed,
Blessings to suffering humanity,
To the envy of the universities!
Trypanosomes, spirochetes,
Amoebas and leukocytes,
Shortly they will be dead!

At home, filled with gratitude,
I propose a toast to Heinrich Hörlein![14]

One of the roles that Hörlein took upon himself as director of the pharmaceutical research division and company manager was liaison between the company and the scientific and medical communities. By his own account, he saw the care of scientific societies within Germany as part of his life's work. At one time or another, he was associated with the German Chemical Society, the *Kaiser Wilhelm Gesellschaft* for the Advancement of Science, the Society of German Scientists and Physicians, the *Adolf Baeyer Gesellschaft* for the Advancement of Chemical Literature, and the *Emil Fischer Gesellschaft* (financed by the Kaiser Wilhelm Institute for Chemistry in Berlin-Dahlem). He also served as chairman of the Justus Liebig Society for the Advancement of Chemical Instruction, which distributed stipends to graduated chemists and to chemistry students.[15]

In his capacity as liaison to the scientific and medical worlds, Hörlein gave several talks to professional meetings in Germany and Britain between 1927 and 1937. In two of these, presented in 1927 and 1932, he gave an expansive picture of his views on the goals, achievements, problems, and prospects of pharmaceutical research. These talks yield insights into the institutional structure of innovation at Elberfeld, and the vision on which that structure—and, not incidentally, Bayer/I.G. Farben's willingness to commit substantial resources to research over a long period—were based.

The keynote of both lectures, and indeed of Hörlein's posture as manager of pharmaceutical research for I.G. Farben, was a robust confidence in the future of research-based medicinal drugs. Hörlein's was not merely the optimism of a salesman speaking to potential buyers, but was based on a well-informed and well-articulated vision of pharmaceutical research as a domain of rational engineering or science-based technology, a synoptic view of the scientific basis, successes, and unrealized potentials of chemically oriented medicine, and a systemic approach to innovation.[16]

Hörlein viewed the pharmaceutical industry as a branch of chemical technology, historically derived from the production of synthetic dyestuffs and distinguished by its partial incorporation of and dependence upon experimental and clinical medicine. He underlined its importance as an element of the German economy and as one source of the scientific, technological, and medical reputation of Germany abroad. Like Thomas Edison, a manager of innovation in a field Hörlein compared to synthetic medicines, he considered his goals and problems from a technical or scientific and an economic point of view simultaneously. He paid close attention to such matters as the cost of selecting one compound out of hundreds for clinical trials, and gave patenting precedence over publication.[17]

Hörlein's explicit and implicit definitions of the fields central to pharmaceutical research emphasized their character as rational engineering rather than as basic science. However much it may draw upon or contribute to knowledge in chemistry, physiology, microbiology, or pathology, research in pharmaceutical chemistry, physiological chemistry, and chemotherapy as Hörlein thought of them was organized around and subordinated to the practical goal of production of medically useful and commercially viable products. Pharmaceutical chemistry harnessed the methods and concepts of organic analysis and synthesis to produce new medicines. Although Hörlein was well aware of the scientific breadth of physiological chemistry as pursued in academic institutes, his own interest narrowed to the "decisive" finding that some compounds produced or taken in by the body—he thought especially of vitamins and hormones—are pharmacologically active and can therefore become medicines. As even its name indicates, chemotherapeutic research had as its primary goal the finding of chemical agents effective against systemic microbial infections. To this practical goal even its aim to understand how the chemical agents work was subordinated. Hörlein's emphasis on the ability of imperfect or deficient animal experimental models to produce valuable results was one expression of this pragmatic or engineering attitude.

Hörlein's attitude was based not simply, or even primarily, on the situation of any particular area of research considered in isolation, but on his comprehensive overview of advance in areas in which chemistry and biomedicine intersected. These areas shared a number of generic problems and solutions, for example, the need to isolate a substance (natural product, synthetic product, body substance) in chemically pure form, the need to synthesize the substance and to do so economically if it was to go on the market, and the need for pharmacological, chemotherapeutic, toxicological, and clinical testing of the substance. Hörlein's efforts to translate success in certain areas (vitamin deficiency disease, chemotherapy of protozoal infections) into optimism about possibilities in other areas (cancer, antibacterial chemotherapy) was characteristic. He regarded the chemical attack on disease as a many-fronted battle in which there was a generally advancing line but also many points at which advance was slow or arrested. In this sense, Hörlein might be said to have thought—as Thomas Hughes has shown that Edison did—in terms of reverse salients and critical problems. Reverse salients are areas of research and development that are lagging in some obvious way behind the general line of advance. Critical problems are the research questions, cast in terms of the concrete particulars of currently available knowledge and technique and of specific exemplars or models (e.g., insulin, chemotherapy of kala-azar and malaria) that are solvable and whose solutions would eliminate the reverse salients.[18]

Hughes describes the components of Edison's electric lighting project as forming a system in the sense that they are interrelated and mutually dependent parts of an integrated whole. The technology that Hörlein describes does not form a system in this sense but is fragmented into distinct and not necessarily related aspects of the relation of chemistry and medicine in its practical manifestations. Hörlein has a synoptic or comprehensive view of these manifestations, but they themselves do not form a system in Hughes's sense.

What was systemic in Hörlein's way of thinking was his concept of the organizational pattern or patterns that will best facilitate the production of valuable results in the areas in which medicine and chemistry interact. A valuable outcome is a result that has practical importance for clinical or preventive medicine and, implicitly, commercial value for industry. Hörlein perceived a need for a set of mutually complementary institutions and trained personnel whose interaction produces the desired results. The organizational pattern that emerges more or less clearly from Hörlein's lectures is closely associated with his view of the typical phases or cycles of development of research in chemotherapy or physiological chemistry. He saw a need for friendly and mutually supportive relations between industrial research and development organizations, academic institutions, and clinicians. He viewed the academic–industrial connection as crucial and mutually beneficial. Underlying this view was his definition and differentiation of the relevant disciplines and his belief in their generally excellent condition in Germany. He saw a need for government support of appropriate institutions, especially research institutes in universities. Within industrial research organizations—and, implicitly, within academic ones—Hörlein called for special institutional arrangements to encourage appropriate interactions between chemistry and biomedicine.

An element of crucial—and to Hörlein, personal—importance in these interactions was the role of the research manager or "team leader." When Hörlein spoke of the research done under his direction as "our work," he used the possessive advisedly to convey a strong sense of his own participation. The research manager had to be active in defining goals, in marshalling means and resources, and in assessing success or failure. He had to intervene where necessary to minimize friction between chemists and medical researchers, an especially important task for chemotherapy as a composite entity. He had to publicize the company's successes—a necessity for what was ultimately a commercial enterprise—and act as liaison between company laboratories and the academic and medical communities. Through it all, he had to take a long view of the value of research, not insisting on immediate results of medical or commercial value.

As a research manager with training and experience in pharmaceutical chemistry, a lively interest in medicine, and rapport with the medical community, Hörlein was well positioned to survey the field where chemistry and medicine joined battle against disease. He could spot the points where the enemy's line was broken, and the reverse salients in his own. What he could not do—or could not do alone—was to direct the day-to-day operations of his troops, that is, to define the critical problems to be solved, to identify the terms of their solution, and to do the work that would carry the day. In the case of chemotherapy, these things could be effected only by the medical researcher and the chemist, each working on his own domain, and cooperatively. For his attack on one of the most important reverse salients—the chemotherapy of bacterial infections—Hörlein called upon the medical researcher Domagk and the chemists Mietzsch and Klarer.

CHAPTER 3

Prontosil

On Christmas Day 1932, I.G. Farben applied for a German patent on procedures to prepare a red crystalline powder with the formidable chemical name of 4-sulfonamido-2,4-diaminoazobenzene. Little was said of the compound's properties, little hint given of the momentous consequences for medicine that might follow from its introduction. Jealously guarded by a small circle within the company, the compound's secrets would not be proclaimed to the world for more than two years. In February 1935, less than two months after the patent was granted, Gerhard Domagk announced the new compound, now called by the trade name Prontosil, in a short communication to a German medical periodical. From that time on, the fate of Prontosil was inextricably bound up with its reception, particularly by the international medical, scientific, and industrial worlds. Before February 1935, however, its history is largely enclosed within the company.

That history is an instance of industrial invention. Prontosil emerged at Elberfeld as the result of a boldly conceived and carefully executed research program carried out in a setting favorable to its realization. The chief architect of the program, as of the setting, was Heinrich Hörlein. In his 1932 lecture on medicine and chemistry, Hörlein had referred to the "endless work" that still lay before researchers on infectious diseases. "The field of bacterial illnesses and those caused by filterable viruses," he had remarked, "still lies absolutely open for a collaboration of medical men and chemists." Five years earlier, Hörlein had already begun to act on that sense of possibility. Against a background of increasing sobriety and even skepticism in the medical and scientific communities on the likelihood of successful bacterial chemotherapy, Hörlein had decided to mount a major effort. He anticipated eventual successes, but was prepared—as he later admitted—for at least ten years of unrewarded labor. Requisite for the success of Hörlein's plan were the selection of key personnel—chemists and medical researchers—and definition by both of critical problems, methods, and strategies in their respective domains.[1]

Building a Research Team

For the chemical part of the work, Hörlein turned to two men, one a veteran of several years with the company, the other newly recruited. Both Fritz Mietzsch and Joseph Klarer came to chemotherapeutic research from dye chemistry. Born in 1896 in Dresden, Mietzsch proceeded from a Dresden gymnasium to studies in that city's *Technische Hochschule*, which he entered in 1915. Mietzsch's training was interrupted by war service. He returned to finish in 1922 with work completed under Walter König. König, who was director of the Dresden Laboratory for Dye Chemistry and Dyeing Technology, left a lasting impression on Mietzsch: in later life he kept at hand in his desk, and consulted, his notebook of König's lectures.[2]

Following a short period as assistant in König's laboratory, Mietzsch, on his mentor's recommendation, joined Bayer at Leverkusen in early 1923. As a newly hired dye chemist, Mietzsch took the mandatory professional development course directed by Richard Kothe and Oscar Dressel, with whom Hörlein had collaborated in his early work at Bayer on dye chemistry. Among the results of the course for Mietzsch would have been a lively awareness of the importance of the azo dyes and their initial and intermediate products. In 1924, a year after Mietzsch joined Bayer, the company's search for a "better quinine" reached a first culmination with the synthesis by the Elberfeld team—Werner Schulemann, Fritz Schönhöfer, and August Wingler—of the compound later termed Plasmoquine, the first purely synthetic antimalarial. By that time, Mietzsch was working in the company's triphenylmethane dye division in Leverkusen. It occurred to him that substances resembling quinine and therefore possibly having antimalarial action might be synthesized from a particular class of dyes. The suggestion caught the attention of Hörlein, and in the fall of 1924 Mietzsch made the decisive move from Leverkusen to Elberfeld, and from dye chemistry to pharmaceutical chemistry.

At Elberfeld, Mietzsch concentrated at first on extension of the approach already used by other Bayer researchers in the synthesis of Plasmoquine to other classes of compounds. This led him first to a compound with a promising action on malaria, and then in 1930 to synthesis of the powerful antimalarial later known by the trade name Atabrine.

Klarer, the son of a Munich manufacturer, was twenty-eight years old when he came to Elberfeld. Following studies at a Munich *Oberrealschule*, he was called to the army in 1916 and served until wounded in 1918. In 1920, he entered the *Technische Hochschule* in Munich and began his studies in chemistry. Even before his diploma examination, he became an assistant to one of his professors, Hans Fischer. Klarer caused a sensation and impressed his teacher when, in his doctoral examination, he succeeded in synthesizing actioporphyrin, which had been shown by Richard Willstätter to be a high-molecular-weight breakdown product of both hemoglobin and chlorophyll. Fischer proposed that Klarer continue his studies with him. Klarer decided instead to accept Hörlein's offer to join the pharmaceutical research division in Elberfeld. Almost as soon as he arrived in 1927, Klarer began work with Mietzsch on a systematic study of the basic alkylated azo dyes. The compounds they prepared were submitted to a variety of *in vitro* (test tube) and animal trials in the laboratories of Elberfeld medical researchers.[3]

Domagk, recruited by Hörlein in the same year as Klarer, came to chemotherapy via medicine and experimental pathology. Born in Lagow in the province of Brandenburg in 1895, the son of a teacher, Domagk was educated at a scientifically oriented grammar school in Liegnitz (now Legnica, Poland). He made an early decision to study medicine but was interrupted in his first term of studies at the University of Kiel by the outbreak of war. A member of a grenadier regiment, he served first on the western front, in Flanders, and then in Russia, where he was wounded in 1915. Transferred to the medical corps, and back to the western front, he was appalled and moved by the helplessness of the medical authorities in the face of epidemics and infections among the troops. Of the thirty-three medical students mobilized with Domagk, only three were still alive when he resumed his studies at Kiel at the end of the war. Domagk himself never fully recovered from his leg wound.[4]

In 1921, Domagk took the state medical examination in Kiel. His M.D. thesis, under the direction of the internist Max Burger, addressed a problem in physiological chemistry, the precipitation of creatinine in humans after muscular exercise. By this time, Domagk felt himself called to medical research, though always, as he later insisted, with the ultimate aim of making medical practice effective by strengthening its scientific foundations. While still at Kiel, he served as assistant to the chemist Ernst Hoppe-Seyler and the pathologist Emmerich, joining his chemical and pathological studies in an analysis of the composition in disease of heart muscle, liver, and kidney. In 1922, he joined Walter Gross as *Privatdozent* in the pathology institute at the University of Greifswald. By this time, Domagk had embraced Rudolf Virchow's injunction that "pathological anatomy must become pathological physiology," and a dynamic or physiological conception of pathology emphasizing the chemical aspects of health and disease became the hallmark of his research. Among his early efforts were studies on the alteration of tissues after exposure to X-rays and experimental investigations of tumors.[5]

An early expression of his movement toward pathological physiology was Domagk's habilitation essay, which examined the defensive role of the reticuloendothelial system—large, white cells that engulf and digest foreign particles in the blood, lymph, or tissues, a process termed phagocytosis—in infections. In a paper published in 1924 based on this research, he described experiments in which mice were injected with living or killed bacteria. Domagk was able to show that, within a few minutes of injection, amyloid precipitates could be detected around the endothelium cells involved in phagocytosis in the liver, spleen, and lungs. He concluded that the amyloid was a degradation product of the phagocytosis, and he was able to strengthen the phagocytosis by sensitization. Several characteristic features of Domagk's later and better known investigations can already be discerned in this work. One of these is his interest in infection as a process, to be analyzed into a discrete set of physiological and pathological events that compose the host organism's response to the pathogen. Noteworthy also is his choice of bacteria, especially staphylococci and streptococci, as pathogens and his use of experimental infections in mice as an investigative model. Much later, just before he died in 1964, Domagk recalled the profound impression of these early studies. His independent observation of phagocytosis—the phenomenon was known but he was not yet aware of it—had moved him almost to tears, fortified his confidence, and directed him toward his future work on bacterial infections and tuberculosis.[6]

This activity in the common area between medicine and chemistry drew the attention of Hörlein, and in 1927 Domagk accepted an offer by I.G. Farben to direct a laboratory in experimental pathology in the company's pharmaceutical research division at Elberfeld. He was thirty-two years old. Domagk, who had followed Gross from Greifswald to Münster in 1925, had already taken the first steps toward an academic career. At first, the connection with I.G. Farben was tentative. He signed a renewable two-year contract and retained his association with the University of Münster, where he was named extraordinary professor of general pathology and pathological anatomy in 1928.[7]

Unlike Mietzsch and Klarer, whose training as dye chemists had prepared them for industrial careers, Domagk began his stint at I.G. Farben with the idea that he was "on furlough" from his academic post. The tensions between his academic values and the realities of his industrial workplace are clear for at least two decades after he began the job. Especially in his first few years at I.G. Farben, Domagk expressed an intense desire to be free to pursue his research and to publish his findings during and after his term of employment. This desire ran head on into the company's need to control the knowledge it produced.[8]

In August 1927, Domagk received from his superiors a document stating his contract period (two years) and his salary (10,500 marks in the first year, 11,500 marks in the second, plus five percent bonuses). The document also specified that he was not to discuss his income with anyone but his immediate family and was not to discuss any matters related to the company with anyone. This was vague enough and does not seem to have frightened him. Ten months later, though, in June 1928, Domagk received a contract supplement listing more than twenty-one kinds of industrial processes. He was asked to agree that for a period of three years after termination of his contract, he would not communicate information about these processes "directly or indirectly, in word or in deed, in any fashion whatsoever, to any establishment in Europe, North, South, or Central America, the British and French dominions, colonies, and protectorates, the Dutch colonies, China, Japan, or Asiatic Russia." This specimen of legal and Germanic thoroughness did alarm him. In a long letter written a few days later, he told the management that he feared his work freedom would be jeopardized if he signed. He had taken a two-year "furlough" from his academic position, he said, only because he was convinced that he could pursue his research and creative work in complete freedom. Under no circumstances could he renounce his right to continue that work and to publish his results after his return to the university. He therefore asked for written guarantees of his research freedom and that universities and research institutes be excepted from the "establishments" with which he could not communicate in the three-year period after leaving I.G. Farben. He wished to be able to negotiate freely in case he received an academic call while under contract to I.G. Farben. Domagk also asked the company to define in writing his relationship to it in case he made a significant discovery and no new contract was concluded at the end of his period of employment. Or, in the event that he did sign a new contract, he wished to know what his share in discoveries would be. The latter questions were astute and show that the secrecy issue had forced him to think through all the implications of his company position.[9]

The records show that the company stalled a bit, but responded within two months with a new work contract. This extended Domagk's employment by another two years but also spelled out his obligations to secrecy in much more detail. Domagk was to make known all results of his work immediately and freely to the company for the company's exclusive use. He was to keep all his findings secret, including to other people in the company except as authorized. Article 4 stated, in part:

> All written materials, . . . especially regarding your own notes relating to business, . . . you will treat as the exclusive property of our firm entrusted to you by us, and you will hold all of this material, together with any copies of it, strictly secret, and turn it over to us at the latest by the end of your period of service, but also at any time earlier on demand.[10]

This document did not respond explicitly to all the questions Domagk had raised. It did put his relationship with the company on a firmer basis and seemed to open the door to a long-term connection. In any case, Domagk signed it. But a year later, in 1929, the company had to draw up a formal letter of clarification. Among other things, this letter made an explicit distinction between Domagk's laboratory notebooks and papers related to his business activity, on the one hand, and "notes on findings resting on his own creative activity," on the other. The former were to be the exclusive property of the company. The latter were to be presented to the firm for inspection at the end of Domagk's term of service but were then to be returned to him for his own use. Exactly what the distinction was is not clear. Whatever it was, it seems to have satisfied Domagk, for the issue never arises again in the existing records.[11] Particularly after his discovery of Prontosil, the company was eager to keep Domagk, and he gained significant royalties from the sale of sulfonamides. Yet his sense of being "on furlough" from academia seems never to have entirely dissipated. On at least two occasions—in 1937 and 1946—he came close to accepting offers from research institutes and universities. In the end, he got his way on some things, such as research staff and facilities, and resigned himself on others, such as lack of academic status and freedom. In the end, Domagk, the scientific professional, came to an uneasy accommodation with his industrial environment.[12]

Domagk took up a variety of research problems in his first years at Elberfeld. One of these began as an assignment to test an antitumor organ extract prepared by the Italian pathologist G. Fichera. Results were negative, but it was characteristic of Domagk that the failure provoked him to further intensive study of cancer. In the near term, this resulted in work showing the possibility of producing resistance in mice to Ehrlich's vaccination carcinoma and to Jensen's sarcoma, using latent infection and cell-free tumor extracts. In the longer term, it set Domagk on a course of cancer research from which he did not waver through the rest of his career and which included studies of the metabolism of tumors, the effects of analogs and precursors of nucleic acids in tumor growth, and action of quinone derivatives on tumors. Also in the domain of experimental pathology, and of Domagk's early research, were studies of the origins of anaphylactic shock and of glomerulonephritis, of the effects of X-rays and of vitamin A overdosage on tissues, and of new techniques for tissue staining.[13]

The Invention of Prontosil

Among these several lines of work, research in the chemotherapy of bacterial infections took an early and prominent place. Domagk was evidently moved in this direction by a convergence of personal inclination and institutional circumstance. His war experience had brought home to him the awful power of infectious disease and the medical profession's helplessness in the face of its ravages. His habilitation research and first publication had examined aspects of bacterial infection and the nature of host responses. By his own later account, the theoretical possibilities of the field had been opened to him by his conviction of the known and potential specificities of bacteria. The early successes of chemotherapy had been won against infections caused by protozoans and spirochetes. In Domagk's view, this was because the former kinds of organisms were relatively more differentiated "and the further developed such a pathogen is, the more points of attack it appears to offer to chemotherapy." Since bacteria could also be differentiated on morphological, physiological, chemical, and physical grounds, however, a bacterial chemotherapy could be imagined. "All of these considerations gave me the certainty," he remarked, "that a chemotherapy of bacterial infections was also in the realm of possibility and that it must be worthwhile to intensively take this field of work in hand, although all prior investigations made this field appear rather hopeless." On this point, Domagk and Hörlein surely concurred, and his superior's enthusiasm for the project both sanctioned and reinforced Domagk's own tendencies.[14]

Expansion of Domagk's activity in bacterial chemotherapeutic research was also made possible, and to some degree impelled, by personnel changes in the Elberfeld research establishment. In March 1929, a year and a half after Domagk's arrival, the director of the laboratory of chemotherapy, Wilhelm Roehl, died suddenly and unexpectedly of a streptococcal infection. Roehl, a medical doctor and student of Paul Ehrlich, had been hired by Hörlein in 1910, in one of Hörlein's first acts as head of pharmaceutical research at Bayer. His task had been to direct the company's newly founded laboratory of chemotherapy. He had since conducted research in several areas, including the chemotherapy of tropical protozoal diseases, leprosy, tuberculosis, and streptococcal infections. Domagk took over temporary direction of Roehl's laboratory. With the arrival of Roehl's successor, Walther Kikuth, a medical researcher from the Tropical Institute in Hamburg, in the fall of 1929, the research territory was redivided. Work on the chemotherapy of streptococcal infections went to Domagk's laboratory, while other areas previously part of Roehl's domain remained with Kikuth. Finally, with the retirement of Georg Wesenberg in 1931, Wesenberg's laboratory of bacteriology, which had been charged since 1914 with studying the antiseptic and disinfectant properties of synthetic compounds, was dissolved. Domagk henceforth directed a renamed Laboratory of Experimental Pathology and Bacteriology.[15]

One of Domagk's first steps was to establish a suitable experimental model. The essential requirement was that host and pathogen be matched in such a way that the investigator succeeded "in infecting animals with certainty in a high percentage of cases." In addition, "the course of the infection must be as much as possible the same in all animals, so that from the observations on the treated animals and the untreated control animals we can draw reliable conclusions." Domagk found that his specifications were best met with streptococcal infections of mice and rabbits, which were almost invariably fatal.[16]

To narrow the field of compounds to be submitted to animal trials, Domagk relied in part on *in vitro* experiments, in which the target strain of bacterium was methodically exposed to a variety of chemicals. Wesenberg, the director of the Elberfeld laboratory of bacteriology, had been conducting such tests since his laboratory was created by Bayer in 1900. For Domagk, however, they had a different meaning. Such "orienting" test-tube trials, he held, could yield at best "general clues" as to which classes of bodies might contain compounds effective against certain bacteria. Domagk emphasized that they could not substitute for animal tests and could even be misleading in the sense that they could not distinguish disinfectants that would kill or damage the hosts as well as the pathogen from true chemotherapeutic agents harmless to the host.[17]

Domagk's target was a deadly one. Streptococci—immobile, spherical bacteria occurring in chains—were known to be causative agents in the most dangerous and common wound infections, childbed fever (puerperal sepsis), tonsillitis, endocarditis, many kidney and joint conditions, appendicitis, and other diseases. For some of these diseases, the mortality was high, as was the cost in human suffering. Domagk described the type used in his animal trials, *Streptococcus pyogenes hemolyticus*, as the most dangerous cause of wound infections in humans. The strain was taken from the blood of a patient who died of blood poisoning, or streptococcal sepsis. To ensure that all the untreated control animals died in twenty-four or, at most, forty-eight hours, he gave 10–100 times the mortal dose of the bacteria to all experimental animals.[18]

With his experimental model established, Domagk proceeded in collaboration with the chemists on a search for chemotherapeutically effective compounds. Selection of classes of compounds for animal trials was not random but was guided—according to Domagk—by "orienting" *in vitro* tests and by a review of the literature. One line of investigation was prompted in part by Domagk's earlier work on the reticuloendothelial system. The idea was to extract from tissues constituting part of the body's natural defenses substances that would be therapeutically active against streptococcal infections. This effort reached the stage of clinical trials but was defeated by side effects produced at therapeutically effective dosages. One of the initiators of this line of attack was Adolf Feldt, who in 1926 had also begun publishing results of treatment of experimental streptococcal infections with organic gold compounds. Feldt had recommended as effective two of these. Domagk confirmed the effectiveness of organic gold compounds but found that, in severe streptococcal infections, they could not be used for extended treatment in high enough doses without danger of gold intoxication, sometimes accompanied by skin conditions and kidney damage. He recommended their use in local treatment of streptococcus-infected wounds.[19]

By Domagk's account, the disadvantages of the gold compounds had led him and his collaborators to consider classes of purely organic substances. Among these were hydroquinine compounds such as the commercial preparations Vucin and Eucupin. These were already known for their effectiveness against streptococci *in vitro* and were used in deep antisepsis, the local treatment of infected tissues such as joints. Unfortunately, Domagk had to report, they failed completely in systemic infections. Much the same had to be said of a group of acridine compounds that surpassed known acridine compounds in effectiveness against streptococci *in vitro* but lost most of this action in infected animals.[20]

While Domagk was pursuing those early efforts, his chemist-collaborators Mietzsch and Klarer were involved in separate investigations, first with Roehl, then with Kikuth, that would eventually be brought to bear on bacterial chemotherapy. By Mietzsch's account, the most important of these was the search for compounds that would complement or improve upon the natural alkaloid quinine in the prevention or treatment of malaria. The search for "a better quinine," as Hörlein put it, had begun during the war and was a major focus of the Elberfeld research effort throughout the 1920s.[21]

A crucial early step in the Bayer antimalarial work had come when the medical researcher Schulemann and chemists Schönhöfer and Wingler had the idea of converting methylene blue—a compound known to be effective in quartan malaria—into a stronger basic derivative. Part of the inspiration for this move had been the prior success of the technique of basic alkylation, in which an alkyl group (general formula: C_nH_{2n+1}) was substituted for a hydrogen, in the derivation of pharmacologically active compounds. Among the early products of basic alkylation were Novocain and other local anesthetics and various compounds with action on the heart and uterus. Schulemann, Schönhöfer, and Wingler's variant of methylene blue had proved more effective than the parent compound. In Mietzsch's view, this work had "thereby opened the era of synthetic antimalarial drugs in Elberfeld." The next step was transfer of basic alkylation to compounds structurally related to quinine, the aminoquinolines. It was by this path, Mietzsch pointed out, that Schulemann, Schönhöfer, and Wingler, working with Roehl, had arrived at the first major synthetic antimalarial, Plasmoquine.[22]

Roehl was aware that neither Plasmoquine nor Quinoplasmine—the other synthetic antimalarial available by 1924—provided a complete solution to the malaria problem. This was because these agents acted on the sexual but not the asexual forms of the parasite. The task therefore was to find a chemical effective against the asexual form. In his work with Ehrlich, Roehl had become familiar with try-paflavine, an acridine compound used as an antiseptic. He conceived the dual ambition of finding another acridine compound effective as an antimalarial—"malaflavine" is the name he coined in confident anticipation—and a third active against streptococcal infections. Roehl's early death prevented his personal achievement of either goal.[23]

Mietzsch collaborated with Roehl on the acridine series from 1924, and in 1926 they were joined by the chemist Hans Mauss. The chemists sought to improve the antimalarial action of acridine compounds by modeling them on selected structural features of quinine and Plasmoquine and by making a systematic study of the effects of changing the nature and positions of substituents in the acridine ring. The compound that emerged from this work in 1930 proved to have an action qualitatively similar to quinine but quantitatively superior. This was Atabrine, a major new synthetic antimalarial, introduced into commerce and medicine in 1932.[24]

By the time that Atabrine was synthesized in 1930, research in bacterial chemotherapy at Elberfeld was moving decisively toward concentration on the azo dyes. Several circumstances favored this direction of work. Roehl's training with Ehrlich predisposed him to the use of dyes as chemotherapeutic agents, and in 1927 he had found an azo dye with activity against malaria in birds. A considerable body of literature from the 1910s and 1920s pointed to the antibacterial effects *in vitro* of azo compounds. By the early 1930s, several azo compounds had been recommended for use in urinary tract disinfection. The azo compounds were also appealing on strictly chemical grounds, since numerous variants could be prepared. Mietzsch recalled that when he began this work with Klarer, they believed that compounds of this type would find chemotherapeutic applications, "without of course at first being able to predict the specific indications," that is, which compounds would act on which pathogen. Azo dyes and the means to prepare them were readily at hand in an industry engaged in their production and sale.[25]

As early as 1927, Mietzsch and Klarer began to prepare azo compounds for chemotherapeutic testing, in close collaboration first with Roehl and Wesenberg and later with Domagk and Kikuth. From the chemists' point of view, the search was an organic chemist's puzzle. "Here also the law of the right man at the right place holds," Mietzsch wrote, "that is, translated into chemical language, the right substituents in the right position on the azo group, when it is a question of bringing out the slumbering chemotherapeutic characteristics in these systems." To narrow the field of possibilities, Mietzsch and Klarer relied on the example of known effective compounds of a different type. The model of Atabrine was especially important and led to the preparation of azo compounds with chemotherapeutic action on trypanosome infections, bird malaria, rat leprosy, and other infections.[26]

At the end of 1931, Mietzsch and Klarer applied for a first patent, in the text of which they noted that "it has been found that it is possible to obtain compounds active against protozoa and bacteria." By that time, they had prepared 300 azo compounds, which they had turned over to Roehl, Wesenberg, Domagk, and

Kikuth for *in vitro* and *in vivo* testing against a variety of pathogens. Of these substances, fourteen had been singled out because they showed activity in at least one of the biological tests. The latter included trials against experimental erysipelas and tuberculosis in animals as well as the tests against trypanosomal and streptococcal infections, bird malaria, rat leprosy, and other infections.[27]

The results with azo dyes obtained by the Elberfeld researchers by the late summer of 1932 were encouraging in that they appeared to lend additional weight to Robert Koch's and Ehrlich's views on the relationship between the staining properties of molecules and their antiparasitic action. The findings to date also suggested a tentative relationship between molecular structure and therapeutic action: placement of radicals in certain positions on the azo compound appeared to enhance activity.[28]

It was just at this juncture that Mietzsch's and Klarer's training in dye chemistry, and the accumulated experience of the Bayer/I.G. Farben research establishment, entered the investigation in a particular and, as events were to show, decisive way. Klarer later recalled that the chemists' working hypothesis was based on the idea of finding compounds that had a selective affinity for fibers and cells and that would thereby damage bacteria either directly or by attacking the conditions of their existence. "In this we could build on the experience of dye chemistry," Klarer noted. Such experience indicated that very definite groups played an important role in this affinity. Accordingly, the chemists systematically built such groups into compounds.[29]

"As we tested in this way all the available substituents," Mietzsch recalled, "we remembered the earlier sulfonamide-containing azo dyes, which had also come out of work at Elberfeld." In one of his earliest research projects at Bayer, Hörlein had collaborated with the chemists Dressel and Kothe in substitution of a sulfonamide radical in azo molecules, thereby improving their qualities of resistance to washing, to weaving, and to light when used to color woolens. The resulting supramine dyes were still in use.[30]

In September 1932, Mietzsch sent Klarer a quantity of an intermediate containing the sulfonamide radical "with a view to synthesis of azo compounds" that were "to be the object of trials on leprosy and tuberculosis." By the end of September, Klarer had reported to his colleagues the synthesis of the first sulfonamide azo compound. Labeled KL695 and turned over to Domagk, who gave it number 3920, this substance was subjected in Domagk's laboratory to test-tube and animal trials against streptococcal infections, tuberculosis, and tumors. KL695/D3920 failed against test-tube cultures of streptococci. In laboratory trials dated October 25, however, the compound showed a striking therapeutic action in mice infected with streptococci. These results were confirmed in Domagk's laboratory on October 31, "and thereby," Mietzsch later noted, "the way to sulfonamide therapy was opened up, a way along which moved all later work at home and abroad."[31]

Domagk and his collaborators now shifted the emphasis of the investigation to the sulfonamide-containing azo compounds. Klarer synthesized a number of these substances. Variations on the new theme began to distinguish what was essential to the therapeutic action from what was not, and in Mietzsch's words, "the path that previously had led from the simply-constructed chrysoidine to the complicated aminoazobenzenes would be retraced backwards." Recalling the known bactericidal action of crysoidine *in vitro*, Klarer synthesized a new molecule very close to it in structure but with a sulfonamide radical substituted in the *para-* position. Labeled KL730 by Klarer, the compound was turned over to Domagk. Relabeled, D4145, this otherwise undistinguished red dye proved ineffective against streptococci in the test tube but *extraordinarily* active against streptococcal infections in mice. In his first published article on this research, Domagk included a table showing the dramatic results of one experiment, dated December 20, 1932, in which the dye was administered to infected mice. Most of the untreated control animals were dead within forty-eight hours of infection, while all treated animals survived.[32]

By now, the magnitude of the breakthrough achieved by Klarer, Mietzsch, and Domagk was apparent. The company added KL695 to the patent taken out at the end of 1931. On Christmas Day, 1932, I.G. Farben applied for a new German patent, No. 607537, on the red dye that Domagk was showing to possess such striking properties. Under the name Streptozon, and later Prontosil, this substance was to open a new era in the chemical treatment of bacterial infections.[33]

The Nature of Chemotherapy

For Domagk and his chemist-collaborators Mietzsch and Klarer, the invention of Prontosil was a momentous event, marking a watershed in their careers as much as in the history of medicine. It is not surprising that all three subsequently wrote accounts of the investigations that resulted in Prontosil. Domagk and Mietzsch, in particular, each wrote about their early collaboration, Domagk in several articles of the mid-1930s, and Mietzsch in a series of publications of the early 1950s. These articles are useful not only for reconstruction of the process that led to Prontosil, but still more for what they reveal about how each party, medical researcher and chemist, viewed the nature of chemotherapeutic research and for what these views, in some ways contrasting and contradictory, tell us about the nature of chemotherapy as an entity and its place in the system of industrial innovation that had emerged at I.G. Farben.

For Domagk, the essential aims of chemotherapeutic research were practical, not theoretical. Though informed by science, its primary goal was not creation of new knowledge of nature but identification of compounds effective in the treatment of bacterial infections. He acknowledged the largely empirical character of the research, in the face of inadequate knowledge of the biology of parasites and hosts. The practical character of the goals shaped the field, for example, leading Domagk to adopt divergent classifications of bacteria and to emphasize those aspects of the biological specificity of bacteria that might suggest targets for chemotherapeutic agents.[34]

Chemotherapeutic research was also, for Domagk, a distinctly medical and biological endeavor. This meant that the researcher needed to focus on the complexities and specificities of the interactions among hosts, the microbes causing disease, and the chemical agents used in treatment. The aim of the physician in chemotherapy was to come to the aid of the body's defenses against infection, not to replace them. Explorations of these interactions required, in Domagk's view, a three-tiered methodology comprising *in vitro*, animal, and clinical tests of prospective chemotherapeutic agents. One aspect of this methodology was Domagk's conviction that failure of a compound *in vitro* did not mean that it would necessarily fail in the animal or human host, a view that was crucial to the discovery of Prontosil. Domagk recognized the essential role of chemistry in chemotherapeutic research but tended to assign to chemists a subordinate role.

For Mietzsch, this order of things was reversed. While he conceded the necessary place of medical researchers in the development of chemotherapy, Mietzsch's view of the field is better captured by Hörlein's description of pharmaceuticals as "a branch of chemical technology." Put differently, Mietzsch thought that the primary engine of chemotherapeutic research was chemistry. He characterized all of the major turning points in the field's history in chemical terms. In particular, in Mietzsch's story the sulfonamides emerged from study of basic alkylated compounds and from use of azo dyes in chemotherapy. Azo dyes were appealing to Mietzsch and Klarer above all for a chemical reason, their ease of variability. The "decisive turning point" for Mietzsch came when a sulfonamide group was introduced in a definite position in the azo dye molecule. Thus, Mietzsch characterized the decisive turning point in the invention of the sulfonamides chemically and located it in the chemical side of chemotherapeutic research at Elberfeld.[35]

Mietzsch was at pains to display the mental effort behind the chemical side of chemotherapeutic research. The research process is not merely trial and error, the blind grinding out and testing of one compound after another. Patterns emerge. A new chemical procedure or phenomenon is found that leads to a useful result in the sense of an effective chemotherapeutic agent. The finding is then applied to other classes of compounds in the hope of getting such a useful result with them. In one series in which it is tried, a promising compound is identified. That leads to more systematic work on that series, which in turn may lead to finding a successful chemotherapeutic agent. Thus, the research process on the chemical side is not random, although it does have a trial-and-error quality. The trial and error takes place within certain boundaries that are determined by some combination of what it is possible to do chemically and previous experience with certain chemical processes or certain classes of compounds regarding identification of successful chemotherapeutic agents. The trial-and-error process appears to have two phases: an initial, relatively loose phase in which promising leads are sought within a fairly broad domain of possibilities, and a second, more intense and systematic phase in which a lead that has been identified is followed up, for example, within a well-defined class of compounds.

For Mietzsch, the search for a chemotherapeutically effective compound therefore involved a narrowing down to the right kind of chemical specificity: the right series, the right position on the compound, the right substituent. For the chemists, the problem was one of chemical variation and chemical specificity, with the goal of achieving a precise match with the target organism.

Central to Mietzsch's message was the conviction that he and other Bayer/I.G. Farben chemists were pursuing not merely a chemical, but a specifically chemotherapeutic research program. Their role was not simply instrumental but involved deliberate judgments and choices based on rational and goal-directed considerations, chemical reasoning in the service of chemotherapeutic goals. Mietzsch saw the chemotherapeutic research process from the standpoint of a chemist's—specifically, a dye chemist's—training, a chemist's way of thinking, and a chemist's vivid intuitive sense of the creative process in the chemical as distinct from the biomedical side of the research.[36]

Taken together, the images of chemotherapeutic research presented by Hörlein, Domagk, and Mietzsch yield a sharper picture of the development of Prontosil as a case of industrialized invention. Among the most important elements of this picture are a systemic approach to innovation, continuities between dyestuff chemistry and pharmaceutical chemistry and between the different chemical lines of pharmaceutical research, and the robust optimism of the Bayer/I.G. Farben industrial team in the midst of a general atmosphere of caution and resignation.

Hörlein viewed bacterial chemotherapy as a reverse salient in a broadly advancing front along which chemistry and medicine joined battle with disease. Working within and expanding a well-developed industrial research organization, he embraced a systemic approach to innovation. He expected technically and scientifically novel results to emerge not from individuals working alone but from groups of specialists working cooperatively under a team leader and supported by a strong research infrastructure. He saw and expected patterns in the work, with innovation occurring in typical steps or phases depending on the fields or kinds of problems involved. He acted the role of research manager to the fullest: setting aims, concentrating resources and personnel, assessing results, and representing his organization's efforts to the medical and scientific communities. It was Hörlein who brought Domagk, Mietzsch, and Klarer into the pharmaceutical research division, and it was in close association with him that their research program in bacterial chemotherapy was formulated and conducted.

For Hörlein's program to succeed, however, critical problems had to be defined and solved by the medical researcher and the chemist, each working in his own domain and with his own concepts, methods, and habits of thought. Both medical researchers and chemists confronted the problem of specificity. The difference was that in one case the specificity was biological, while in the other case it was chemical. Biological specificity meant identification of the difference between host and pathogen, such that a means was available to attack the pathogen without harming the host. It meant, in addition, definition of differences between the kinds of bacteria, differences that could manifest in subtle metabolic, nutritional, or other aspects of the organism. Chemical specificity meant conceiving and synthesizing all possible variants on a given kind of compound, that is, by starting with a nucleus of some sort and building around it; or, in a more general sense, the division and subdivision of chemical compounds—in this case, mainly or exclusively organic ones—into classes and subclasses.

Both the medical researcher and the chemist ostensibly had the same goal: to identify a specific compound that would attack a specific pathogen that was harming a specific host. But to reach the goal, two complementary but distinct efforts had to be mounted in which each investigator wrestled with his own problems of specificity. The medical researcher had to find an experimental model that was adequate to the pathogen in the sense that experimental infections could be consistently produced with that type of pathogen, and that was adequate to the host in the sense that it was the same pathogen that attacked the human host and against which a chemotherapy was sought. He also had to take into account the reaction of the host organism, both to the pathogen and the changes it induced and to any chemical agent introduced as a therapeutic measure. The medical researcher also had to consider specificity in the sense of the particular locale (tissue, organ, cells) attacked by the pathogen and the pattern of distribution of the chemical agent in the host organism.

The chemist had to decide—with or without the aid of the medical researcher—which class or classes of compounds to try against the kinds of infections in question. His criteria for doing so might be chemical, for example, ease of variability by changes in coupling components or substituents, or prompted in some way by prior experience with living organisms, such as *in vitro* activity against bacteria. Once a promising compound was identified by the medical researcher, the chemist's task was to produce variations around this starting point with the aim of increasing the specificity of the match between the chemical agent, the pathogen, and the host. Here, indeed, was a signal difference between the two components of chemotherapeutic research. Whereas the medical researcher took the variability given in nature, tried to analyze it in detail, and identified points where chemical therapy might find a purchase, the chemists produced variability by synthetic manipulation.

Chemotherapy so conceived and practiced cannot be regarded as a unitary scientific discipline in the academic sense. The nature of its problems necessitates cooperation between chemists and medical researchers, the latter variously identifying themselves as pathologists, bacteriologists, physiologists, or in other ways. Neither the chemist nor the medical researcher by himself has the necessary experience to conduct research in the field. Chemotherapy in Hörlein's conception therefore is defined not as much by a move for autonomy vis-à-vis other disciplines—for example, physiological chemistry or biochemistry vis-à-vis physiology—as by the necessary cooperative linkage of two or more disciplines that continue to retain distinct identities while interacting at specific sites on their boundaries. That is, chemotherapeutic research can be characterized as a permanent cooperative association of two or more disciplines around certain problems.

The problems were first defined by Ehrlich. To some degree, as Hörlein pointed out, Ehrlich embodied in himself the two necessary components of the field, the medical and the chemical, although even in his case he relied on chemists for part of the work. But the fine chemicals industry, because of its prior commitment to pharmaceuticals, already had in place one of the institutional arrangements required by Ehrlich's program, that is, an organization in which chemists and medical researchers were in cooperative association. What was needed was the addition of a new component that would emphasize the particular aspect of the medical–chemical interaction defined by Ehrlich. At Bayer, for example, this took the form of the new chemotherapy laboratory added in 1910, or of Domagk's laboratory established in 1927 and expanded in 1930. In the setting of the fine chemicals industry, the components of Ehrlich's program were more clearly differentiated in both methodology and organization. Thus, the primary aim of chemotherapeutic research—essentially an engineering goal—could be most effectively realized in a setting that was interdisciplinary, in the sense of juxtaposing more than one field in a single institutional setting, and industrial, because of the massive resources that could be brought to bear to set up and maintain a differentiated research infrastructure and—in the case of the fine chemicals industry—to make available thousands of synthetically produced chemicals and the expertise to vary these compounds in determinate ways to achieve the ends in view.

The Industrialization of Innovation

Pharmaceutical research at Bayer/I.G. Farben, and chemotherapeutic research in particular, was a product of, and was incorporated into, a system of innovation elaborated over several decades in the German fine chemicals industry. The research and development enterprise of Bayer/I.G. Farben consisted of an aggregate of devices, artifacts (e.g., compounds), organizational structures, trained personnel, and other resources in which substantial capital had been invested. The direction of the research enterprise was a product both of goals imagined and set by researchers and managers and of responses to opportunities opened up by the results of prior research and development efforts. The endeavor was driven in part by economic motives that favored diversification to maximize return on capital investment and to cushion fluctuations in demand for any one kind of product. As Georg Meyer-Thurow has shown, the perceived need for diversification was one factor behind the institutionalization of research within Bayer from the 1880s.[37] Finally, a powerful component of the momentum of the research enterprise within Bayer/I.G. Farben was the culture that had developed around it by the early twentieth century. Many individuals and institutions in the medical and academic scientific communities were committed in one way or another to its goals, methods, and products.

The movement from synthetic dyestuffs to pharmaceuticals to chemotherapy to bacterial chemotherapy may be regarded as a series of steps in the diversification of an industrial enterprise and its research establishment. Continuity from dyestuffs chemistry was expressed in personnel, in concepts and methods, and in the use of specific products. Hörlein, Mietzsch and Klarer were trained in dyestuffs chemistry and practiced it before moving to pharmaceuticals. On its chemical side, chemotherapeutic research involved methods of synthesis and concepts of specificity and variability taken over from dyestuffs chemistry. Hörlein drew a direct analogy between the natural/synthetic dichotomy in dyestuffs and the natural/synthetic dichotomy in medicinal substances. The azo dyes were tried as medicines, and one of them became Prontosil. According to Mietzsch, there was a thread of continuity in the research at Elberfeld running from the basic alkylated compounds through the sulfonamides to the later sulfones and thiosemi-carbazones, with each development drawing on previous ones. Hörlein was acutely aware of the need for a culture of pharmaceutical research both in the sense of a network of supporting institutions and in the sense of a strong constituency in the medical and scientific communities, a constituency that he worked assiduously to build.

Analysis of pharmaceutical research at Bayer/I.G. Farben in terms of such an industrial system of pharmaceutical innovation goes far to explain the optimism about bacterial chemotherapy that prevailed within the Elberfeld group in the 1920s and early 1930s. That mood is in need of explanation since, as described here, the prevailing attitude in the medical and scientific communities by the early 1930s ranged from cautious optimism coupled with critical scrutiny of research goals and methods, to outright frustration and resignation.[38] Hörlein could be optimistic because he approached bacterial chemotherapy not as an individual working on a discrete problem within a single discipline, but as a manager of a well-developed research organization with a systemic approach to innovation, a wide-ranging vision of the possibilities of chemistry in medicine, and a record of success with closely related problems.

Comparison of Hörlein's research organization with that of Hugh Young at Johns Hopkins is revealing.[39] There are a number of similarities. Ehrlich's ideas and optimism played a role, direct or indirect, in the initiation of both research programs. Both employed a variety of trained personnel, including medical doctors, bacteriologists, and organic chemists, working cooperatively in spatial proximity to one another. In both cases, individual leadership was important in initiating the research, mobilizing resources, and mediating between the research effort and the larger organization of which it was a part.

There the similarities end, however. And the differences are telling. The Brady Institute was committed to a general disinfectant model of chemotherapeutic research, while the Elberfeld group took over a specific therapy model already institutionalized in the pharmaceutical research division and extended and refined by Domagk. The Brady Institute team gave little weight to in vitro trials, and even less to animal tests, instead relying heavily on uncontrolled clinical trials. The Elberfeld group, in contrast, relied heavily on controlled trials of compounds against experimental infections in animals, in fact, on carefully designed "experimental models," with auxiliary use of in vitro trials.

Hugh Young's emphasis on clinical case reports flowed in part from the aims and structure of the Brady Urological Institute. The work of the institute and of the Journal of Urology, which Young founded and edited, was to contribute to the building of urology as a specialized field of medicine. Chemotherapeutic research was a part of this larger project. Clinical practice dominated architectural space and action. Whereas chemotherapeutic research at Elberfeld enjoyed stable and generous funding, such research at the Brady Institute had lower priority than clinical practice and teaching, a fact placed in stark relief when endowment income or private donations declined. Young and his co-workers did not set up a continuous or broadly based program of chemotherapeutic research and did not establish a system of innovation in chemotherapy.

It was just such a system of innovation, embedded in a corporate setting, that shaped and sustained the research on bacterial chemotherapy at Elberfeld. Hörlein's overriding purpose was to identify compounds that were at the same time effective medicines and viable commercial products. He saw and encouraged possibilities for developing such compounds across a broad front that included vitamins, hormones, and various antimicrobial chemotherapies, including those aimed at bacterial infections. Such a setting ensured concentration and continuity of effort on the search for effective compounds without pressure for immediate clinical application. It allowed for and facilitated transfer of expertise and of synthesized compounds from one research program to another, and full exploitation of any positive results obtained. These comparisons indicate that Carl Voegtlin's criteria for successful research in chemotherapy had much to recommend them, especially as amended by the Elberfeld model.[40]

When he decided in 1927 to mount a major research effort in bacterial chemotherapy, Hörlein had expected to reach his goal in ten years. That he succeeded in less than six is testimony not only to the energy and talents of his research team but also to the effectiveness of the system of invention he had built. By the time I.G. Farben applied for a patent on Prontosil in December 1932, that system seemed firmly in place. It was not. Within two months, one of its essential elements would be seriously challenged from a new and unexpected direction by the National Socialist accession to power.

PART II

The Making of the First
Miracle Drugs

CHAPTER 4

Into the Maelstrom

L ittle more than a month elapsed between I.G. Farben's application for a patent on the compound that became Prontosil and Adolf Hitler's assumption of office as Reich Chancellor on January 30, 1933. By the time that Hitler took his own life in his Berlin bunker in April 1945, Prontosil and its descendants of the second generation of sulfa drugs, produced by an international effort of research and development, had transformed medical management of bacterial infections. Gerhard Domagk had been awarded a Nobel Prize. Both Allied and Axis armies had made extensive use of sulfa drugs, with considerable impact on morbidity and mortality on both sides.

With the entry of penicillin into the Allied war effort in late 1943, the sulfa drugs began to be displaced from a central position in treatment of bacterial infections, a process that was to continue after the war with the introduction of other antibiotics. Never entirely eclipsed, and still in use today, sulfa drugs henceforth enjoyed a secondary status in the physician's armamentarium. Chronologically, therefore, the heyday of the sulfa drugs corresponds almost exactly to the rise and fall of the Third Reich. The global story of the sulfa drugs in this period comprises several distinguishable but closely related stories, among them the laboratory and clinical testing of Prontosil, the recognition and early testing of Prontosil's first offspring, sulfanilamide, the reception of both medicines by the medical community and their introduction into medical practice, the development of a new generation of sulfa drugs as derivatives of sulfanilamide by the pharmaceutical industries of several countries, the mobilization of production and use of the sulfas in World War II, and the first efforts to understand how the sulfa drugs worked.

Among these stories, there is reason to begin with, and to consider separately, the fate of the new medicines under the Nazi regime. Prontosil was developed in

Germany, and Germany was the site of its initial laboratory and clinical testing, patenting, and the first efforts to develop related compounds. Consideration of the first sulfa drugs and their makers can contribute to our developing picture of the place of the sciences, in particular, the biomedical sciences, in the Third Reich. Several questions, some of them recently under discussion by other scholars, may be addressed anew in the light of the sulfa drugs story. What was the content of the National Socialist critique of scientific medicine, and of pharmaceuticals and chemotherapy in particular? What effects did this critique have on the conduct of research or on therapeutic practices in the German medical community? What effect did the regime's patent policy have on pharmaceutical research and development? What measures were taken by the regime to intervene in or suspend the internationalism of science, including its international reward system, and what degree of success did they achieve? What forms were taken by the use of human subjects in medical research, and in what ways did these forms break with prior practices in the medical and scientific communities? In what ways and to what degree were biomedical scientists and research establishments involved in development of weapons for gas or biological warfare? Finally, what were the modalities of the relationships established between scientists, doctors, biomedical research institutions, and the Nazi regime?[1]

Medical Research under Attack

Part of the answer to the last question may be found in the struggle over use of animal experimentation in medical research that spanned much of the regime's first year in power. On one side were Nazi zealots and animal protection societies for whom scientific medicine was, at best, of dubious value and, at worst, part of a vicious conspiracy to rob and corrupt the German *Volk*. On the other side were representatives of German science, medicine, and industry, including, notably, Heinrich Hörlein, for whom the threat of a total ban on animal experimentation struck at the foundations of medical research. In the middle, ostensibly listening to both sides and in possession of final decision-making authority, were Hermann Göring as Prussian Minister of the Interior and officials of the Prussian Interior Ministry's medical division.

Opening rounds were fired in the winter of 1932. Almost on the eve of I.G. Farben's filing of a patent application for Prontosil, the National Socialist contingent of the Prussian *Landtag* moved to entirely prohibit vivisection and to make it punishable. Exception was to be made only for three scientific institutes to be named by the government and whose activities were to be placed under permanent public supervision. Had it been enacted, such legislation would have gone beyond existing Prussian ministerial regulations issued in 1930, which already confined experiments on animals to important research under prescribed conditions.[2]

Hörlein saw in such proposals, which were soon followed by the National Socialist takeover of power, the possibility of an imminent end of animal experiment and thus of the whole medical research enterprise in Germany. Later, he recalled that "as leader of the largest German pharmaceutical research establishment

I held it to be my duty to combat these tendencies, and therefore tried to make contact with people in the party who I assumed had direct contact with Hitler." The local *Gauleiter*, one Florian-Düsseldorf, was not interested. Two local officials of the SA (*Sturmabteilung* or Storm Troopers), on the other hand, put Hörlein in touch with Julius Uhl, one of SA leader Ernst Röhm's adjutants. In the spring of 1933, Uhl visited Elberfeld and was given a tour that included demonstrations of the I.G. Farben pharmaceutical Germanin (Bayer 205), a medicine against sleeping sickness, and the antimalarials Plasmoquine and Atabrine. Uhl seemed friendly and recommended that Hörlein take the matter up with the *Generalarzt* of the SA, whom he thought to be the most influential physician in Germany. When he traveled to Munich a few weeks later to follow this advice, Hörlein found Uhl "as if transformed." Uhl "explained to me in the most unfriendly way that he wanted to have no more to do with us, that we were not only an international Jewish enterprise, but also simply traitors, since in spite of the taking away of the German colonies by the treaty of Versailles," I.G. Farben had introduced Germanin, Plasmoquine, and Atabrine, products that exclusively benefited Germany's former enemies. It was fortunate for I.G. Farben that all of this had happened before 1933, Uhl continued, adding ominously that in future such cases the company would be dealt with in other ways. Finally, Uhl stated that animal experiment as well as ritual slaughter was to be forbidden, and that Hörlein would hear more about it soon.[3]

Hörlein was convinced that Uhl's newly hostile attitude came directly from Hitler. That view is made plausible by our knowledge of a clash that occurred in May 1933 between Hitler and Carl Bosch, chairman of the executive board (*Vorstand*) of I.G. Farbenindustrie. Bosch, who opposed Nazi antisemitism, had by his own account tried to convey to Hitler the damaging effects of official racism on German science, industry, and trade. Furious, Hitler had lectured Bosch on the latter's ignorance of politics and on Germany's ability to "work one hundred years without physics and chemistry" if necessary, and had shown him the door.[4]

Uhl's prediction of imminent action seemed to be fulfilled on August 17, when Göring issued an order to go into effect immediately that

> vivisection of animals of whatsoever species is prohibited in all parts of Prussian territory. The chairman of the cabinet has instructed the ministries to present to him without delay the text of a law incorporating this provision. Until the promulgation of this law, persons who engage in vivisection of animals of any kind will be removed to a concentration camp.

By this time, Bavaria, too, had adopted similar prohibitions. It was understood at the time that Göring's edict was to be in effect temporarily, pending issuance of a federal animal protection law. In the meantime, routine diagnostic and other tests using animals would be allowed, but medical research would be suspended. An Interior Ministry statement promised that "consideration will be given to the requirements of science."[5]

I.G. Farben's whole research and development effort in pharmaceuticals and pesticides was now placed in question. Hörlein recalled that this, together with simultaneous attacks on mineral fertilizers in favor of "biological-dynamic" or organic fertilizers, made him temporarily so discouraged that he considered immigration to the United States. On his second American visit, in 1932, Hörlein had been offered the directorship of the scientific laboratories of the Bayer Company in Albany, New York, in the event that revolutionary change occurred in Germany. The offer came from W.E. Weiss, general manager of Sterling Products, which had purchased the Bayer Company in the United States from the Alien Property Custodian after the war. American Bayer had already acquired one of its leaders, Wilhelm Hiemenz, from among the Elberfeld executives. "But finally I decided," Hörlein reported, "to remain in Germany and to take up the fight for freedom of science."[6]

The chance to fight came almost immediately. Acting in Göring's name, an official of the Prussian Interior Ministry, Frey, convened a meeting on August 29 that included representatives of German animal protection societies and representatives of German science. Prominent among the former were an SS doctor from Hannover, Albert Eckhard, who was chairman of the Association of German Antivivisectionist Physicians (*Verband vivisektionsgegnerischer Aerzte Deutschlands*), and Caesar Rhan, chairman of the Association of Antivivisectionist Organizations (*Verband vivisektionsgegnerischer Vereine*). Eckhard had a special standing in the animal protection movement. Not only was he a medical doctor and member of the SS, but he also was in possession of a personal letter from Hitler promising support for his cause. In 1929, Hitler had written to Eckhard, "Many thanks for sending your animal protection brochure, which I have only just read! As you might think, with deep indignation. . . . You can be sure that in the coming National Socialist state these conditions will be very quickly ended!" Among the representatives of science were leaders of state medical and scientific institutes in Berlin, and Hörlein. Some sense of the confrontational quality of the meeting may be gathered from the partisan accounts published after it by Eckhard and by an antivivisectionist organization to which Rhan reported.[7]

The ostensible purpose of the meeting was to allow a full airing of the positions of both sides so as to inform the ministry in its preparation of a draft of the *Reich* animal protection law. Discussion went on for seven hours. It was presided over by Minister Frey, who, Eckhard conceded, tried to be fair to all. Both Eckhard and Rhan, however, found reason to be dissatisfied with the proceedings. By Rhan's account, Eckhard, who as a medical doctor found himself doing most of the work for the animal protectionist side, was in an extremely difficult position. Faced with some twenty or twenty-five opponents, "he resisted bravely, but the odds were too uneven." Most difficult for the animal protectionists was the issue of the animal trial (*Tierversuch*) in medical research. Eckhard and Rhan had wanted to challenge the effectiveness of serums and toxins (*Giften* [*sic*], perhaps a deliberate substitute for antitoxins) and to argue that they could be dispensed with in favor of natural treatment in both human and animal diseases. Not only did everyone else present take the effectiveness of these agents as given, but the animal protectionists could not bring in an antivivisectionist veterinarian to challenge conventional treatments of animal diseases. Frey would not give a definite answer to Rhan's question whether animal protectionist groups would be given a role in the final drawing up of the new law, and an official of the Agricultural

Ministry rebuffed the animal protectionist demands to have a role in oversight of vivisection sites.[8]

Reflecting on the meeting several days afterward, the opponents of animal experiment found other cause for complaint. The heads of at least seven German animal protection societies had not been invited to the meeting. The group to which Rhan reported, the World League for the Protection of Animals and Against Vivisection (*Weltbundes zum Schutze der Tiere und gegen die Vivisektion*), was also excluded by Frey on the grounds that it was an international organization and that its views would be well represented by Eckhard. Members of the World League, which regarded itself as a leading German antivivisection organization, were indignant and promptly voted to change the group's name to German Reich League for Animal Rights and Against Vivisection (*Deutscher Reichsbund für Tierrecht und gegen Vivisektion*). Rhan attacked press reports of the meeting that described it as an "agreement" or "reconciliation" (*Vereinbarung*). Not only did the meeting expose irreconcilable differences, but his understanding was that it was a non-binding discussion, for which minutes were not taken. He was also disturbed that members of the animal protection societies were scattered around the meeting hall and so were unable to consult on points under debate.[9]

Both Rhan and Eckhard reserved their harshest language for Hörlein. Hörlein had taken a prominent part in the discussions, several times launching "extremely irritating attacks" on the animal protectionists, to which both Rhan and Eckhard had to respond. Among these were Hörlein's energetic rejection of Rhan's proposal to prohibit use of large animals in research, his charge that Eckhard had deliberately made false statements, and his prediction that prohibition of animal experiment in research would cost the jobs of 800–1,000 workers at I.G. Farben. In their written accounts of the meeting, neither Eckhard nor Rhan addressed the substance of Hörlein's remarks on medicine, but instead made every effort to delegitimize Hörlein as spokesman on such matters by political and racialist innuendo. Hörlein was not a real physician but only an honorary doctor of medicine who had received that title "during the time of the Marxist government," Eckhard wrote, playing misleadingly on the name of the Center Party leader, Wilhelm Marx, whose government was in place during part of 1926, when Hörlein received his honorary degree from Munich. Hörlein, the "handsomely paid member of the executive board of I.G. Farben," had questioned the veracity of Eckhard, who described himself as the leader of "a great idealistic movement." Before threats of job losses were made, Eckhard insisted, the salaries of I.G. Farben leaders and the monies going to foreign representatives of I.G. Farben should be investigated. The initials I.G., Eckhard claimed, stood for "internationalen Gesellschaft für Farbenindustrie [*sic*]," a false assertion that played on the negative valuation of "international" in National Socialist ideology. Eckhard also found "interesting and informative" the names of members of the executive board listed in I.G. Farben's 1932 report. "I believe it would be rewarding to look a bit into the 'Aryan' descent of these men," Eckhard remarked. "Thus it was generally noticeable in our meeting in Berlin," he continued, "that Prof. Dr. Hörlein so warmly supported the Jewish professor Rosenfeld." Eckhard immediately went on to call for takeover of the pharmaceutical industry by the National Socialist state as the best and swiftest way to reduce animal experiment to the unavoidable minimum and to separate the practice from capitalist profit interests.[10]

Animal protectionist fears were soon confirmed. On September 5, 1933, less than a week after the Berlin discussions sponsored by the Interior Ministry, Göring issued temporary regulations to govern vivisection pending issuance of the federal law. Referring to "agreements" reached in the Berlin discussions, the statement of interior regulations drew a sharp line between vivisection, which was to be prohibited, and the use of animal experiments in "serious scientific research, in the interest of the health and life of men and animals." Animal experimentation would not be regarded as vivisection if certain conditions were met. Experiments were to be performed "only in institutes under scientific management, and only on the responsibility of the director of the institute." There had to be prospect of definite and original results. Discomfort of the animal subjects was to be minimized, with use of local or general anesthetics whenever possible. Use of higher animals was to be avoided, and the numbers of animals used were to be kept to the minimum necessary. To conduct animal experiments, scientific institutes were either to have a concession from the state, commune, or municipality or to obtain special ministerial approval. Animal experiments for purposes of instruction would be permitted only under special circumstances and with state permission.[11]

The issuance of the interior regulations so soon after August 29 and the simultaneous statement that a draft of the federal animal protection law was already in existence suggest that these documents were drawn up in the wake of and under the influence of the Interior Ministry debates. Such was the recollection of Clemens Giese, an Interior Ministry official closely involved in the discussions of the draft law. By Giese's report, the "thoroughly moderate" character of the interior regulations, which then became the basis of the federal law, was heavily indebted to Hörlein's vigorous arguments at the August 29 meeting. Whatever the restrictions placed on animal experiment by the regulations, Hörlein and his allies, including Giese, felt that they could live with them. Animal protection groups, in contrast, felt that their demands had been only partially met, and this by a state that they presumed to be highly sympathetic to their cause. This divergence, together with the uncertainty created by the interim character of the regulations, opened the way for a heated polemical and legal struggle during the two and one-half months between September 5 and the promulgation of the Reich animal protection law on November 23, 1933.[12]

Hörlein and I.G. Farben now came under violent attack in National Socialist publications such as *Deutsche Volksgesundheit aus Blut und Boden!* and Nazi-oriented animal protection journals. In these assaults, hostility to scientific medicine, including but by no means limited to use of animal experiment in research, was fused with antisemitism and attacks on international big capital. Under the title "What Is Up with 'Germanin'?" one article in *Deutsche Volksgesundheit* lambasted the famous remedy for sleeping sickness. Citing Hitler's letter to Eckhard, the author predicted that the sufferings inflicted on animals in "so-called scientific investigations" would soon be ended by law. Adduced by representatives of I.G. Farben as their "trump card" showing the necessity of animal experiment, Germanin was no such thing, the writer claimed. Far from being "nearly miraculous," "reminiscent of Biblical cures," "unprecedented," or "staggering," the author warned, Germanin might well go the way of other "shimmering illusions" such as tuberculin, the diphtherium serum of "the Jew Behring," or the Salvarsan of "the Jew Ehrlich." Citing the failure of Germanin against a St. Louis outbreak of a disease resembling sleeping sickness but apparently caused by a filterable virus, the author mocked the pretensions of pharmaceutical research. Even if the "causative agent" were isolated in pure form, he asked, would this mean there was a certain remedy? "Certainly the bacteriologists of I.G. would bring it out! For variety, and in honor of the spirit of the place, as 'Americanin'? And certainly at once it will have effects 'reminiscent of Biblical cures'!" In any case, the author warned, a dubious medicine such as Germanin should not be invoked in defense of vivisection or in attacks on its critics as traitors to the German economy or even as traitors to the country. The representatives of the pharmaceutical industry "should not confuse the economy of their business with the economy of the German *Volk!*"[13]

Cartoons conveyed this kind of vitriol in its most concentrated form. One series that appeared in *Deutsche Volksgesundheit* in the fall of 1933 under the title "The Life and Deeds of Isidor G. Färber" (a fiction whose name plays off the company name I.G. Farben, a contraction of Interessengemeinschaft Farbenindustrie, or dye industry combine) portrays a grossly caricatured Jewish businessman as the manipulative power behind a large chemical industry that produces pharmaceuticals such as serums and vaccines. He acts through boards of directors, doctors, and so on, but the real power is in his hands. His medicines are tested on hapless animals and human patients. He wields powerful influence on the government from behind the scenes. He feels threatened by natural healers and by National Socialism, which is represented as "the spirit of the times." In another cartoon, not part of this series, a figure looking like Isidor G. Färber but labeled "stockholder" is shown with his foot on the neck of a prostrate man labeled "natural healing." In the background, beneath a Star of David labeled "Jewish-influenced medicine," stand two men in laboratory coats. One holds a bottle labeled "chemical medicine," the other a huge hypodermic needle. The cartoon's caption asks, "How long will the Jewish spirit suppress German reform?" The associated article is headed "Stop the Thief: The Role of the Jews in Medicine."[14]

The same blended motifs of hostility to scientific medicine, antisemitism, and more or less direct attacks on the chemical and pharmaceutical industry, are visible in the animal protectionist literature. In the lead article of the December 1933–January 1934 issue of *The German Friend of Animals* (*Der Deutsche Tierfreund*), the editor, Finus, identified the primary enemy and target of his movement as I.G. Farbenindustrie. Applauding the swift action of the National Socialist government in outlawing ritual slaughter, Finus lamented that the same undiluted success had not accompanied action against vivisection. Although at the time he went to press he did not yet know the wording of the Reich animal protection law, Finus feared that, along with restrictions on animal experiment, the law also contained compromises. The greatest user of animal trials, "chemical big capital," had, he thought, created difficulties for the government, which he presumed to be otherwise sympathetic to a complete ban. Failure to achieve such a ban meant that the movement would have to continue its struggle and especially try to reach the younger generation.[15]

Finus was particularly incensed because I.G. Farben had brought against him a formal document of complaint (*Klageschrift*) in which he and his cause were denied the attribute of idealism. I.G. Farben had accused Finus of striking at the very existence of the pharmaceutical industry, which, it maintained, could not operate without animal trials. Finus reported derisively that the company had asked that he be forbidden to assert that "Jesuitical and Jewish capital" was behind I.G. Farbenindustrie, that the chemical industry was the mortal enemy of helpless animals, that vivisection at I.G. Farben was driven by insane seeking for power and profit, and that I.G. Farben produced narcotic medicines and other preparations dangerous to health, propositions that he evidently considered to be self-evident. He singled out Hörlein, the well-paid head of the division of I.G. Farben making most use of animal trials, for special censure. "If the inheritance of the German race is to be saved, then we will forbid the use of poisonous medicines and the injection of serums alien to the species into healthy German blood. Then, to be sure, there would be fewer dividends to distribute, but we would get a flourishing of the people's health as a blessing to the nation!"[16]

As Finus's angry denunciations indicate, Hörlein had not remained idle in the face of attacks on I.G. Farben. Always pugnacious, he opened a running battle with the offending publications on two fronts. With the help of company counsel Schramm, he took several journals, including Finus's, to court. So as to give courage to the judges, "who were at that time already somewhat anxious," Hörlein worked through a local party legal official, the *Gaurechtsführer* for Düsseldorf, Schroer. The company was able to get from the courts temporary decrees, confiscations, and other measures, which brought about a gradual diminishing of the slander campaign. Other tactics were necessary against *Deutsche Volksgesundheit aus Blut und Boden!*, which was published first by a Nuremberg party physician, *Gauärzteführer* Will, and subsequently by party-influential Julius Streicher. Schroer advised Hörlein that legal action against Streicher would be impossible and that he should work through high representatives of the party or the state. This route proved successful. Hörlein was able to get one prohibition of offensive material through Reich Physicians Leader Gerhard Wagner, who was the highest medical official in the Nazi government, and a second and final one through Joseph Goebbels's medical advisor in the Reich Propaganda Ministry, Dr. Curt Thomalla.[17]

Finus's fears of government "compromise" were borne out by the text of the new law, which was firmly based on the interim regulations. By early 1934, the Interior Ministry had published detailed instructions, to become effective on February 1, on the permits to be issued to scientific laboratories and how the law was to be administered. Each laboratory receiving a permit to conduct experiments on animals would be subject to semiannual inspections, which would be unannounced and would be conducted jointly by physicians and veterinarians. Irregularities were to be reported immediately to the competent ministry. Penalties for infractions of the law were stiff and could include fines and imprisonment of up to two years. In conjunction with the new law, the Reich Interior Ministry moved to bring

the animal protection movement under its control by officially merging its 679 societies to form the Reich Animal Protection League (*Reichstierschutzbund*).[18]

No doubt the regulations were an irritant, but Hörlein was satisfied that, with
the help of Interior Ministry officials Giese and Frey, he had "succeeded in effecting the freedom of animal experiment to an adequate extent against hard resistance." Even after the law was in place, opposition continued in the form of
attacks on synthetic medicines and the pharmaceutical industry in the National
Socialist press. The lead article in *Deutsche Volksgesundheit* for May 1935, for
example, launched a vituperative assault on Emil von Behring and serum therapy
under the title "Science as Business." Beginning with a physiognomical analysis
that purported to discern in Behring's facial features a susceptibility to "Jesuitical
and Jewish" ways of thinking, the author went on to portray the Nobel Prize–winning
developer of serum therapy as a willing instrument of a Jewish plot to weaken and
bring about the degeneration of non-Jews. The damage done to the German *Volk*
through Behring's serums, the author wrote, was boundless and not to be described in words. Countless numbers of people had been killed by serum who
might have been saved by German folk healing, he maintained. *Deutsche Volksgesundheit* also ran a column "From the Medical World" that claimed to extract
"from the specialized medical literature cases of damage which could have been
avoided through treatment by German folk healing."[19]

The battles surrounding animal experiment in medical research fought in the
first year of the National Socialist regime place in relief one mode of the Nazi relationship to medical science that has been well discussed in separate studies by
Michael Kater and Robert Proctor. This is the hostility of a substantial, vocal, and
influential element of the Nazi movement toward laboratory medical science and
its associated phenomena of chemical and surgical intervention and professional
specialism. Opposed to this form of scientific medicine was the ideal of a "natural" or organic medicine drawing on traditions of German folk healing. On the
philosophical level, Nazi medical writers articulating this ideal attacked what
they saw as a mechanistic, reductionist, analytical, laboratory-based approach to
the phenomena of life that strove to achieve a universal, objective, value-free science. In its place, they would substitute a holistic, synthetic vision of life that recognized and accepted a role for subjectivity and intuition in achieving medical
knowledge. As one writer put it, what was needed was "more Goethe, less Newton." Recognition of the role of subjectivity, they thought, would allow for development of a national medicine open to the specific ways of thinking and practice
of the German *Volk*, conceived as a differentiable biological and cultural entity.
Thus, the organic medicine favored by National Socialist thinkers would put an
end to the "cosmopolitan internationalist" medicine fostered by both capitalist
and socialist ways of thought and replace it with a truly German science of healing. On the level of practice, organic medicine favored the rural generalist physician over the urban specialist. In the domain of social policy, it merged easily
with a wider movement to return the German people to more "natural" ways of
living, which included such elements as discouragement of makeup for women,
anti-tobacco and anti-alcohol campaigns, preference for midwifery over physician-
assisted births, advocacy of whole-grain over refined white bread, support for

conservation of natural resources and protection of rare or valuable species, and antivivisection sentiments. As Kater has put it, "*volkisch* physicians strove for a return, medically speaking, to a pre-industrial state, where the forces of nature such as sun rays or fresh air or herbs, rather than synthetic pharmacological products and the technology of a laboratory or operating room, were enlisted to aid the human body in maintaining or recovering its balance."[20]

At every point, the organic medicine advocated by National Socialist writers embodied an antisemitism grounded in the doctrine of racial biology that was at the center of Nazi ideology. The alien Jewish presence held particular consequences for medicine, in this view. Philosophically, it was a "Jewish-international" conception of science as objective, value-free, and universal that threatened to efface the ideal of a national medicine grounded in the *Volk*. Professionally, Jewish physicians represented the urban specialist, in contrast to the *völkisch* ideal of the rural general practitioner, or they represented the academic researcher standing aloof from the organic community of the people (*Volksgemeinschaft*). At several points, the Nazi critiques of scientific medicine drew upon, and gave fresh forms to, older currents of antisemitism. The association of animal experiment and ritual slaughter played on the ancient theme of Jewish sacrifice of the blood of the innocents. Accusations that synthetic pharmaceuticals, some developed by Jewish scientists (e.g., Paul Ehrlich) or by "Jewish-influenced science" (e.g., chemotherapy, serum therapy), were poisoning the blood of the German *Volk* took part of their force from resonance with old indictments of the Jews as poisoners who intentionally caused epidemics. Such accusations linked the National Socialist critique of synthetic pharmaceuticals to a more general preoccupation with blood purity, which also took the form of racial hygiene measures to protect the German race through sterilizations, marriage law, euthanasia, and, eventually, mass killings. Finally, the hostility of National Socialist medical writers toward big capital, most pointedly in the form of the chemical and pharmaceutical industry, incorporated and exploited the notion of Jews as manipulators of international finance who were engaged in a hidden conspiracy to control the world.[21]

Several prominent Nazi leaders supported the natural health movement and organic medicine. Hitler was a vegetarian, did not use alcohol or tobacco, and endorsed antivivisectionism. Rudolf Hess favored homeopathy, while Heinrich Himmler backed organic medicine. Streicher, who published the violently antisemitic *Der Stürmer*, also put out *Deutsche Volksgesundheit aus Blut und Boden!* and headed the popular People's Health Movement.[22]

Pharmaceutical research within I.G. Farben engaged, and was vulnerable to the attacks of, Nazi ideologues at many points. Its products were overtly and nakedly synthetic, not "organic" products of nature. At best, they were derivative of or were modeled on natural products, in the way that quinine served as the model for synthetic antimalarials. They were produced by laboratory science that relied on both synthetic organic chemistry and animal experiment, and in which animals were frankly a means to an end, although the end did include pharmaceuticals for use in veterinary medicine. The pharmaceutical division of I.G. Farben was indebted to Jewish scientists such as Ehrlich for part of its program and for some of its products (e.g., Salvarsan) and included Jews on its research staff. The products and laboratory methods of pharmaceutical research dealt directly with the blood. Sera, vaccines, and chemotherapeutic agents introduced into the circulatory system could have toxic effects. I.G. Farben was perhaps the most prominent example of a huge capitalist combine joining several companies, with many international connections and interests. Its supervisory board (*Aufsichtsrat*) included seven Jews early in the Nazi regime. To these ample grounds for hostility must be added Hörlein's vigorous struggle with the National Socialist–oriented antivivisection movement over the Reich animal protection law, and persistent tensions generated by Nazi party fears that the pharmaceutical division might betray German technical and economic information to foreign enemies and competitors.[23]

It was in the midst of these tensions and struggles, in June 1934, that Hörlein joined the Nazi party (NSDAP). By his own later account and those of others who knew him before and after, his decision was based not on political conviction but on the calculation that party membership would strengthen his ability to protect the interests of his industrial group and of scientific research in Germany. Such a claim can be evaluated only in the context of Hörlein's whole career, which I address further below. For the moment, several circumstances surrounding the decision must be noted. Prior to his application for membership in the spring of 1934, Hörlein had no connection to the NSDAP. He had been among the founders of the German Democratic Party in Wuppertal-Vohwinkel and, although not active in party politics, remained democratic in his views. He had resisted the NSDAP's intensive recruitment campaign in the spring of 1933 but, despite this, had been named to the municipal council of Wuppertal. In 1934, he was notified by the mayor of Wuppertal that a new law required members of the council to be members of the NSDAP. Although not politically ambitious, Hörlein evidently believed that his position in local government gave him influence that was valuable in the protection of his company and research establishment. He later testified that he did not at that time foresee the violent directions in which National Socialism would develop, and that even then he recognized that there were some matters, for example, antisemitism, on which he could never agree with the party.[24]

A Corporate Cover-up?

Hörlein's struggles in the summer and fall of 1933 had helped assure enactment of a moderate animal protection law that allowed animal experiments, and therefore medical and pharmaceutical research, to continue in Germany. From November 1933, compliance with the law at Elberfeld was the responsibility of individual heads of institutes such as Domagk.

Domagk's laboratory, and that of Fritz Mietzsch and Joseph Klarer, his chemist-collaborators, was now heavily but not exclusively committed to research on Prontosil and related compounds. As far as the sulfa drugs are concerned, research at Elberfeld may be divided into two phases. In the first, running from the patent application of December 25, 1932, to Domagk's first publication on Prontosil in February 1935, development was largely enclosed within the company. Apart from a few physicians with whom the company made arrangements for clinical trials, and French researchers who took note of Prontosil after publication of the French patent in June 1934, a policy of secrecy was successfully maintained. With publication of the German patent on January 2, 1935, and especially with Domagk's first article of February 1935, the situation was fundamentally altered. Prontosil went on the market and was widely available for therapeutic testing and use. Interested researchers outside of Germany, notably in France, Britain, and the United States, began to plan and carry out independent laboratory and clinical trials.[25]

Within months came dramatic news from Paris that a team at the Pasteur Institute had shown a constituent of the Prontosil molecule, a compound later to be known as sulfanilamide, to be at least as effective as Prontosil in animal and clinical trials. The finding was of fundamental importance for several reasons. Prontosil, an azo dye, could have the unfortunate effect of turning the patient red during the course of treatment. Sulfanilamide was colorless. Sulfanilamide, a simpler molecule than Prontosil, could be manufactured more easily and more cheaply. Not the least important was that sulfanilamide, unlike Prontosil, was not covered by patents. Or rather, the process for making it had been patented by Bayer soon after its synthesis by the Austrian chemist Paul Gelmo in 1908, and Bayer had made use of sulfanilamide as an intermediate in the synthesis of dyestuffs, never suspecting its therapeutic potential; in due course, the patent had expired. Finally, recognition of the therapeutic efficacy of sulfanilamide demonstrated the irrelevance of the azo bond, and of the dye character, of Prontosil. Chemotherapeutic research could begin afresh, taking the sulfanilamide molecule as nucleus and building around it variations that might expand the therapeutic spectrum, reduce the toxicity, or improve on the intensity of action of sulfanilamide. Sulfanilamide opened the way for a new generation of sulfa drugs.[26]

Publication of the Pasteur Institute findings in November 1935 and the subsequent displacement of Prontosil by sulfanilamide in medical use, in the pharmaceuticals market, and as starting point for development of new chemotherapeutic agents have raised persistent questions about the actions of Elberfeld researchers between December 1932 and November 1935. Did the Elberfeld team know about the action of sulfanilamide before the Pasteur Institute publication but choose to conceal it because the compound could not be protected by patents and would therefore be less profitable? The question has been put most sharply by British bacteriologist Ronald Hare, who was strongly inclined to answer in the affirmative. In a book on penicillin published in 1970, Hare devoted one chapter to the sulfa drugs. He asked why there had been a delay of two years and three months between the discovery of the first effective compounds in 1932 and Domagk's first publication in 1935. Hörlein had said in 1937 in a talk to British doctors that the time had been needed to complete intensive experimental and clinical trials. The problem with this, as Hare saw it, was that many clinical studies were already completed in 1933, and that Domagk's February 1935 article did not say what animal studies were done after 1932, or when they were done. So Hare offered an alternative explanation. Bayer chemists, he reasoned, quickly realized that only a part of the Prontosil molecule was required for therapeutic action, and that part was unpatentable. So the company feverishly set out—so Hare conjectures—to find a related compound that was equally or more effective and different enough to patent. Meanwhile, they stalled for time and refused to send samples of Prontosil abroad for outside testing.[27]

The plausibility of the Hare thesis, as this argument may conveniently be called, depends heavily on chemical reasoning. Hare gave four reasons why he found it "very difficult to believe" that the Elberfeld group did not recognize the therapeutic efficacy of sulfanilamide at an early date. One of these was that, by early 1933, the German researchers had not one but three compounds in hand that were chemotherapeutically active. One of these was the one eventually called Prontosil but at first called Streptozon in batches released to clinical investigators. The second was the compound Hare calls the precursor of Prontosil, the first sulfonamide azo compound synthesized by Klarer and Mietzsch. This substance, referred to as KL695/D3920, had been prepared by the chemists by September 1932. It was supplanted by Prontosil and did not go into clinical use. The third was Prontosil Soluble, at first known as Streptozon S, which was available for clinical trials by early 1933. Also a sulfonamide azo compound, it had a more complex structure than Prontosil but was more soluble.

Second, Hare pointed out, inspection of the structural formulas of these three compounds would have immediately revealed a common feature:

Precursor of Prontosil (KL695/D3920)

Prontosil or Streptozon

Prontosil Soluble or Streptozon S

In all three compounds, the left-hand benzene ring has a sulfonamide group attached in the *para*-position relative to an azo bond ($-N=N-$) that links the ring to another benzene ring on the right.

A third reason why, in Hare's view, the Elberfeld team should have suspected that sulfanilamide was the therapeutically active component was that the synthesis of all these compounds began with operations on sulfanilamide. It was both a common structural element and the first building block of all these therapeutically active compounds. Finally, Hare reasoned, the Elberfeld chemists must have known that a simple reduction of any of these compounds in the animal or human body could break the double bond and release free sulfanilamide into the circulation. All of this made it very improbable, in Hare's view, that the Germans had not known at an early date that sulfanilamide was the real chemotherapeutic agent.[28]

Despite the plausibility that commercial motives, timing, secrecy, and chemical reasoning lend to the Hare thesis, its conclusions have been rejected by Daniel Bovet, who was a member of the Pasteur Institute team that recognized the therapeutic efficacy of sulfanilamide and who published a history of the sulfa drugs. Bovet felt that he had incontrovertible proof that the Elberfeld researchers did not know of sulfanilamide's therapeutic virtues until they read the Pasteur Institute team's publication of November 28, 1935. Bovet's strongest evidence comes from Mietzsch and Klarer's monthly reports during 1935 and 1936. These show that the chemists were trying a number of ways to produce new chemotherapeutic agents by varying the Prontosil model, such as substitutions for the azo bond $-N=N-$, but that they did not begin to consider "colorless products," including sulfanilamide, until March 1936. Equally revealing is Domagk's laboratory journal, in which the formula for sulfanilamide appears, without comment, only in January 1936. Bovet points out that prior to the Pasteur Institute team's publication, the Elberfeld group was committed to the idea that therapeutic activity was linked to coloring properties in the dye molecules under test. For this reason alone, Mietzsch and Klarer, who had prepared sulfanilamide in their own laboratories by 1932, saw it only as an intermediate in the preparation of dyes and did not send it to the bacteriological laboratories until 1936. I.G. Farben did not begin clinical trials of sulfanilamide until March 1936, and it went on the German market under the name Prontosil Album (the Latin-derived *Album* indicating its lack of color) only later in that year.[29]

For Bovet, the case against the Hare thesis is clinched by two personal recollections. One is that of Mietzsch, who in a 1955 article stated that the irrelevance of the azo bridge in the Prontosil molecule for its therapeutic activity had been demonstrated by Jacques Tréfouël and his colleagues. The other comes from Ernst Auhagen, who had joined the Elberfeld physiology laboratory in 1933. In a conversation with Bovet in 1981, Auhagen recalled that, apart from the quality and variety of tests to which prospective chemotherapeutic agents were submitted, the hallmark of the Elberfeld team's research was the "myth and fascination of color," the notion that a dye would be found with therapeutic activity. Auhagen recalled very well the shock felt in the Elberfeld group on learning of the action of the colorless sulfanilamide. He was indignant at the suggestion of a prior knowledge and a cover-up and stated categorically that Hörlein would never have stood for such a thing.[30]

Bovet's evidence, if not the definitive proof that he considered it to be, adds weight to a strong case that can be made against the Hare thesis on other grounds. Domagk's internal report on the activities of his laboratory during 1934, submitted to the company in late January 1935, reveals a variegated research agenda that included vigorous attempts to follow up the success of Prontosil against streptococcal infections, but no indication that Domagk or his colleagues were aware of the action of sulfanilamide. Hörlein later told a British audience in 1937 that since 1932 the Elberfeld laboratories had synthesized more than 1,000 compounds related to Prontosil and that their action in various bacterial infections had been tested in "tens of thousands of experiments." Domagk's 1934 report makes clear that many of these compounds had been synthesized, and many of the experiments performed, before Domagk's first publication on Prontosil in February 1935.[31]

In 1934, Domagk's laboratory was occupied with a variety of problems, among which the most prominent were cancer research, disinfection, and the chemotherapy of bacterial infections. Nearly two-thirds of the 1934 laboratory report was taken up with results of animal trials of compounds in streptococcal, staphylococcal, pneumococcal, and gonococcal infections. Also important to Domagk, however, was the work on tumors, to which he devoted a long introductory section. Domagk believed that research to date had shown that active immunization of humans against tumors was possible. He also sought substances that would inhibit tumor growth, and to this end received in 1934 twenty-one sterol compounds from the organic chemist Adolf Windaus. In April, Christian Hackmann, a medical doctor, joined the laboratory and devoted all his efforts to tumor research.[32]

Domagk's 1934 laboratory report weighs heavily against the Hare thesis. It contains no hint of an awareness that sulfanilamide is the therapeutically effective part of Prontosil. On the contrary, there is every indication that Domagk and his collaborators were vigorously pursuing, and expected to continue to pursue, work on azo compounds more or less modeled on Prontosil. The one clear success in this effort so far, Prontosil Soluble (Streptozon S), fell into this pattern. The numbers of active compounds sharing the sulfonamide group in the *para*-position relative to the azo bond evidently suggested to Domagk and his colleagues not that the intermediate product sulfanilamide was the active part, but that greater intensity and range of chemotherapeutic action was to be sought by variation of the rest of the molecule. Even then, the Elberfeld group did not confine themselves to azo compounds but extended their tests to include acridine, azo-acridine, and other types of substances, many with no relation to sulfanilamide. The scope of the research, and the time consumed by it, was being extended not only by the addition of hundreds of compounds but also by the decision to seek chemotherapies for bacterial infections other than streptococcal ones, and by the need to develop and refine animal experimental models. In the midst of this, Domagk was committing a part of his own time, and of the resources of his laboratory, to other problems, especially cancer research.

First Trials of Prontosil

While Domagk and his laboratory were so engaged, a handful of German doctors were quietly conducting the first clinical trials of Prontosil. In early 1933, selected physicians received from I.G. Farben samples of the compound under the label Streptozon or D4145. Patients suffering from streptococcal, staphylococcal, and other bacterial infections began to receive treatment with Streptozon almost immediately. Apart from mention of a single case at a medical society meeting in May 1933, however, no clinical results were published until February 1935. In that month, three clinical reports appeared in the same issue and immediately following Domagk's first publication on Prontosil in the *Deutsche medizinische Wochenschrift*. A fourth paper, also reporting results of clinical tests begun in 1933, appeared in the same journal in October 1935. Scrutiny of these reports permits evaluation of Hare's claim that clinical tests of Prontosil had been largely completed in 1933.[33]

One of the first physicians to receive Prontosil was Philipp Klee, who headed the medical clinic at nearby Wuppertal Hospital and was also a professor at Munich. Klee and his assistant, a young physician named Herbert Römer, had used Prontosil in treatment of an unspecified but apparently substantial number of cases of streptococcal infection between early 1933 and February 1935. In "numerous preliminary trials," they found Prontosil to be harmless and well tolerated. In one of these, a case of septic miscarriage that occurred not in the clinic but in Klee's private practice, the cessation of fever and recovery had been so rapid and striking as to propel them into sustained testing of the medicine. Unfortunately, this success had not been repeated in serious septic infections of the uterus, they reported, and, "as expected," Prontosil had not worked in cases of advanced septicemia. Undeterred, Klee and Römer had used Prontosil in treatment of streptococcal sore throats, tonsillar abscesses, tonsillar thrombophlebitis and lymphedenitis, jugular vein thrombosis, septic perimetritis, erysipelas, acute and ulcerative endocarditis, sepsis lenta, and acute and chronic polyarthritis. Confirmed cases of endocarditis lenta (inflammation of the interior lining of the heart) proved resistant to Prontosil. In contrast, Klee and Römer reported excellent results in treatment of septic sore throat and some of its most serious complications. In the past two years, they said, they had had no deaths from these conditions, a notable departure from previous experience. They did not feel that the precise role of Prontosil in treatment of septic sore throat and its complications was yet established, and urged physicians to attend carefully to the particulars of each case and not to neglect more conventional therapeutic measures. They did feel confident enough to recommend immediate use of Prontosil whenever the clinical picture suggested septic complications of sore throat.[34]

Klee and Römer gave details of three of their cases by way of example. One of these was offered as evidence that Prontosil also worked well in older patients:

> 62 year old engineer. Already in 1929 had severe thrombosis in leg after tibial fracture. Pain in swallowing and chills for 5 days. Temperature between 39 and 40 degrees. Gradually increasing difficulty of speech. In the last days pain in the neck on both sides over the jugular, then from today reddening and swelling. Hospitalization because of suspicion of jugular vein thrombosis. Threatening clinical picture. Confused. Dry tongue. Mucous membrane and throat edematous. Palatine arch in both sides arched outward and swollen. Entry to the throat narrowed. Tonsils

not visible. Slight lockjaw. Speech barely understandable. On the neck and over the jugulars on both sides a slight edematous swelling with very great sensitivity to pressure. Over the left jugular hand-sized redness and edema. Treatment 2 times a day with 10 cc., later once a day with 10 cc. Prontosil intravenously and 3 times a day 0.6 g. by mouth. Already on the third day considerable improvement, gradual decline of the swelling and fever, after a further 9 days completely free of fever, after a further 14 days free of complaints and discharged cured.[35]

Success came also with use of Prontosil in cases of erysipelas of the face and head. A streptococcal infection of the skin and subcutaneous tissue, erysipelas is characterized by a spreading inflammation and redness in the affected areas. "The critical cessation of fever in erysipelas cases and the rapid restoration of skin processes was in some cases so striking," Klee and Römer reported, "that we could scarcely doubt a connection with the therapy, although the judgment in erysipelas is, as is known, always especially difficult." Less certain was the effect of Prontosil on polyarthritic disorders, where the picture was clouded by use of Prontosil in combination with other modes of therapy. Uncertainty also surrounded the mode of administration. Klee and Römer believed that Prontosil was well absorbed in the intestine but had also found that better results often came from giving a much smaller dose intravenously, a procedure they recommended in all serious cases.[36]

Klee and Römer reported that Prontosil was "harmless, free of undesirable side effects, easily tolerated, and effective" and recommended its use especially in serious forms of streptococcal sore throat and its complications, and in erysipelas. Although they remained uncertain as to why intravenous administration was more effective, they had found that a suitable dosage was 10–20 cc of the 0.25 percent solution once or twice a day intravenously and 0.3–0.6 g. three times a day orally. They concluded that "we see in the use of the azo compound Prontosil an enrichment of our therapy."[37]

Similar good results were reported by H.T. Schreus, director of the Düsseldorf Medical Academy's Dermatological Clinic. In March 1933, Schreus and his assistant, Richard Foerster, had in their care an infant one and one-half years old on the verge of death from staphylococcal septicemia. The child suffered from serious weight loss and elevated temperature, and the whole body was covered with abscesses. Several weeks of treatment with existing chemotherapies had been to no avail. In these desperate circumstances, the doctors began to give the infant 0.05 g of Prontosil by mouth twice a day. They observed no immediate change, but on the third day the child's temperature dropped from 40°C to 39°C in the morning, then suddenly to 37°C in the evening. Thereafter, the temperature fell gradually to normal, the abscesses softened and could be opened by incision, the skin improved, the child began to gain weight, and a fundamental change in the child's condition was evident. Schreus reported that "the success in this case made an exceedingly deep impression on those who participated."[38]

Deep impression or not, Schreus found that he could not replicate the dramatic results of the first case on other patients with staphylococcal infections. Nor could he get satisfactory results with use of Prontosil in gonorrhea, although in early 1935 he was still using Prontosil against both gonorrhea and staphylococcal infections. The real success came with erysipelas. The clinic treated an unspecified but large number of cases, mostly of facial erysipelas of various durations and severities. The standard measures before Prontosil included injection of the compounds Streptosan and Omnadin, and topical treatments. Most cases responded favorably in three to eight days, but some resulted in serious and even fatal complications. "Now, after the introduction of Prontosil treatment, a completely unmistakable change occurred," Schreus wrote enthusiastically. In one and one-half years of Prontosil treatment, the clinic had not had a single case of therapy-resistant erysipelas. "The rule is that already on the next day, at the latest on the second day after administration of two to six grams of Prontosil by mouth, the temperature drops to normal and the erysipelas is brought to a stop. We have seen this striking success in cases that were already treated elsewhere for a long time without results," he reported. Schreus was forthright in his conclusion, writing that "we have in Prontosil for the first time an agent that undoubtedly permits a causal treatment of erysipelas and indeed is to be spoken of as a true chemotherapeutic agent . . . [and] its specific action in erysipelas alone justifies its introduction into practice."[39]

Puerperal (childbed) fever, too, was apparently yielding to treatment with Prontosil. Eugen Anselm, an assistant in Max Henkel's University Women's Clinic in Jena, had received from I.G. Farben ampules of 10 cc and 20 cc of 0.25 percent Prontosil solution and also containers of 20 tablets of 0.3 g Prontosil each. With Domagk's animal trials in mind, he had used Prontosil as the exclusive therapy in two cases of bacteriologically confirmed streptococcal sepsis following miscarriage. Both patients were given intravenous doses of 20 cc Prontosil solution each day. In both cases, the temperature dropped after the first dose, and both patients were well and released after six doses, without evident side effects. Favorable results in what later proved to be mixed cases of streptococcal and staphylococcal infection led Anselm to conjecture that Prontosil not only exerted an elective action on streptococci but also had a general bactericidal action, or acted to mobilize the body's defenses including the reticuloendothelial system. On this basis, he tried Prontosil in those cases of confirmed mixed streptococcal and staphylococcal infection and purely staphylococcal infection, all with successful outcome. After such "unequivocal success," Anselm "henceforth as a matter of principle treated *every case of puerperal fever* immediately after admission exclusively with Prontosil without regard to the time-consuming and costly bacteriological confirmation of the infective agent." Thirteen cases treated successfully in this way led Anselm to give "the best recommendation of Prontosil for treatment of every form of pueperal fever."[40]

A more cautious but still positive evaluation of Prontosil in puerperal sepsis was published later in 1935 by Kurt Fuge, an assistant in L. Nürnberger's University Women's Clinic in Halle. The clinic had begun receiving Prontosil from I.G. Farben in 1933 and since then had treated 120 women for fever following birth or miscarriage, of whom fourteen were cases of sepsis, with very positive results. Given the background of skepticism in the medical community, however, Fuge felt it necessary to justify even making a trial of Prontosil. "In view of the fact that the chemotherapy of sepsis has enjoyed the unlimited and perhaps justified rejection of all authors who have had the opportunity of testing the results of all medicines recommended against sepsis," he admitted, "it may appear incomprehensible that we have nevertheless tried to improve the therapy of sepsis with this new medicine." Fuge held that past failures did not justify the rejection of new medicines on principle, and that they should be tried provided they did the patient no harm. In his view, the latter condition, which Prontosil satisfied, was critical since the body's powers of resistance had to be strengthened in every way possible: "the etiological treatment of sepsis [i.e., chemotherapy] is always only a support to this general treatment." All this said, he conceded that he was not as optimistic about Prontosil's prospects as some authors, and that his final judgment would have to await further clinical trials.[41]

The early German clinical trials of Prontosil fell into a clear pattern. Soon after filing its patent application on Prontosil, I.G. Farben began to release samples of the compound in liquid and tablet form to a handful of physicians, all of whom were on the staff of clinics independent of the company in which numbers of patients were treated for streptococcal and other bacterial infections. Clinical trials of Prontosil proceeded on a case-by-case basis at the discretion of individual physicians. Three of the four studies of Prontosil described above began with dramatic successes in one or two individual cases. These early successes appear to have played an important role in prompting continuation of the trials against a background of numerous previous failures of other drugs and some skepticism, a background sharply underlined by Fuge.

Investigating physicians typically gave close attention to the particulars of their cases, including the precise nature of the illness, the patient's tolerance of the medication, effective dosages, mode of administration, and failures. If patient consent to treatment with an experimental drug was asked for or obtained, the fact was nowhere recorded in any of these reports. None of the doctors mentioned large-scale or controlled clinical trials or appeared to be aware of their necessity or desirability. Lack of awareness of the utility of controls is all the more striking in view of the recurrent problems raised in the clinical trials. The physicians testing Prontosil confessed themselves unable to distinguish with certainty in all cases between the effects due to Prontosil and the ordinary variability in the course of untreated infections. Multiple therapies, including Prontosil, applied to the same case raised even more complex problems of interpretation. So, too, did cases of mixed infection, even where Prontosil was the sole therapy used.

Given these sources of confusion, the number of different kinds of streptococcal infections, not to mention staphylococcal or other types, on which the action of Prontosil had to be assessed, and the atmosphere of skepticism in which they worked, it is hardly surprising that physicians carrying out the first clinical trials of Prontosil remained tentative or uncertain on many points. Nor is it surprising that the preliminary trials occupied the greater part of two years, although that time exceeded by about a year the average laid down in the company's 1930 internal report for the clinical testing of a new compound. Hare's contention that many clinical trials were completed in 1933 and his conjecture that the company simply sat on the results for an additional year or more therefore appear implausible at best. More remarkable is that, in spite of limitations of methodology and the complexity of the phenomena under study, the physicians testing Prontosil were able to confidently recommend its use in erysipelas, puerperal fever, and the complications of streptococcal sore throat and that the company was prepared to act on these conclusions, advanced by a small number of clinicians on the basis of a small number of cases, by early 1935.[42]

This account is consistent with the position taken later by Domagk. Speaking in 1961 to the French Society of Chemotherapy and Serology, Domagk responded indignantly to characterizations of the delay between the first laboratory results in 1932 and the first publication in 1935 as "incomprehensible and mysterious" and underlined the need to confirm the clinical results so as not to raise false hopes among doctors and patients.[43]

Despite its initial plausibility, therefore, Hare's thesis is supported neither by the record of the laboratory development of Prontosil nor by that of its early clinical testing. Against Hare's views, finally, we must place several errors in his reasoning and a number of characteristics of the Elberfeld research endeavor that are misconstrued or not taken into account by his argument. Hare appears to have little sense of the background of chemotherapeutic research at Elberfeld. Thus, the significance of such predominant ideas as the principle of basic alkylation, the kind of analogical reasoning that made Atabrine a source of inspiration to Mietzsch and Klarer, and the mystique of color referred to by Auhagen does not enter into his interpretation of the actions of Elberfeld researchers. At the same time, Hare imputes to these investigators questions and procedures of dubious relevance. So, for example, he supposes that the testing of intermediate products for therapeutic action was routine at Elberfeld, which does not appear to have been the case. Apparently determined to make recognition of sulfanilamide's therapeutic qualities appear inexorable, he misrepresents the significance of what he takes to be Walter Jacobs and Michael Heidelberger's 1919 finding in research at the Rockefeller Institute that a sulfonamide-containing azo-cinchona compound had antibacterial action *in vitro*. [44]

The Mystique of Color

In making his assessment of the time taken by Elberfeld researchers to bring Prontosil to market, Hare does not know of, or chooses to ignore, the background of skepticism regarding the possibilities of bacterial chemotherapy that was widespread in the medical community in the early 1930s. Nor, apparently, is he aware of Hörlein's characteristic caution in introducing new drugs into medical practice.[45] More seriously, Hare's analysis reflects no awareness of the framework of thinking that guided Elberfeld researchers and that made it unlikely that they would even raise the question of sulfanilamide's effectiveness. Part of this framework is captured in Auhagen's reference to the "myth and fascination of color" that led the Elberfeld group to seek a dye with therapeutic action. Color in this context meant the azo bond, and the genealogy of Prontosil indeed placed it among azo dyes with medicinal effect, such as chrysoidine, phenazopyridine, and neotropine. Even the member of the Elberfeld research establishment most likely to raise the question of sulfanilamide's therapeutic qualities saw Prontosil in this way. Gerhard Hecht, a pharmacologist in Hörlein's organization, recognized that, in general, the azo bond was not necessary for therapeutic action, citing as example the sleeping sickness remedy Germanin (Bayer 205), which was colorless. Hecht also emphasized the importance of using constituents and intermediate products of dyes in the synthesis of medicines. Nowhere, however, did Hecht suggest that dyes in general, or basic azo dyes in particular, became therapeutically active when broken down in the body. When he mentioned Prontosil up to 1935, it was as a basic azo dye related to chrysoidine but with a particular substitution that made it effective against septic illnesses caused by streptococci.

Even after the Pasteur Institute publication and general recognition of the therapeutic action of sulfanilamide, the Elberfeld group continued to present sulfanilamide as a product of the breakdown of Prontosil, a "fragment" compound, an attitude given expression in the I.G. Farben trade name, Prontosil Album, or colorless Prontosil. This name has the form of a binomial, indicating that the substance is merely one species within the genus Prontosil. Such language suggests not only the temporal priority of Prontosil but also a way of thinking according to which the dye molecule was regarded as a whole, and sulfanilamide as a mere part. This is not a language or way of thinking that would have encouraged testing of sulfanilamide, although it could be and was adapted after the fact to acknowledge recognition of the "fragment" compound's action. As late as 1937, Domagk was voicing doubts about the views "expressed by certain French and British authors" that Prontosil and related compounds were effective only when broken down by a reductive process in the body. That Domagk attributed this idea to the French and British and had to be convinced of its validity renders it unlikely that he had the notion independently or pursued its implications in laboratory or clinical tests.[46]

In the last analysis, the plausibility of the Hare thesis depends on hindsight, a capacity that may distort as well as illuminate. How could the German researchers *not* have realized what soon became common knowledge and the starting point for new generations of sulfa drugs? The answer to this question emerges when Prontosil is viewed not from the standpoint of later developments but as the product of an older research program both driven and bounded by the world of its own concepts and practices.

By the time that Prontosil entered the German market and medical practice in 1935, the Elberfeld pharmaceutical research establishment had weathered early challenges from Nazi ideologues and had made a start at pushing beyond Prontosil to identify compounds with better or different qualities as antibacterial agents. In the next decade, it would continue its work in the face of new and varied pressures, first from the regime, then from a long and devastating war.

CHAPTER 5

Accommodation and Survival

B eginning in 1935, research on sulfonamides at Elberfeld proceeded in a changed environment. With the wraps off Prontosil, I.G. Farben's product was exposed to international competition both in the marketplace and in research laboratories. In France, where German patents were not recognized, a copy of Prontosil soon went on the market under the trade name Rubiazol. After the therapeutic action of sulfanilamide was made known by the Pasteur Institute team in November 1935, the new "fragment" compound could be used in place of its parent, and the way was opened for development of a second generation of sulfonamides no longer modeled on Prontosil. The search for new derivatives was taken up in France, Britain, Switzerland, the United States, and elsewhere, forcing the Elberfeld research establishment into repeated reassessments of the needs and priorities of research. A National Socialist regime that emphasized military preparedness and the push for autarky brought increasing pressure on industry to protect German commercial advantage and strategic interests by preventing access to vital technical and scientific information by potential enemies.[1]

Beyond Prontosil

B y 1935, enough clinical experience was available to show Prontosil effective against severe streptococcal sore throat, erysipelas, scarlet fever, puerperal sepsis, and other streptococcal infections. Striking as these successes were, they also put in relief the conditions in which Prontosil was useless or of uncertain activity, including infections caused by staphylococcal, pneumococcal, gonococcal, and anaerobic bacteria.[2]

92

Research continued at Elberfeld on the uses of Prontosil and related azo compounds, but by early 1936 Gerhard Domagk, Joseph Klarer, and Fritz Mietzsch were also turning to sulfanilamide and the other colorless compounds that could be derived from it. Sulfanilamide, described in chapter 4, is a relatively simple compound, with structural formula:

$$H_2NO_2S{-}\hspace{-0.5em}\bigcirc\hspace{-0.5em}{-}NH_2$$

Researchers began with the premise that therapeutic action depended not only on the presence of the sulfonamide group, SO_2NH_2, but also on its location in the *para*-position relative to the amino group, NH_2, or, in azo compounds such as Prontosil, to the azo bond, $-N{=}N-$. Starting with sulfanilamide, then, variation of the compound could proceed in three directions. Substitutions could be made in the sulfonamide group, in the amino group, or in both groups at once. Prontosil and Prontosil Soluble could be viewed as products of substitution in the amino group. It was in the other direction, however, through substitution in the sulfonamide group, that effective new compounds began to be identified. By some time in 1936, Klarer and Mietzsch had synthesized a compound, at first called DB90, that Domagk found in animal trials to be as effective as Prontosil or Prontosil Soluble against streptococcal infections and more effective against infections caused by staphylococcal, gonococcal, and some anaerobic bacteria.[3]

The apparent effectiveness of the new compound against staphylococcal, gonococcal, and some anaerobic infections made it an obvious candidate for patenting and clinical trials. In the ideological and legal circumstances of the Third Reich, however, the process could not be straightforward. Already in 1933, the regime had made betrayal of military secrets a crime punishable by death, and Heinrich Hörlein, as a representative of I.G. Farben, had heard the company castigated by party officials for its manufacture of medicines for tropical diseases, products that purportedly benefited only the former enemies of Germany. I.G. Farben had been attacked in the National Socialist press for its international interests and connections. By April 1934, legal changes introduced by the National Socialist government required I.G. Farben to submit to the Reich War Ministry any patent applications for a product that might fall under the definition of state secret. Until October 1935, the I.G. Farben patent office in Leverkusen dealt directly with the various parts of the military. Beginning in that month, the Reich War Ministry created a central office for patent secrecy questions, and I.G. Farben funneled these matters through its Army Liaison Office (*Vermittlungstelle W*) in Berlin. An exception was anything having to do with weapons, about which Elberfeld and Leverkusen dealt directly with the Army General Headquarters (*Oberkommando des Heeres*).[4]

Hörlein, who regarded the secrecy requirements as a mortgage (*Hypothek*) that had to be borne in order to continue scientific work at Elberfeld, felt himself forced into dependence on military authorities for protection. He found such a contact for pharmaceuticals in the Army Health Inspector (*Heeressanitätsinspektor*), a Prof. Dr. Waldmann, and for toxic substances, which might be viewed by the Army as potential weapons, in Army Ordnance (*Heereswaffenamt*).[5]

The new compound, which soon took the trade name Uliron, was the occasion of Hörlein's first encounter with the Army Health Inspector. What made Uliron a potential secrecy problem was its action against anaerobic bacteria. Hörlein was aware that among these organisms were those responsible for gas gangrene, to which he attributed the deaths of 100,000 soldiers on the German side alone during the 1914–1918 war. Uliron was submitted for review and was not released for marketing and medical use until receipt of Waldmann's approval on May 21, 1937.[6]

Success with Uliron reinforced a sense of urgency at Elberfeld that was already fueled by a keen awareness of international competition in chemotherapeutic research and a conviction that further breakthroughs in the field of the sulfonamides were imminent. Two months after the approval of Uliron, in July 1937, Hörlein wrote a letter politely declining an offer by Richard Kuhn to make Domagk director of the Pathology Division of the Kaiser Wilhelm Institute for Medical Research in Heidelberg. While conceding Domagk's qualifications for the position, Hörlein was loath to see him removed from a collaborative effort that had already produced such substantial results in the field of bacterial infections, and from which still more was to be expected. Referring to Uliron, though not yet by name, he wrote that a medicine was soon to be introduced that shared the antistreptococcal action of Prontosil and Prontosil Album (sulfanilamide) but that was also a specific treatment for staphylococcal infections and was effective against gonococci and the causative agents of gas gangrene. Hörlein saw indications that the same or similar substances would be effective against all possible bacterial infections. "The whole world has been awakened by the success with Prontosil," he noted, "and in America, England, and France, they are working feverishly in this field. I believe that we can remain in the forefront if we let the apparatus we erected work as quietly as possible."[7]

Domagk stayed at Elberfeld, and the apparatus worked on. On March 29, 1938, Klarer sent to Domagk a compound for chemotherapeutic testing that differed from the Prontosil and Uliron groups of substances in breaking with the prior assumption that the amino group had to be directly bound to the benzene ring. In the new compound, in contrast, the amino group was joined to the ring with the aid of an aliphatic residue, CH_2. On August 19, 1938, Domagk reported that the compound showed activity against blackleg or symptomatic anthrax (*Pararauschbrand*), an anaerobic bacterial infection. Since further chemotherapeutic tests went well, the company applied on January 27, 1939, for a patent on the procedure for making the compound (application number J 63 929; later patent number DRP 726 386). Since the new compound did not appear to show advantages over other sulfonamides in bacterial infections other than those caused by anaerobes, the patent application singled out the latter, which included gas gangrene.[8]

Mention of anaerobic infections set off the same alarm bells that had rung for Uliron, with the result that Army General Headquarters required the patent application for the new compound to be kept secret. Hörlein, who opposed secrecy for

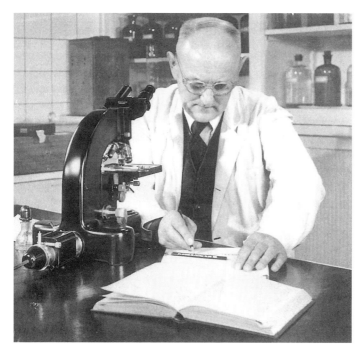

Figure 5.1. Gerhard Domagk (1895–1964) at his desk (reprinted courtesy of the Bayer Archive).

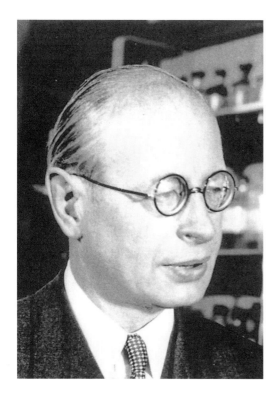

Figure 5.2. Fritz Mietzsch (1896–1958), one of Gerhard Domagk's principal chemist collaborators in research on sulfonamides (reprinted courtesy of the Bayer Archive).

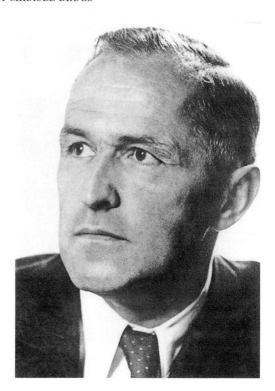

Figure 5.3. Joseph Klarer
(1898–1953), one of Gerhard
Domagk's principal chemist collaborators in research on sulfonamides (reprinted courtesy of
the Bayer Archive).

new pharmaceutical products on principle, urged the Elberfeld researchers to find
applications for the new compound that would be important in peacetime and that
would thereby improve the company's chances for approval of the application.
Animal studies in Domagk's laboratory showed that the substance had activity
against gonococcal infections. Mesudin, as the compound was called for testing
purposes, was sent to H.T. Schreus in Düsseldorf and H. Löhe in Berlin for clinical trials. Löhe's results were published in the *Klinische Wochenschrift* in 1940
but, because of the secrecy order, did not include the chemical formula of the
compound. On February 9, 1940, Mietzsch and Werner Knauff, from I.G. Farben's patent office in Leverkusen, met with officials of the Reich Patent Office in
Berlin. I.G. Farben was asked to "enrich" the patent application with statements
about animal trials in gonococcal infections in place of earlier statements on
anaerobic infections, now declared secret. Domagk accordingly conducted new
animal trials, and on the basis of these the company submitted a revised application for Mesudin on June 6, 1940. Even this was not enough, and over the suc-
ceeding months Hörlein appeared personally on several occasions before the
Pharmacological Administrative Department (*Pharmakologischen Dienststellen*)
at Army General Headquarters to petition for release of the application. Approval
of the revised application, which now included the chemical formula, finally came

on October 7, 1941, and Klarer published the formula for the compound, now given the trade name Marfanil, in the *Klinische Wochenschrift* on December 13, 1941.[9]

Although Elberfeld researchers had recognized the special properties of the compound that became Marfanil long before the beginning of the war in September 1939, the war lent new urgency to the compound's testing, to the patent and secrecy issues, and to specification of the conditions of its use by doctors.

The war also had an increasing and largely detrimental effect on the wider research enterprise at Elberfeld. Before the war, and even in its early phases, Domagk's laboratory benefited from an expansion linked to the present success and bright future prospects of the sulfonamides. A medical doctor joined the staff in 1934, and between 1937 and 1942 another medical doctor and two bacteriologists were added. In 1939, Domagk's laboratory was expanding with the addition of more rooms. Domagk, his staff, and his chemist-collaborators pushed ahead with research on the chemotherapy of bacterial infections. Prompted by success with Mesudin, they placed special emphasis on anaerobic infections, but other targets were not neglected. Elected an honorary member of the German Society to Combat Sexually Transmitted Diseases (*Deutschen Gesellschaft zur Bekämpfung der Geschlechtskrankheiten*), Domagk used the occasion to call attention to experimental and clinical successes in the treatment of gonorrhea with Uliron and other compounds. By early 1940, the first favorable clinical reports on use of Mesudin against gonorrhea had come in. Research was also proceeding in Domagk's laboratory on chemotherapy of pneumococcal infections, and Domagk was optimistic that compounds would be found to surpass sulfapyridine, which had been introduced with great fanfare in 1938 by the British firm of May & Baker. Domagk published two papers in 1939 on the chemotherapy of bacterial infections.[10]

Despite these positive notes, it is clear that already in 1939 the Elberfeld research establishment was beginning to feel the pressure of the war. In Domagk's laboratory, turnover of personnel accelerated, leading to a noticeable slowing of the pace of work. The war accomplished in part what animal protection groups could not. There were now shortages of laboratory mice, and the deficiency could not be made up by the few mice produced in the plant's own breeding facilities. "If the war should last longer," Domagk wrote in early 1940, "we must try for a substantial increase [in production of mice] by next winter."[11]

By 1942 the effect of the war, and of war-related activity, played a preponderant role in Domagk's laboratory. The rapid turnover of personnel continued. Of twenty-three outgoing staff, eight, or more than a third, went to the military. The main effort of the laboratory was devoted to war-related tasks, above all the further development of the chemotherapy of wound infections. Intensive research on the treatment of gas gangrene centered on animal tests to determine the most appropriate use of Marfanil powder. So as to better approximate real conditions of use, Domagk and his staff induced experimental infections using bacteria-bearing soil samples received from the various theaters of war. *In vitro* and animal tests led Domagk to conclude that Marfanil was far superior to all other sulfonamides in the treatment of gas gangrene. On the basis of animal studies, he formulated guidelines for treatment of wound infections that were tested and confirmed in clinical trials on patients wounded by bomb or flak fragments or in serious traffic accidents. He prepared a report on these results for the Army Health Inspector and for distribution to military doctors and demonstrated some of his findings for military officials when summoned to Brussels in June 1942. Domagk's report did not take for granted the acceptance of his recommendations by military surgeons. Pointing out that the treatment of serious wound infections constituted a major part of war surgery, he noted that although very few surgeons questioned the value of serum therapy for tetanus, the value of serum therapy in gas gangrene and of sulfonamide therapy of wound infections was still controversial. This was so, he thought, because practicing surgeons were not yet familiar enough with the experimental foundations of these therapies, and he very strongly urged conformity to the experimental experience embodied in the guidelines as a guarantee of therapeutic success.[12]

Research also continued during 1942 on chemotherapy of other kinds of bacterial infections, but under increasingly difficult conditions. Few new compounds were delivered for testing against streptococcal infections because Domagk's chemist-collaborators were heavily occupied with production and patent questions and by ongoing work on compounds already in hand. Both new and old compounds were tested against staphylococcal infections, some of them wound infections. Domagk had little to report about research on typhus or paratyphus infections, except that sulfapyridine and sulfathiazole, both products of British research, had so far proved the most effective against paratyphus infections in mice. Animal trials of several compounds in typhus, paratyphus, and other infections had to be suspended in November 1942 because of a shortage of mice.[13]

Four months after submission of the annual report for 1942, in May 1943, Domagk's frustration with the deteriorating conditions of research at Elberfeld boiled over in a letter he addressed to the directors of I.G. Farben via his superiors, Hörlein in Elberfeld and Max Brüggemann in Leverkusen. Evidently responding to questions raised about the value of research in wartime, Domagk emphatically rejected the idea that "further decisive work" be deferred until after the end of the war. Such work must continue, he wrote, even under difficult conditions, when no immediate financial advantage is to be gained from it, and when there are obstacles to the building of new institutes. He complained in very strong terms of the minute regulations placed by the company on the time of researchers under conditions of total war. Such regulations damaged not only morale but also productivity, Domagk asserted, since to be productive researchers needed to dispose freely of their time. Dangerous conditions had been created by the regulations in laboratories in which human pathogens were handled, Domagk wrote, because of the fatigue suffered by staff. Conditions were especially dangerous where tuberculosis was under study, he noted, pointing out that there had already been several accidental infections among the staff. He reminded the management acidly that "research laboratories are not factories." Domagk was eager to push forward with research on the chemotherapy of tuberculosis, a project he had begun in 1941 and had proposed expanding in reports submitted to the company in January 1942, January 1943, and April 1943. His efforts had been hindered, he said, not only by the regulations on time use but also by the inability of the chemists to hold up their end of the work, that is, the synthesis of new compounds, because of their absorption in efforts to improve production.[14]

One month later, the war intruded in a more direct and devastating way. On June 24 and 25, 1943, Allied bombers attacked Wuppertal-Elberfeld. The building housing Domagk's laboratories was undamaged except for broken glass, but the division's working strength was seriously affected. Sixteen staff members lost all of their homes and belongings. One of the staff was killed, and others wounded. Many weeks of staff time were lost. For six to eight weeks after the bombing, only the most pressing work could be done, since animal breeding facilities and incubators were unusable and there was no gas. The plant was not fully operational again until September.[15]

Despite the losses and delays, research continued during 1943. Domagk's laboratory conducted animal trials of new compounds against streptococcal infections before and after the June bombing attacks. Studies proceeded on various disinfectants, and although apparently little new work was done on them in 1943, pneumococcal and staphylococcal infections were on the laboratory's agenda. Chemotherapy of gas gangrene infections remained a high priority, with medicines composed of combinations of different compounds proving most effective. On October 6, 1943, Domagk presented results on the latest methods of treatment to an audience of 900 surgeons in Dresden, and a Marfanil-Prontalbin (Prontosil Album, Sulfanilamide) combination went into use in the German army.[16]

Domagk assigned increasing significance to tuberculosis, probably because of its threat to public health, and work on chemotherapy of the disease intensified during 1943. Through painstaking histological studies, Domagk was able to establish that a few sulfonamide compounds, including sulfathiazole, had a limited effect on tuberculosis. His major finding, however, one already included in a previous year's report, was that the sulfonamide group was not necessary for the antitubercular effect, at least not by itself. In particular, Domagk established that the compound thiosemicarbazide had an antitubercular action without presence of a sulfonamide group in the molecule. Domagk had received the first thiosemicarbazide compound, prepared by the Elberfeld chemist Robert Behnisch, on November 28, 1941. At first slow to respond to Domagk's finding, the chemists were now pursuing the lead more intensively. Unfortunately, Domagk noted in January 1944, research on the chemotherapy of tuberculosis was hindered by difficulties, several of which he had mentioned in his letter of May 1943. Animal trials were slowed by the lack of mice and consequent need to use guinea pigs and rabbits in their place. Space, including the room for dissections necessary in a full set of trials of antitubercular agents, was inadequate. Domagk pointed out that, in part because of the danger of the work, a room set aside for dissection of tuberculosis cadavers or animals should be set up like a large, well-lighted operating theater and should be capable of being completely disinfected. Staff should be well nourished and well rested. Under present circumstances, he reported, overwork and fatigue were common. He had proposed that food be set aside for staff working on tuberculosis, but the matter had not yet been decided. In spite of these problems, Domagk's report indicates that more than seventy compounds had been tested for antitubercular action in his laboratory during 1943.[17]

Domagk's associate Christian Hackmann also managed to push ahead with his research on the chemotherapy of cancer. During 1943, Hackmann's laboratory tested 247 compounds against tumors. Most were without effect, but a few had slight effect. Hackmann also continued earlier studies of tumor immunity.[18]

A Nobel Prize, and Jail Time

One of the complaints voiced by Domagk in his letter of May 26, 1943, to I.G. Farben management concerned credit for the development of Prontosil and thus for initiation of research on and use of the sulfa drugs. Domagk's letter, and articles in the German medical press about this time, reflect tensions between Domagk, who insisted on the medical research findings as decisive, and Mietzsch and Klarer, who claimed at least an equal role as those responsible for the synthesis of the compounds. At stake were both reputation outside the company and monetary recompense within it. Although the war reduced the possibilities of both kinds of reward, the chemists already had ample grounds for sensitivity on the issue. By the beginning of the war, Domagk had gained the lion's share of credit in the eyes of the world outside the company for introduction of the sulfa drugs. The outbreak of the war in September 1939 interrupted Domagk's preparations to travel to Edinburgh in October to accept the University's Cameron Prize and to deliver the associated lectures, and on October 26 he learned of the Nobel committee's decision to award him the 1939 Prize in Physiology or Medicine "for recognition of the antibacterial properties of Prontosil."[19]

Domagk's Nobel award created yet another point of friction between the National Socialist state and the Elberfeld research establishment. In 1936, the German pacifist writer Carl von Ossietzky, then in a concentration camp for opposition to the regime, had been awarded the Nobel Peace Prize. Infuriated, Hitler had issued a decree forbidding any German to accept a Nobel Prize. Ossietzky died in the camp in 1938, but the decree remained in force. In that year, Domagk was nominated by French and American scientists for the prize in physiology or medicine. At least in the case of the French nominator, P. Maré of the Pasteur Institute, a second, non-German name was also submitted in view of the widely publicized prohibition by the German government. The Nobel committee deferred a decision on Domagk, in part because of insufficient clinical documentation on use of the sulfa drugs in Sweden, in part in the hope that talks then under way between Hitler and representatives of other states would lead to an improvement in the international situation. Those hopes were dashed in 1939. The president of the Nobel committee, G. Liljestrand, sounded out German colleagues regarding the prohibition but received only private expressions of regret. The committee's vice president, F. Henschen, who had known Domagk personally for fifteen years, wrote directly to Hermann Göring asking him to use his influence on Domagk's behalf. The result of this appeal, and of news of the situation passed to the German ambassador in Stockholm, was a telegram from the German minister of education to the Swedish foreign minister stating that the award of a Nobel Prize to a German citizen was "entirely unwelcome" (*durchaus unerwunscht*). After consulting the Swedish foreign minister, the Nobel committee met on October 26 and decided in spite of the position of the German government to award the 1939 prize to Domagk. Two Germans, Kuhn and Adolf Butenandt, also shared the 1939 Nobel Prize for Chemistry.[20]

Domagk learned of the Nobel committee's decision the same day, first by a call from a Swedish journalist in Berlin, then by an official telegram from Stockholm. By his own account he was taken completely by surprise, as was the government. A few hours later the German Foreign Office called, asking whether he had indeed received the Nobel Prize and whether he had accepted it. Congratulations and messages from well-wishers began to flow in from all over the world. Only in Germany, where the news could not be reported, was there silence, with the exception of a few individuals who had heard of Domagk's award from foreign radio broadcasts.[21]

Domagk now found himself in a dilemma. He consulted Hörlein, who reminded him of the prohibition against acceptance of a Nobel Prize, and who advised him how to apply to the Education Ministry. Domagk did so, asking the ministry if the prohibition applied to science prizes as well as to the peace prize. At the same time, acting as a member of the faculty of the University of Münster, Domagk informed the rector and the medical faculty of the award of the prize to him and within a few days received the faculty's official congratulations. When, by November 3, he had no response from the Education Ministry, Domagk sent a carefully worded letter of thanks to Gunnar Holmgren, the rector of the Caroline Institute:

> I most gratefully acknowledge your telegram and the subsequent letter of confirmation from Professor Liljestrand informing me that the 1939 Nobel Prize for Physiology and [*sic*] Medicine has been awarded to me for my research in the field of the chemotherapy of bacterial infections. This recognition of my work has pleased me very much, and I warmly thank you and the members of the Caroline Institute in Stockholm. Since, so far as I know, existing law does not permit German citizens to accept the Prize, I must first inquire about the particulars, and attend to the exact basis of this law. Since this is taking longer than I hoped, I must ask you to excuse the delay in my reply. Apart from that, I still hope that at some time I will have the opportunity in Stockholm of speaking to Swedish circles interested in my field of work, and thereby rendering small thanks for the recognition accorded my work. Whether it will be possible for me to come to Stockholm already on December 10, I cannot now say. I will give you more information as soon as I am able.
>
> With best collegial greetings.
> Yours respectfully,
> G. Domagk[22]

Domagk had been warned by Hörlein that such a letter might have grave consequences but had not taken the advice too seriously and had written other letters of thanks to those who had sent congratulations. On November 17, his house was suddenly surrounded by Gestapo agents, with weapons drawn. Two agents entered the house, placed Domagk under arrest without explanation, and confiscated all his papers having to do with the Nobel Prize, including foreign newspaper clippings. Domagk was taken to the Wuppertal police station, his personal belongings were taken from him, and he was placed in an isolated cell. In the midst of his fear and anger, the absurdity of the situation was brought home by an incident that occurred during the first night of captivity. One of the jailers, making his rounds, asked Domagk why he was there. Domagk replied, "Because I have received the Nobel Prize." The guard said nothing, but on meeting a fellow guard near Domagk's cell, said to him "In that cell we have a crazy man." The next day Domagk was interrogated at length, in the presence of a high officer of the SS from Düsseldorf, regarding the events leading up to the award of the Nobel Prize. Domagk spent a week in jail, during which he was befriended by the local police commissioner, who arranged for a more comfortable cell and for Domagk's wife to bring him food. Hörlein worked with his usual energy to obtain Domagk's freedom. He was released with only the vague explanation for his arrest that his letter to Sweden had been too friendly. Later he learned from a physician acquaintance with contacts in the NSDAP, a Professor Wirtz in Munich, that Hitler had been incensed by Domagk's Nobel award. When none of his medical entourage could inform him about Domagk's work, Hitler assumed that he had gained the prize through some kind of forbidden international connections and ordered his immediate arrest.[23]

The Gestapo was not through with Domagk. Shortly after his release from jail, he was arrested again as he arrived in Berlin to speak about his research to an international medical congress. In police presence, he was forced to sign a document forbidding him to give the lecture. His intended audience was told that the speaker was incapacitated by illness. To obtain his release he was also forced to sign a second document, this time a letter to the Caroline Institute refusing the Nobel Prize. This letter differed sharply from the first in wording and tone:

23 November 1939
In my letter of the third of this month I already mentioned that as far as I know German citizens are not permitted by law to accept a Nobel Prize. When I wrote this letter, however, the situation of this prohibition and the circumstances leading to it were not yet known to me. Only now have I become aware that in fall 1936 the Nobel committee in Oslo awarded the peace prize to Carl von Ossietzky, who had been convicted of treason, and that the international demonstration against National Socialist Germany contained in this award was the occasion for a special order of the Führer and Reich Chancellor in which the above-mentioned prohibition was made known.

Under these circumstances I must ask that you look upon my letter of the third of this month, which was sent without knowledge of the actual state of affairs, as not having been written. I regret that I can no longer view the decision of the Caroline Institute as an honorific recognition of my work, but must rather assume that the Institute, which was undoubtedly aware of the basis of the German prohibition, expected me simply to disregard this prohibition. Such a disregard would be for every German like an act of disloyalty, which I must obviously put far from myself. I therefore feel myself compelled hereby to refuse acceptance of the Prize.

G. Domagk

Although this letter was presented to Domagk in the Education Ministry in Berlin, he was required to post it in police headquarters in Wuppertal so as to preserve the appearance of a voluntary act. From this time until the end of the war, Domagk lived with the consciousness that he was always under surveillance and that further suspicions of his actions might endanger both himself and his family.[24]

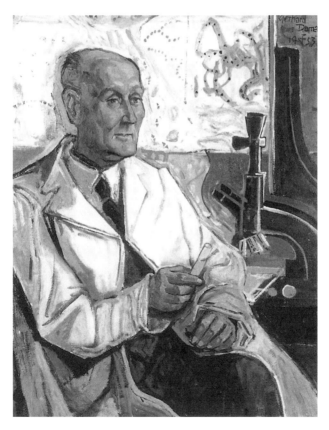

Figure 5.4. Gerhard Domagk, oil portrait by his friend, the painter Otto Dix, 1953 (reprinted courtesy of the Bayer Archive).

The Sulfa Drugs Enter Medical Practice

After the war, Domagk gave an interview in which he complained bitterly that in 1939 his contributions to therapeutics were more highly valued outside of Germany than they were in his own country. He attributed this disproportion to the serious difficulties experienced by scientific medicine under the Nazi regime, during which all possible types of mystical natural healing methods were propagated. The inability of Hitler's medical entourage to describe the basis of Domagk's Nobel award, the appeal of alternative healing methods of various kinds to high officials in the NSDAP, including Hitler himself, and the harsh attacks on scientific medicine, and on pharmaceuticals in particular, from certain quarters of the National Socialist movement, as described above, all lend credence to Domagk's remarks. This picture must be compared, however, to an assessment of actual use of sulfa drugs in Germany during the Nazi era. Figures on manufacture and sales, the content and quality of reportage on the sulfas in the German medical press, and statistics on the effects of sulfas use on mortality are among the circumstances that need to be taken into account. The case of the sulfa drugs can be viewed as a litmus test of the fate of scientific medicine during the Third Reich precisely because, while they were effecting a revolution in therapeutics that could scarcely be ignored by practicing physicians, they were also the product of a scientific medicine that was, at least on occasion, the object of ideological hostility or indifference on the part of the National Socialist movement and state.[25]

Prontosil was a commercial success from the beginning. In 1935, its first year on the market, sales of Prontosil by I.G. Farben reached 175,000 marks. In 1936, sales rose steeply to more than one million marks, and in 1937 to five million. By 1937, Prontosil had risen to third place in sales, surpassed only by Neosalvarsan and aspirin, on the list of 464 pharmaceutical products offered by I.G. Farben.[26]

Use of Prontosil by physicians had evidently surged ahead of the attention given Prontosil in the German medical press. To take only one example of a periodical widely circulated among the German medical profession, the *Klinische Wochenschrift*, 1935 witnessed only about fifteen references to Prontosil, including articles, reviews, notices of articles in other German medical journals, and reports of the proceedings of professional meetings. The corresponding figures in 1936 and 1937 were nine and fifteen items, respectively. Only in 1938 did the volume of attention accorded Prontosil and more recently released sulfonamides begin to catch up with the volume of medical use of these compounds. From 1938 through 1940, the annual number of references to sulfa drugs in the *Klinische Wochenschrift* ranged from fifty to sixty. In 1941, it jumped to around 100. In each of the years 1942 and 1943, in the midst of the war, more than sixty items on the sulfa drugs appeared in this journal. A review of this material reveals a largely favorable response to Prontosil and later sulfonamides on the part of German physicians who made evaluations of the new medicines and who chose to speak or write about their views. Criticism and reservations were common but, as in the examples of early clinical reports described above, were characteristically directed to defining the limits of a medicine's effectiveness under widely varying conditions of use, including assessment of possible side effects. If criticism of bacterial chemotherapy based on the tenets of organic medicine or natural healing methods played a role in the reception of the sulfa drugs, its effects were at best muted, implicit, or indirect in the record of the *Klinische Wochenschrift*.[27]

One example among many of the early spread of use of Prontosil by German physicians may be added to those described above. It is the experience of A. Roth, a staff doctor at the General Hospital of the city of Hagen. Prompted by an earlier publication by L. Gmelin citing favorable results in erysipelas, Roth decided to try Prontosil in cases of streptococcal infection. Roth emphasized in his own published report that he regarded chemotherapy as merely an adjunct of surgical treatment of the foci of an infection, where this was possible. Nevertheless, he had tried Prontosil in a case of sepsis in which surgery was ruled out, with favorable results. He also reported success with use of Prontosil in cases of rheumatic endocarditis, erysipelas, and endocarditis lenta, and possibly also in a case of lung abscess in which other drugs were also used. Without changing his view of the priority to be given surgical treatment, Roth still concluded that "after what we have seen so far, we would not treat any serious streptococcal illness without Prontosil, since it appears to be superior to any chemotherapeutic agent available up to now."[28]

About the time that Roth was reporting his results, Domagk himself had a harrowing experience that brought home in a personal way the uses of Prontosil. In the *Klinische Wochenschrift* for October 1936, he wrote:

> I will briefly describe only one case of a severe streptococcal infection following a wound, which I myself observed and treated, since it concerned my own daughter and I was able to follow the course of the illness in the most exact way. The child wounded herself on December 4, 1935 with a needle as she was occupied with a piece of Christmas handicraft. She came down the stairs with the needle in her right hand to have her mother thread it, so that when she fell, the large needle, eye first, went into the hand up to the wrist bone and broke off. A half hour later in the clinic the child was x-rayed and the needle was removed. The next day she had a rising temperature, which at first was attributed to the flaring up of a sore throat the child had had a few days earlier. When the dressing was changed after a few days there was marked swelling of the hand, and despite removal of all the stitches the fever continued to rise rapidly. In spite of numerous incisions the inflammation phlegmon extended to the under-arm. A serious worsening of the general condition and dizziness occurred, so that we were gravely worried about the child. Since further surgical intervention was not possible, I asked the permission of the treating surgeon to use Prontosil, after I had also established by culture that streptococci were the cause of the illness. At the beginning of the treatment on the morning of December 8 the axillary temperature was 39.3 degrees. The child was dizzy, and without her taking notice of it I pressed the Prontosil tablets into her mouth, and in the afternoon I gave her 15cc., and in the evening 10cc. of Prontosil Soluble rectally. Already the same evening the temperature fell to 38.7 degrees,

on the morning of the next day to 38.2 degrees, and on December 10 to 37.7 degrees. On this day, after another incision when the dressing was changed, the temperature rose again in the evening to 38.2 degrees. In place of the previously diffuse serous fluid the operating surgeon now found "bonum et laudibile" pus. On December 12 the temperature had dropped to normal.

When the temperature began to rise again on December 14, 15, and 18, Domagk responded with large doses of Prontosil and Prontosil Soluble. On December 19, the temperature fell to normal and stayed there and recovery proceeded. Domagk remarked that he varied the dosages according to his daughter's temperature and general condition. When her temperature rose he gave larger doses until the temperature dropped and there was marked improvement. When her temperature dropped to normal he continued "for some time" with daily doses of three 0.3 g tablets. Domagk used the occasion of publication of the story to make general recommendations to clinicians on the administration of Prontosil under varied conditions.[29]

Some idea of the position of the sulfa drugs in German medical practice by the middle of World War II may be gained by a look at the leading textbook on infectious diseases, edited by Max Gundel, the second edition of which appeared in 1942. Domagk contributed a section on the foundations of modern chemotherapy of bacterial infections that painted a picture of success and promise in stark contrast to the resignation bordering on pessimism expressed by Gundel in the first edition of 1935. Very few physicians any longer doubted the value of sulfonamides in the treatment of erysipelas, Domagk reported. Septic sore throat was now usually cured with small doses of Prontosil or Prontalbin, and sulfonamides also helped prevent more serious complications resulting from these conditions that might otherwise prove fatal. Childbed fever, usually caused by streptococci, was "more and more losing its terrors," Domagk wrote. He cited statistics gathered by Reichert showing that mortality from childbed fever had dropped by sixty-six percent between 1932 and 1938, thanks to chemotherapy. Domagk quoted advice now given to physicians by the Reich Health Office (*Reichsgesundheitsamt*) recommending the early use of Prontosil Soluble and Prontosil in tablet form in cases of childbed fever. He cited figures from British and American as well as German literature indicating that sulfonamide treatment had reduced mortality from pneumonia from twenty to thirty percent to five to ten percent. He referred to G. Säker's survey of world medical literature to document an even steeper drop in mortality in epidemic meningitis, from around ninety percent to less than ten percent, again thanks to sulfonamide treatment. Citing a long list of predominantly German medical writers, Domagk reported the use of sulfas in treatment or prophylaxis of infections of the inner ear, gall bladder, and urinary tract, in arthritic conditions associated with bacterial infections, and in dentistry. Sulfas had also been used with some success, he noted, in treatment of Malta fever, actinomycosis, and dysentery, in conjunction with serum therapy in diphtheria, and in other conditions. All clinicians were now agreed, Domagk reported, that chemotherapy with sulfonamides had effected extraordinary progress in the treatment of gonorrhea, which only a few years ago had been difficult and discouraging. Finally, on the topic "now of greatest interest" because of the war, Domagk wrote that wound infections could be effectively treated with sulfonamides. Citing clinical observations gathered by several German physicians, he formulated rules for treatment of wound infections, quoting with approval one physician's recommendation to join surgical treatment with the use of a Marfanil-Prontalbin combination chemotherapy and serum therapy.[30]

Domagk's section in Gundel's textbook was one of thirteen of his publications on the sulfonamides that appeared between 1941 and 1943. Another of these, titled "The Sulfonamide Therapy of Bacterial Infections in Experiment and Practice," originated as a talk to the teaching staff of the veterinary *Hochschule* in Hannover. Domagk was introduced to the teachers league, which was affiliated with the NSDAP, by one of its officials, a Professor R. Götze, who was also director of the school. Götze described the cultivation of research and scientific discussion as one of the purposes of the organization. His introductory remarks included a ringing endorsement of chemotherapy and of the industrial research that had produced much of it. He spoke of the breach opened by chemistry and medicine in the citadel of the pathogenic bacteria. He spoke of the sulfonamides as "true wonder drugs" and of Domagk's "tireless experimental work" that had contributed to their development. Götze's remarks were politically correct in a National Socialist sense in that he emphasized the importance of German contributions to chemotherapy and assigned its origins to Robert Koch but not to Paul Ehrlich, an elision of the role of the Jewish scientist that appears to have been common in medical writings during the Third Reich. Just for this reason, it is noteworthy that Götze's statement betrays no trace of the hostility to scientific medicine, or to the chemical industry, voiced by earlier National Socialist writers on the basis of tenets of *völkisch* medicine or animal protectionist doctrines. Noteworthy also is that Domagk's published article in the *Deutsche Tierärztliche Wochenschrift* was followed by three papers on the applications of sulfa drugs in veterinary practice. Among these was one by Götze in which he wrote that he had been in direct contact with the Elberfeld researchers since the first successes with sulfonamides had been made known and had worked in close cooperation with them to use the sulfas experimentally and clinically in veterinary medicine.[31]

Prontosil, Uliron, and Marfanil were made and sold in quantity. In the war years 1940–1945 alone, I.G. Farben took in more than 48.5 million marks on sales of Prontosil, exclusive of veterinary medicine; 21.9 million of this was profit. In the same period, the equivalent figures for Uliron were 10 million marks, of which 3.8 million was profit, and for Marfanil 1.8 million marks, of which 0.26 million was profit. The company manufactured Marfanil powder, which was used in the treatment of wounds, in quantities of up to ten tons per month. Some of this powder fell into Allied hands in North Africa, but before the chemical formula had been published.[32]

It appears that the war did not introduce any significant discontinuity either in the attitudes of German doctors toward the sulfa drugs or in their use of those medicines. If anything, medical attention to the capabilities of the sulfa drugs and use of them intensified as incidence of wound infections, gonorrhea, and other war-related infections rose sharply. On the whole, for the period 1935–1945, the sulfas appear to have been accepted by German physicians, including the medical press, on clear-cut utilitarian grounds and with little or no ideological debate or commentary about the relative virtues of natural healing methods. This is consistent with the conclusion, also suggested by Robert Proctor's findings on the continuities in the German medical press from 1930 to 1950, that substantial areas of German medical research and practice proceeded without either affecting or being directly affected by the political and ideological currents of the Third Reich.[33]

On Trial at Nuremberg

The Elberfeld research and production establishment survived the war largely intact. The German pharmaceutical industry, insofar as it can be separated from the chemical industry, had not been a major target of Allied bombing. Some facilities had been destroyed, but the overall damage was uneven. Even the June 1943 attack on Wuppertal-Elberfeld, mentioned above, had resulted in only temporary stoppages. More serious were indirect effects brought about by interruptions of supplies of basic chemicals through bombing of other chemical sites or by destruction of railroad or canal transport. When Leverkusen was bombed, for example, Elberfeld was deprived of supplies of sulfuric and chlorosulfuric acid necessary for manufacture of its medicines, including sulfa drugs. Such breakdowns in the system proved temporary, however, and the Elberfeld plant was able to maintain most of its production throughout the war.[34]

Occupation of the area by U.S. forces achieved what the war could not. All production was halted at Elberfeld. On May 16, 1945, Hörlein and his co-director, Clemens Lutter, appealed to the military government to permit reopening of the Elberfeld plant. They stressed the urgency of supplying dispensaries and military hospitals with pharmaceuticals, including aspirin, hypnotics, narcotics, sulfa drugs, scabies treatments, vitamins B_1 and D, and disinfectants. To that end, they requested minimal supplies of fuel, raw materials, including especially basic chemicals, and transport. Perhaps prompted by this request, an Allied intelligence team from the Combined Intelligence Objectives Sub-Committee, CIOS Group 3, visited the Elberfeld laboratories and plant from May 21 through May 29. The CIOS team interrogated all members of the research staff, including Hörlein and Lutter, and gathered information on "factory methods of production of medicinals made at that plant, researches completed and in progress, testing methods and results on tropical diseases and a list of pending patents." On May 24, the local commanding officer of the military government granted temporary permission to I.G. Farben to reopen the Elberfeld plant. Finally, on May 31, in response to a request from the office of the U.S. Army Chief Surgeon citing the urgent need for pharmaceuticals to treat prisoners of war and displaced persons, authority to resume production at Elberfeld was granted by the Production Control Agency of the Supreme Headquarters Allied Expeditionary Force.[35]

Pharmaceutical production was an urgent and uncontroversial necessity. Germany's defeat meant, however, that the larger entity of which Elberfeld was a part, the I.G. Farbenindustrie industrial combine, came under severe scrutiny by the Allies for its role in the war and in the crimes of the Nazi regime. As a member of the executive board (*Vorstand*) and a leading figure in I.G. Farben's pharmaceutical and plant protection divisions, Hörlein was swept up in the net cast for those held to be responsible for I.G. Farben's actions. In August 1945, he was placed under arrest by the U.S. military government. After two years of detention, he went on trial, along with twenty-three other high executives of I.G. Farben, before the U.S Military Tribunal VI in Nuremberg, charged with war crimes and crimes against humanity. Each of the defendants in *United States of America v. Carl Krauch et al.*, also known as the I.G. Farben case, was charged individually. Collectively, the accusations were staggering. They included planning of a war of aggression, coordination with military planning of the German High Command, directing mobilization for war, equipping the Nazi military machine, espionage, participation in plunder and spoilation of occupied countries, enslavement, and mass murder. Charges against the defendants and sentences passed on them varied widely. Thirteen were convicted of various charges and received prison sentences ranging from one and one-half to eight years. The remainder, including Hörlein, were acquitted of all charges.[36]

National Archives records of the I.G. Farben trial, one of twelve separate proceedings held before U.S. military tribunals at Nuremberg against citizens or officials of the Third Reich, occupy 113 rolls of microfilm. They include trial transcripts that alone fill forty-three bound volumes, prosecution and defense briefs and statements, prosecution and defense exhibits and document books, and other material. Even the small fraction of this material directly related to Hörlein is substantial. Among the issues raised in Hörlein's trial were the nature of his relationship to the Nazi regime, its ideology, policies, and practices; the extent of participation of I.G. Farben pharmaceutical units in preparations for a war of aggression; the existence and extent of Elberfeld and Leverkusen managers' knowledge of experiments on human subjects in concentration camps; and participation of Elberfeld in weapons research and development. Testimony evoked by the trial places in sharper relief aspects of Hörlein's, and the Elberfeld establishment's, relationships to the Nazi party and regime.[37]

Hörlein had joined the NSDAP in 1934. His party membership was bound to become an issue in his trial. It provoked the defense to gather extensive testimony to clarify Hörlein's relationship to the regime, and especially to support a distinction between formal party membership and real attitudes and behavior. Those giving testimony, frequently in the form of sworn affidavits, were usually people who had known Hörlein over a period of years. They were not members of the Nazi party and often were its victims. Many were prepared to give witness to Hörlein's humane character and liberal political inclinations, his inward hostility to many of the policies and practices of the National Socialist government, and his efforts to aid and protect individuals both inside and outside the Elberfeld research establishment from the consequences of these policies and practices.

In its cumulative effect this testimony is persuasive and supports three conclusions about Hörlein. First, his party membership represented tactical accommodation rather than ideological conviction. He did not share the regime's political goals

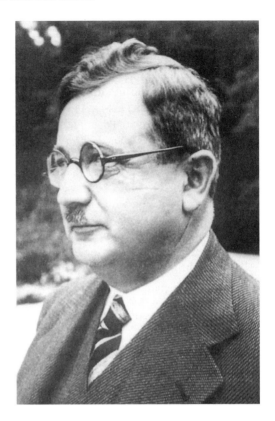

Figure 5.5. Heinrich Hörlein (reprinted courtesy of the Bayer Archive).

or racism and was primarily concerned to preserve the domain of research and production he had built. Second, he worked throughout the Nazi era to shield German science and scientists from the ill effects of the regime. Third, although not medically trained, he infused his research and development efforts with a medical ethos that gave priority to the welfare of patients in the introduction of new drugs.

Hörlein had first joined the party as a condition for remaining on the city council of Wuppertal. Adelheid Schulte, a resident of Wuppertal-Elberfeld who had been retired from her job as student counselor in 1934 because of her political convictions, had known Hörlein as one of the founders of the German Democratic Party in Wuppertal-Vohwinkel in 1919. She had perceived no change in his "free and human attitude" after he joined the NSDAP and thought that party membership had enabled him to exert a strong influence in the economic affairs of the city. Hörlein's influence evidently extended to other local matters, as well. When, after the June 1943 bombing of Wuppertal, the party moved to requisition the city's churches for its own use, a local Catholic priest, Heinrich Rembold, had appealed to Hörlein for help. Hörlein had responded by renting Rembold's church on behalf of Elberfeld workers whose homes had been destroyed and by contributing 10,000 marks toward its repair.[38]

Many of the professional employees of I.G. Farben at Elberfeld testified that Hörlein's party membership should not be taken at face value. Thirty-two Elberfeld staff members who had not been party members stated that they had not thought of Hörlein as a convinced National Socialist but had always thought that he had joined the party so as to keep the damage to the Elberfeld establishment from party programs to a minimum. In weekly meetings, Hörlein had made no secret of his critical attitude toward party members, directives, and organization, they noted. Party representation in the plant was formally acknowledged but was always under a certain ridicule. Hörlein, they said, protected colleagues persecuted for racial or political reasons as long as he could or tried to establish them in comparable positions in other countries. In a separate statement signed by twelve other professional staff members, including Domagk and Klarer, the writers testified that they were astonished to learn of the charges against Hörlein. Describing themselves as opponents of National Socialism, the signatories thanked Hörlein for resisting the demands of party doctrine in the plant and for making it possible for them to avoid joining the party. They attributed the relatively good atmosphere of the Elberfeld plant to Hörlein's actions, for example, his protection of colleagues from attacks by the party.[39]

Several witnesses attested to the persistence of Hörlein's liberal, democratic political orientation and negative attitude toward Nazi policies and practices through the early years of the regime. Clemens Giese, the Prussian Interior Ministry official who had worked with Hörlein to achieve an animal protection law tolerable to medical science, described Hörlein as "anything but a National Socialist" and as someone who never made any secret to Giese of his negative opinion of the NSDAP.[40]

A similar impression was given by Irene Claasen Young, a woman of German origin who had settled in the United States with her American husband in 1931. Young had worked as secretary for German and English correspondence and translator for the Winthrop Chemical Company in Rensselaer, New York, an American partner of I.G. Farben. A large part of Young's job involved handling technical reports from I.G. Farben pharmaceutical plants, especially Elberfeld but also others such as Höchst and Wolfen. Young recalled that several years before the war Hörlein had sent Winthrop directions for manufacture of the antimalarial Atabrine, "including the various steps of production, listing the raw materials required and giving detailed test methods for each intermediate as well as for the finished product." Winthrop had decided for financial reasons to purchase one of the intermediaries from I.G. Farben but, after the war broke out, was able to move rapidly to manufacture "from the ground up" of the strategically important medicine because of the data supplied earlier by Hörlein. Hörlein had also supplied Winthrop before the war with all data required for manufacture of the various sulfa drugs. Young recalled a conversation she had overheard while taking dictation during a visit Hörlein had made to Rensselaer. Hörlein, she said, had expressed "disgust with the then existing Nazi regime in Germany." His words had been "to the effect that we could be glad to be so fortunate as to be in the United States, that in Germany neither business nor life itself were any longer worthwhile since the Nazi government meddled in every single transaction and there was no freedom of action or thought."[41]

Paul György, a German biochemist who had immigrated to the United States in 1937, warmly recalled Hörlein's "invaluable assistance" to himself and Kuhn in their studies that led to the breakdown of the vitamin B_2 complex into its first two members, riboflavin and pyridoxine. György recalled that

> on the few occasions he and I discussed political matters, he struck me as a liberal, democratic individual. I saw him last time in 1937 in Cologne. He appeared to be very depressed and pessimistic with regard to Germany's future and the reckless policy of the Nazi government. He appeared to be sincere in wishing me good luck in America and in expressing the opinion that the future is decidedly with the United States.

György recalled Hörlein's strong will and was convinced that "through all the war years he must have remained in his inner soul faithful to his old convictions."[42]

Other testimony at Nuremberg revealed that Hörlein had actively intervened to protect individuals from actions of the party. Among these cases, one of the more surprising is that of Jacques Tréfouël, the director of the Pasteur Institute in Paris. Tréfouël had written a letter to the British doctor Leonard Colebrook in which he made violent remarks about Adolf Hitler. Colebrook had left the letter with other documents in Paris in June 1940. The Colebrook documents had reached the German authorities, who had passed them on to Hörlein to examine for their chemotherapeutic interest. Finding the letter in question, Hörlein had withdrawn it from the dossier and had passed it to Marcel Bô, assistant director of the Pasteur Institute, so that it would not fall into the hands of the Gestapo.[43]

Several German Jews testified to Hörlein's lack of prejudice both before and after Hitler came to power, and in some cases to his help in making arrangements to safely leave Germany and to secure positions abroad. One such case was Erich Danziger, who had joined I.G. Farben at Elberfeld as a chemist in 1916 and who had eventually risen to head the Analytical Department there. Danziger recalled that Hörlein's "kind and cooperative" behavior toward him had not changed in 1933 and that Hörlein had continued to trust him with confidential work. After the situation for Jews worsened in 1935, Hörlein arranged for Danziger to be hired by the Winthrop Chemical Company in the United States, where he began work in June 1937. Siegfried Thannhauser, a physiological chemist, had headed a medical clinic at the University of Freiburg before he was forced out of his position by the Nazi regime and immigrated to the United States in 1934. He recalled Hörlein as "a man of extremely high intellectual and scientific qualities" who was "very democratic and unbiased" and who, up to the time of his last personal contact with him in 1937, had "remained the same and was not touched politically by the Hitler poison." Another prominent physiological chemist, Bernhard Zondek, recalled that in the twenty years he had known Hörlein he had never known him to be involved in any activity hostile to Jews. After his forced departure from Germany in 1933, Zondek stated, Hörlein had maintained friendly contact with him even though this could have placed Hörlein in danger. Ludwig Taub, a chemist who had worked with Hörlein at Elberfeld for thirty years before leaving in 1936, recalled that Hörlein had treated all colleagues the same "regardless of person or race" and that this had not changed under the Nazi regime. In 1939, Hörlein had helped Taub immigrate to Palestine.[44]

A somewhat different situation was reported by Benno Reifenberg, who was dismissed from his job at the *Frankfurter Zeitung* after 25 years of work, under pressure from the Propaganda Ministry, because he was a "half-Jew" in Nazi terminology. In desperate circumstances and fearing for the safety of himself and his family in Frankfurt, Reifenberg accepted an unpaid post as assistant in Professor Oskar Vogt's institute for brain research in Neustadt. Hörlein heard of Reifenberg's plight and, having failed to secure funds in his capacity as treasurer of the Kaiser Wilhelm Society, arranged for a stipend to go from I.G. Farben through Vogt to Reifenberg. Reifenberg credited his survival in the last year of the war to this support.[45]

Well before 1933, Hörlein had seen it as part of his task as research manager to support and encourage German science, especially chemistry and the medical sciences, both inside and outside of industry. This activity continued after January 1933, but with the added burden for Hörlein of frequently having to work against the policies or practices of the National Socialist state. Hörlein aided individual scientists in their difficulties with the regime, worked against politicization of academic appointments, and resisted pressures from the party and state to place excessive emphasis on utilitarian goals, including military ones, in research. When he went on trial at Nuremberg, a number of German scientists came forward to clarify his actions before and during the Third Reich. Among these were Nobel Prize winners Adolf Windaus, Otto Hahn, Heinrich Wieland, and Butenandt.[46]

Karl Freudenberg, who was professor of chemistry and director of the Chemical Institute at the University of Heidelberg, recalled Hörlein's many services to German and international chemistry through his support of research, teaching, and publications. Hörlein's scientific disposition and tireless activity on behalf of chemistry had won him the trust of academic chemists, Freudenberg noted. Freudenberg viewed Hörlein's entry into the NSDAP not as an expression of inner convictions but as a sacrifice made for tactical reasons so that Hörlein could work against high party officials hostile to science, such as Julius Streicher. The chemistry professors, Freudenberg recalled, had increasingly looked to Hörlein to resist the "cultural bully" Rudolf Mentzel, an SS man in the Education Ministry, especially the latter's efforts to place unqualified National Socialists in teaching positions.[47]

Hahn, a 1944 Nobel laureate, had known Hörlein for many years as the treasurer of the Emil Fischer Society, through which private funds were distributed in support of chemical research. The greater part of the society's funds went to the Kaiser Wilhelm Institute for Chemistry, of which Hahn was the director in the 1930s and 1940s. In the last years of the war, the annual subvention had been more than 200,000 marks. Hahn testified that although most of this money came from I.G. Farben, neither Hörlein nor the company had made any attempt to influence the direction of the institute's research. In particular, they had never given the institute war-related work, even after Hahn's discovery of uranium fission in

1938. Hahn also recalled that Hörlein had helped him secure housing for Lise Meitner's successor at the institute, Joseph Mattauch, after the latter gained the enmity of the NSDAP for opposing the regime in Vienna.[48]

Windaus, Hahn, and Wieland, a 1927 Nobel laureate in chemistry, signed other statements, in which Hörlein's name appeared several times, attesting to the role of I.G. Farben in funding scientific research outside the company, in supporting freedom of research, in helping researchers persecuted for political or racial reasons, and in contributing to technical and medical progress for the benefit of humanity.[49]

The same themes were given more specific content by Butenandt, who from 1936 to 1945 had directed the Kaiser Wilhelm Institute for Biochemistry in Berlin-Dahlem before moving to the University of Tübingen as professor and director of the Institute for Physiological Chemistry. Butenandt, a 1939 Nobel laureate who had known Hörlein throughout the Hitler years, affirmed that Hörlein had used all his influence to maintain the German tradition of science and research and had resisted political encroachments on science from the NSDAP. As member of the board of the German Chemical Society, Hörlein had sought to preserve the purely scientific goals of the organization from party influence and to maintain traditional contacts with foreign scientists and scientific societies. He had tried to help scientists who were under pressure from the party or regime when he was convinced of the value of their work.[50]

As evidence for the last point, Butenandt described his own case. While teaching organic chemistry at the *Technische Hochschule* in Danzig from 1933 to 1936, Butenandt had experienced difficulties with the Education Ministry and the NSDAP because of his political views. At first, these were expressed in shortages of funds for his research. In 1935, when the government was on the point of closing the school entirely, Butenandt received an offer of a professorship at Harvard. When he asked the Education Ministry whether it could guarantee employment equivalent to his current position if he declined the Harvard offer, he was told that he should accept the offer because his political attitude made it impossible for him to receive such a guarantee. Hearing of this situation, Hörlein offered to set up at Elberfeld a well-endowed research section in which Butenandt and his assistants could proceed freely with their research without industrial obligations. That Hörlein was motivated solely by dedication to German science Butenandt concluded from the Elberfeld director's knowledge that Butenandt had already made arrangements with a competing firm to make use of any industrially valuable results of his research. With Hörlein's offer in hand, Butenandt declined the position at Harvard, and further negotiations with the Education Ministry led to his appointment as director of the Kaiser Wilhelm Institute for Biochemistry in 1936.[51]

In Berlin-Dahlem, Butenandt once more found himself the beneficiary of Hörlein's support, this time in a direct financial way. In 1938, on Hörlein's initiative, funds were provided by I.G. Farben to the Kaiser Wilhelm Institute for Biochemistry for the establishment of a division of virus research. Later, this unit was joined to a similar one in the Institute for Biology to form an interdisciplinary workshop (*Arbeitsstätte*) on viruses, which carried on significant research through the war years. Butenandt doubted that the workshop would have been founded without the financial support arranged by Hörlein, and he cited it as one example of Hörlein's commitment to basic research throughout the National Socialist period.[52]

Other witnesses who had been in a position to know Hörlein over a period of years testified to his humane motives and sense of responsibility toward patients and consumers of I.G. Farben products, a medical ethos that took precedence over commercial considerations. Eberhard Gross stated that Hörlein had given full support to occupational health activities at Elberfeld and had backed I.G. Farben's medical-scientific personnel in placing limits on activities of the commercial divisions of the company, for example, by restricting the chemical content of foodstuffs. Paul Loth, who handled the quality control laboratory for pharmaceutical products manufactured at Elberfeld and Leverkusen, emphasized the importance Hörlein attached to his work in providing protection for users of I.G. Farben pharmaceuticals all over the world and in maintaining the company's good name. Loth recalled the conclusion of a company meeting at which Hörlein had stated that he saw the meaning of his work in the help he brought to suffering humanity and that he expected the same attitude from his co-workers.[53]

According to Helmut Weese, who as head of pharmacology at Elberfeld was responsible for testing every compound for toxicity before releasing it for clinical trials arranged by Leverkusen, Hörlein insisted on personally scrutinizing all his reports before they were released. As partial evidence for Hörlein's caution in releasing compounds for clinical trials, Weese cited the case of Helmut Thielicke. In 1933 Thielicke, a theology student, suffered damage to his parathyroid gland in the course of a goiter operation. As a consequence, his blood concentration of calcium fell below normal. At the time, it was not possible to obtain the needed compensatory hormone in Germany, and Thielicke was placed in mortal danger. Elberfeld had a compound, called AT 10, that in animal experiments restored blood calcium concentration to normal but that at high doses caused damage to blood vessels. Hörlein had not approved its release for clinical trials, fearing the same ill effects in humans. Hearing of Thielicke's case, he met with the student, explained the hazards, and with the patient's consent approved use of AT 10 under closely controlled conditions. An effective and safe dosage level was established, and Thielicke went on to lead a full life. Dismissed from his teaching position in 1940 because of conflict with the Nazi party in Heidelberg, Thielicke was forbidden to travel or speak publicly during the war. After the war, now a professor of theology at Tübingen, Thielicke gratefully recalled Hörlein's humane and physician-like handling of his case.[54]

Testimony such as that of Gross, Loth, Weese, and Thielicke was evoked in part in response to charges by the prosecution that Hörlein, and others at I.G. Farben, had knowingly supplied medicines used in criminal experiments on prisoners in concentration camps during the war. In Hörlein's case, special attention was given to his knowledge of one Hellmuth Vetter, a doctor in the Waffen-SS (combat arm of the SS) who before the war had been employed in the pharmaceutical scientific department at Leverkusen and who was convicted by the Nuremberg tribunal of crimes against humanity. Vetter had joined I.G. Farben in 1938, had worked in Leverkusen especially on matters related to hormones, and had left the company to join the SS in 1939.[55]

In January 1942, Vetter came to Leverkusen and spoke with Karl Koenig, who was then the director of the Pharmaceutical Scientific Department II. Koenig's department was responsible for collecting, analyzing, and distributing information on the use of medicines manufactured by I.G. Farben in the treatment of tropical diseases, including typhus. Vetter explained to Koenig that he was a physician to SS soldiers at Auschwitz and that he was in urgent need of medicines to use in treatment of typhus, of which there were many cases. Vetter did not tell Koenig that Auschwitz was the site of a concentration camp or that Vetter was treating concentration camp inmates. On Koenig's authority, Vetter was supplied with a compound called B 1034, which was then in clinical trials as a treatment for typhus and which had been developed and was manufactured at Elberfeld. Vetter reported back to Leverkusen on his results with B 1034 and another compound, Periston, also made at Elberfeld. It was not until December 1943, however, that Koenig inferred from the body weights of Vetter's patients that he was treating concentration camp prisoners. What neither Koenig nor others suspected until it was brought out at Nuremberg after the war was that some of Vetter's patients had been inmates deliberately infected with typhus, an act of murder for which Vetter was condemned to death by the tribunal.[56]

The prosecution tried but failed to establish Hörlein's knowledge of, and indirect complicity in, Vetter's criminal experiments on prisoners. The weakness of the prosecution case resulted not only from a lack of documentary or testimonial evidence but also from the convincing picture of Hörlein's good character, humane concerns for patients, and rigorous standards for developing and testing new medicines that emerged from the defense presentation. One point of medical language became especially important in this part of Hörlein's trial. In the translation of German documents, for example, Vetter's reports on his results with new medicines, the term *Versuch* was routinely rendered as experiment. Thus, it appeared that Hörlein, Koenig, and others had been in possession of documents that explicitly referred to experiments on human subjects. In response, the defense brought forward a number of witnesses, including research staff at Elberfeld and Leverkusen, to explain that *Versuch* meant clinical trial and that the distinction was crucial to the case. The difference was put most clearly by Koenig, who stated that

> in the exclusive sense used by us, the term "*Versuch*" means a curative endeavor of a physician towards a patient, suffering from a disease, by the application of a new remedy which previously, and as a result of profound and extensive scientific research work, has been declared by the medical experts of the laboratories as non-toxic in the prescribed doses and as to the best of their judgment possessing a real curative effect. The disease of the patient in question must have been naturally contracted (not intentionally induced) and the exclusive aim, when applying the new medicine, is to cure the disease or to improve the conditions of the patient.

. . . In contrast to this, the characteristic of a medical experiment is the intentional creation of the experimental condition. That means that in an experiment the human being or the animal is an experimental object on whom the experimenter afflicts [*sic*] by willful intervention an alteration on his or its bodily condition, i.e. mostly a damage corresponding to a disease which in the further procedure of the experiment has to be influenced or simply observed in its further development.

As examples of medical experiments, Koenig cited intentional infection with germs producing a disease, deprivation or excess of heat to change body temperature, or deprivation or abnormal consumption of food and drink. Vetter had indeed carried out medical experiments in this sense by deliberately infecting individuals with typhus, but had represented himself to managers at Leverkusen and Elberfeld as performing clinical trials.[57]

The prosecution also attempted to associate Hörlein with the production of Zyklon B, a granular vaporizing pesticide that was used in the mass killing of Jews at Auschwitz. Zyklon B, generically known as hydrocyanic or prussic acid, was manufactured by the German Pesticide Corporation (*Deutsche Gesellschaft für Schädlingsbekamfungsmittel* or *Degesch mbH*), a subsidiary of I.G. Farben, and had been widely used since World War I as a delousing agent in settings such as military barracks and prison camps. As owner of 42.5 percent of Degesch's stock, I.G. Farben was entitled to three seats on the company's administration committee. Hörlein formally occupied one of these starting in 1937. It came out in the trial, however, that Hörlein had not attended any meetings of this committee and had had no active role in the affairs of the company. The administrative committee itself had not met after 1940. Since Zyklon B was widely employed and was supplied by the company to many sites, its delivery to Auschwitz did not in itself reveal the murderous uses to which it was put. Rumors of mass killings at Auschwitz probably reached some members of I.G. Farben's executive board in 1943, although no proof of first-hand knowledge was brought forward in trials after the war. If Hörlein came by such information, it was indirectly, as one member of I.G. Farben's executive board, and not as a manager of a subsidiary who knowingly supplied poison gas to concentration camps for the murder of their inmates.[58]

Along with other I.G. Farben executives, Hörlein was accused of participation in planning for a war of aggression. His acquittal was based in part on records of meetings of I.G. Farben's pharmaceutical major conference, of which Hörlein served as chair *primus inter pares* on the basis of seniority. At the seventy-fifth meeting of the conference on July 19, 1939, for example, its members were discussing business in France as though peace would continue indefinitely. The same implicit view of relations with Russia was expressed in conference proceedings for the eighty-third meeting on October 11, 1940. Hörlein had tried to maintain international contacts almost to the eve of the outbreak of war. In late July 1939, for example, he had helped to host the visit to Cologne and Leverkusen of 150 staff from the London, Manchester, and Dublin offices of Bayer Products, Ltd. Five of this group visited Hörlein at Elberfeld. On June 30, 1941, only days after the German invasion of Russia, Hörlein resigned as director of the Elberfeld factory, while retaining his position on I.G. Farben's executive board and his responsibilities related to research at Elberfeld. Later he cited as reason for his resignation his distaste for the whole internal and external political situation, with the invasion of Russia as the last straw. His secretaries recalled that he had also mentioned difficulties with the NSDAP.[59]

The prosecution at Nuremberg also attempted to show that Hörlein, and the Elberfeld research establishment, had participated in the development of gas weapons. Here there was some basis for the charge, although the extent of Hörlein's and Elberfeld's role was limited. In 1935, Hörlein and the then second director of the Elberfeld plant, Werner Schulemann, met with representatives of Army Ordnance (*Heereswaffenamt*), including Leopold von Sicherer. After this meeting, Hörlein was required to turn over to Army Ordnance information on toxic substances that were encountered in research and that met defined criteria. Much of the preliminary screening was done in Gross's occupational hygiene laboratory in Elberfeld. Gross prepared reports on these substances and passed the reports to Hörlein, who sent them on to Army Ordnance, sometimes with copies to the parts of I.G. Farben from which the compounds had originated. The aim of the work at this stage was to identify compounds that might be of interest to Army Ordnance and to obtain that office's clearance to proceed with patent applications and peaceful industrial use for as many of the screened compounds as possible, as quickly as possible. By this means, several substances were selected by Army Ordnance for further development as chemical weapons. Among these were two phosphorus compounds first prepared by the Elberfeld chemist Gerhard Schrader and subsequently developed as poison gases by the Army under the names Tabun and Sarin. From 1937 to 1944, Gross conducted animal experiments at Elberfeld on the effects of Tabun. As the German military position deteriorated by later 1944, Hitler seriously considered use of the nerve gas Tabun and was dissuaded only by the argument, later found to be mistaken, that the Allies also had the gas and could reply in kind.[60]

Screening of toxic substances was a routine part of peacetime research and development at Elberfeld. Compounds needed to be tested for toxicity because they might pose an occupational health hazard, and some of those identified as toxic might be sent to Leverkusen for further development as pesticides. That many compounds after 1935 had to be sent to Army Ordnance before they could be developed for peaceful uses represented both an additional burden on I.G. Farben's research and development effort and a degree of participation, albeit compulsory, in weapons development priorities, and it appears that Hörlein tried to keep to a minimum Elberfeld's association with Army Ordnance. Elberfeld never did directed research, held a contract, or received money from Army Ordnance, and no weapons were ever manufactured at Elberfeld. By his own account and by the separate testimony of two employees of the Army Ordnance research section (*Heereswaffenamt Prüfwesen 9*), the chemist von Sicherer and the pharmacologist Wolfgang Wirth, Hörlein saw weapons development as antithetical to his life's work and to the fundamental mission of Elberfeld to supply medicines to the whole world. In September 1944, Hörlein ordered the destruction of all substances and documents in Elberfeld related to weapons.[61]

As the American army approached in March 1945, Nazi party officials threatened to destroy the works and research holdings at Elberfeld, in fulfillment of Hitler's scorched earth policy. The works foreman, one Liebold, stated that when the Americans arrived they would find not a single stone of any building still standing. Hörlein ordered the head of works security, Amandus Hoffman, to billet his well-armed staff inside the works and to resist with force any attempt to destroy the buildings. Hörlein hoped that if it came to a fight he could delay the party's action long enough to mobilize the whole staff in defense of its workplace.[62]

It did not come to a fight, and amid the ruins of a defeated Germany the Elberfeld research and production establishment remained standing. Its last-minute defense and persistence may serve as metaphor for Hörlein's posture and actions throughout the Nazi era. Hörlein's fundamental purpose was to preserve what he conceived of as the freedom of science in Germany and, in particular and especially, the existence and integrity of the pharmaceutical research and production establishment he had built. To this end, he was prepared to do whatever was necessary. On occasion, this meant fighting or preparing to fight, as in the struggle over animal experimentation at the beginning of the regime or the defense of the Elberfeld buildings at its end. On occasion, it meant quietly extending help to victims of the regime from the scientific or medical communities.

Doing whatever was necessary also meant, for Hörlein, outward political accommodation to the regime and lack of resistance to it outside of the limited sphere within which he saw the vital interests of his life work at stake. It is in this light that his joining of the NSDAP in 1934 must be seen. Hörlein was not a National Socialist in any ideological sense. His overriding values were scientific, medical, technical, and commercial. His life work, to which he was intensely dedicated, was the building and maintenance of a pharmaceutical research and production organization in an industrial setting, with close ties to the scientific and medical communities. Politically, his own tendencies were liberal. He did not subscribe to party doctrine, did not envision a greater Germany, and did not think in racial hygiene terms. Once the regime was in place, however, he joined the party in order to gain leverage in protection of his own domain, which he identified with a high purpose.

Whatever judgment is made of Hörlein must take into consideration the whole picture of his actions before and during the Nazi regime. Apart from the limited and compulsory role played by Elberfeld in the development of gas weapons, Hörlein did not initiate, endorse, or participate in the worst aspects of the Hitler regime, including militarism, expansionist aggression against neighboring states and peoples, domestic political repression, persecution on racial grounds, experiments on concentration camp inmates, or mass murder. Yet, once the regime was in power, he chose to stay in Germany, to create at least a façade of acceptance of the regime, and to try as far as possible to conduct business as usual. Hörlein said that he was working for the good of humanity. There is no reason to doubt that this was his view of himself and that such sentiments composed part of his motivation, along with career ambition, an entrepreneurial zest for institution building and the commercial struggle, and scientific and medical curiosity. Was it tenable for him to think that he could encapsulate a zone of scientific freedom and humane values within a society and regime that was militaristic, racist, and repressive? From our vantage point, knowing all that we know, the answer must be no. From the standpoint of 1933, or the years that followed before the war, the answer was not so obvious. As Alan Beyerchen has pointed out, perceptions of National Socialism both within and outside Germany were different before the war than they were during and after it.[63]

Beyerchen's pioneering study of German physicists in the Third Reich and more recent scholarship have shown that Hörlein was far from alone in his determination to preserve German science in the face of a regime that he regarded as hostile to or destructive of its real interests. Perhaps the best known such case is Max Planck, who as head of the Prussian Academy of Sciences and the Kaiser Wilhelm Society worked quietly behind the scenes to help colleagues and to salvage what he could of the institutions of German science. John Heilbron's study of Planck shows that, like Hörlein, the physicist practiced outward compliance with the regime, though, unlike Hörlein, without joining the NSDAP, and that he refrained from public protest of its worst injustices. Like Hörlein, too, Planck "tried to build enclaves within the system in which relatively normal life and work could be pursued."[64]

Kristie Macrakis's study of the Kaiser Wilhelm Society has shown that those scientists who remained in Germany during the Third Reich represented a spectrum of beliefs. Many of them, though lacking Planck's eminence or position, were hostile or indifferent to National Socialism and were determined to try to continue their work, often by outward accommodation to the regime. Although certain areas of German biology, especially eugenics and racial hygiene, were not only politically sensitive but also central to Nazi ideology, Macrakis shows that other areas of fundamental biology, for example, virus research, bore little or no relationship to political doctrine.[65]

The present study indicates that the same may be said of substantial areas of medical science. Although Hörlein ran head on into the *völkisch* critique of scientific medicine, and in particular chemical medicine, early in the regime, the subsequent reception of the sulfa drugs by German physicians does not appear to reflect ideologically grounded hostility. Chemotherapy in the form of the sulfa drugs was not problematic for most German physicians except in the ways that it was for physicians in other countries. That is, initial skepticism based on past failures of bacterial chemotherapy was replaced by increasing acceptance, and even enthusiasm, tempered by the recognition that much remained to be sorted out about the extent, limits, and modalities of the uses of sulfa drugs in medical practice. The reception of the sulfa drugs in Germany appears to exemplify the continuity and apolitical character of much of the German technical medical press before, during, and after the Nazi regime. Many German physicians joined the party, but much of German medical science did not.[66]

Whatever judgment is made on Hörlein's actions, it is also the case that Hörlein and I.G. Farben were able to maintain a measure of continuity in pharmaceutical research and production operations throughout the Nazi period. Research, including that of Domagk and his collaborators Mietzsch and Klarer, went on. New drugs were developed, clinically tested, and put on the market. Laboratory and clinical reports on the sulfas were published in the medical press. Production and use of sulfa drugs rose. Sulfa drugs were used extensively by German military and civilian physicians during the war. Anticipating shortages, I.G. Farben stockpiled essential medicines toward the end of the war and was able to bridge the gap in production that followed Allied occupation. Already by June 1945, pharmaceutical production had been resumed at Elberfeld, meeting the needs of a population vulnerable to disease in the midst of immediate postwar hardships.

For all this, there were costs. Hörlein had to struggle to preserve the conditions for pharmaceutical research from the very beginning of the Nazi regime. I.G. Farben staff were lost to political or antisemitic oppression. Especially after the war began, research staff was lost to military service, and later to Allied bombing. Research and development had to be curtailed for lack of funds or necessary materials. Contact with the international medical and scientific community was inhibited, and then cut off. At the end of the war, production temporarily ceased altogether. Once the war was over, the former I.G. Farben pharmaceutical establishment faced the task of reconnecting with the international medical and scientific community, in an environment in which competition in pharmaceutical research and development was significantly greater than it had been before the mid-1930s. For all that, the Elberfeld research organization remained intact. As part of a Bayer company reconstituted in the wake of Allied dismantlement of I.G. Farbenindustrie, it became a key element in the postwar reconstruction of pharmaceutical research in Germany.

CHAPTER 6

Pathways of Recognition

Most histories of medicine correctly credit the first sulfa drugs, Prontosil and sulfanilamide, with initiation of a revolution in therapeutics. Some also say or imply that the transformation was sudden and irresistible, that the new medicines were so clearly superior to existing treatments that they immediately marked off the past of medical practice from its future. That such was not the case is indicated by the German experience described in chapters 4 and 5. Even in the land of its birth, Prontosil was not an instant success. Physicians rendered skeptical by failures of earlier chemotherapies for bacterial infections gave Prontosil a positive, but cautious and critical, reception, and sales of the compound did not reach their full potential until three years after its introduction. Outside of Germany, too, in France, Britain, and the United States, Prontosil and sulfanilamide became "miracle drugs" only through a process that extended over more than two years after the introduction of Prontosil. The process involved a complex interaction of laboratory and clinical investigations, physician use, and scientific, medical, and popular representations. Its end points were roughly Gerhard Domagk's first publication in February 1935, and the Paris International Exposition and American Medical Association Atlantic City meeting in 1937.

The results were similar. By the middle of 1937, most physicians in France, Britain, and the United States were convinced of the value of the sulfa drugs in the treatment of a variety of bacterial infections, and some were already hailing a new age for medicine. The process of becoming, however, was different for each country. The reception of the first sulfa drugs reveals national differences in the way new drugs were evaluated, in the relations between the pharmaceutical industry and the medical community, and in the status of foreign, in this case German, patent law. It also places in relief the relative closeness with which pharmaceutical developments in Germany were followed in the three countries, the credence given claims made for new drugs in general and those from Germany in particular, and the roles of professional and popular media in publicizing and creating demand for new medicines.

Entering a New Age

P rontosil first came into the French pharmaceutical market on May 8, 1935, in the guise of a copy with the trade name Rubiazol, manufactured by the Roussel Laboratories in Paris. Information on the preparation of Prontosil had been available in France nearly a year earlier. On December 24, 1933, a year after the filing of the German patent application, I.G. Farben had registered a corresponding French patent. This was issued on April 9, 1934, and published on June 21, more than six months before publication of the German patent and almost eight months before Domagk's first publication on Prontosil. Since at this time French patents protecting chemical products did not extend to medicines, Roussel was unobstructed in its efforts to reproduce Prontosil. This accomplished, the compound was turned over to two medical researchers, Constantin Levaditi and Aron Vaisman, at the Institut Alfred Fournier in Paris, for animal trials. Levaditi and Vaisman's paper, published on May 13, 1935, just five days after Rubiazol went on the market, was the first confirmation of Domagk's laboratory results to appear in France. By July, the first reports of clinical trials began to appear, confirming earlier German claims about the effectiveness of Prontosil/Rubiazol in treatment of erysipelas and puerperal fever.[1]

Roussel Laboratories, Levaditi, and Vaisman were not alone in their rapid response to the news of Prontosil. Within ten days of publication of Domagk's article in February 1935, a copy was in the hands of Ernest Fourneau, director of the Pasteur Institute's section of therapeutic chemistry. Fourneau had already taken note of the French patent eight months earlier, and at that time had written to Edmond Blaise, the scientific director of the chemical and pharmaceutical firm Rhône-Poulenc. Now, with Domagk's paper before him, he acted quickly, speaking to two of his own research staff, Jacques Tréfouël and Daniel Bovet, the same day and soon thereafter conferring with Blaise on a joint course of action. Fourneau and Blaise agreed to pursue a coordinated program of research on compounds related to Prontosil at the Pasteur Institute and at Rhône-Poulenc's laboratories near its factory at Vitry.[2]

In so doing, Fourneau and Blaise were continuing and extending a commitment to research in chemical therapy and its support by French industry that had its origins in the early years of the century and in which Fourneau had been closely involved. The Pasteur Institute had set up a section of therapeutic chemistry in 1901 as part of an expansion directed by Pasteur's successor, Émile Duclaux. Work on chemotherapy, notably that of Charles Laveran and Félix Mesnil on trypanosome infections, figured in the institute's *Annales* even before Paul Ehrlich coined the term in 1906. Fourneau began as a student of pharmacy in Paris, learning organic chemistry from Charles Moureu. A chance meeting with

Emil Fischer, who was staying at his parents' hotel in Biarritz, led Fourneau to a three-year sojourn in Germany, where he continued the study of organic chemistry with Fischer and L. Gatterman in Berlin and with Richard Willstätter in Munich.[3]

Fourneau returned from Germany convinced that new chemical therapies could best be sought in collaboration with the chemical industry, which was in a position to supply the number and variety of compounds necessary for testing. He entered into an arrangement with the Établissements Poulenc Frères, one of the two parent companies of Rhône-Poulenc, to conduct research with the company's support. Out of this laboratory, which Fourneau headed from 1903 to 1911, came one of the first synthetic local anesthetics, named Stovaine in a pun on the English translation of Fourneau (*le fourneau*, stove).[4]

In 1910, the director of the Pasteur Institute, Émile Roux, prompted by Ehrlich's recent breakthrough with Salvarsan and by Fourneau's growing reputation, offered Fourneau the directorship of the institute's section of therapeutic chemistry. Fourneau agreed on the condition that his section maintain the ties he had previously established with Établissements Poulenc Frères. The connection meant both financial support and a continuing flow of intermediates and new compounds. In return, Fourneau agreed with Roux that all his research would be published, contrary to the usual industrial practices of the day. In addition, the company did not attempt to impose research problems, and Fourneau had a free hand to do as he pleased. In practice, this meant not only the search for new synthetic medicines in competition with leading German pharmaceutical research, but also outright copying of existing German products, which were not covered by patents in France, so as to free French pharmaceutical manufacturing from dependence on Germany. The urgency of the latter task increased dramatically with the outbreak of war in 1914.[5]

Fourneau's service scored early successes, including an oral treatment for syphilis called 190F or Stovarsol, and a sleeping sickness medicine, 270F or Orsanine. When the Bayer Company kept secret the formula of its sleeping sickness remedy, Bayer 205 or Germanin, Fourneau's team succeeded in synthesizing it independently. Under the name 309F, the compound was distributed to doctors in the French colonies through the overseas Pasteur Institutes and was received enthusiastically.[6]

The successes of Fourneau's service flowed not only from his leadership and the special combination of steady support and freedom of action built into the arrangement with Établissements Poulenc Frères—what Fourneau proudly called "the mechanism that I created"—but also from the close teamwork he imposed between chemists, medical researchers and clinicians.[7] In all of these respects, Fourneau may be compared with Heinrich Hörlein, with the notable difference that Hörlein acted as executive of the industrial corporation that supported his research enterprise.

In 1928, Établissements Poulenc Frères was absorbed by the Société chimique des Usines de Rhône to form a new and larger entity, Rhône-Poulenc. Both parent companies had their origins in the first half of the nineteenth century, and both had begun to manufacture synthetic organic chemicals in the second half of the century. During or after the World War, Les Usines de Rhône began to manufacture aspirin, and it was their common interest in the aspirin market that brought the two companies together. The leadership of Les Usines de Rhône was composed mainly of men of finance, while that of Les Établissements Poulenc included a majority of pharmacists and doctors of pharmacy. The merger opened new possibilities for pharmaceutical research and development. In addition to its continuing support of Fourneau's service at the Pasteur Institute, where in 1935 Rhône-Poulenc supplied almost half of the budget of what was one of the largest sections of the institute, the company also maintained at the factory at Vitry a staff of about ten chemists and two medical researchers. One of the latter was R.L. Mayer, a German bacteriologist of Alsatian origin, and the other was Bernard Halpern, a Polish doctor who would later occupy the chair of experimental medicine at the Collège de France.[8]

In February 1935, Fourneau and Blaise initiated a research program that aimed to prepare and test azo compounds that might match or improve upon Prontosil's therapeutic action. Chemical and animal experimental work was to proceed simultaneously at Vitry and the Pasteur Institute. They assigned the first stage of the chemical work, the preparation of *p*-aminobenzenesulfonamide as intermediate, to the Rhône-Poulenc laboratories at Vitry because of its proximity to the factory and greater potential for quantity production. Marcel Delépine, the director of the Vitry laboratories, was a professor at the Collège de France and a long-time friend of both Fourneau and Blaise. A chemist at Vitry delivered the first sample on March 30, and by April 15 had accumulated 200 g. By June, the intermediate was in the hands of chemists P. Goissedet at Vitry and Jacques Tréfouël at the Pasteur Institute.[9]

Meanwhile, Bovet at the Pasteur Institute strove to replicate Domagk's animal experimental model and to reproduce the results of Domagk's animal trials of Prontosil. To do so, he enlisted the aid of Frédéric Nitti, a bacteriologist working with pathogenic microbes in A. Salimbeni's vaccine service one floor above Bovet's laboratory. Swiss by origin, trained in zoology at Geneva, Bovet had come to Paris in 1929 to work in Rhône-Poulenc's laboratories at Vitry. Instead, a temporary assignment to Fourneau's service turned into a permanent position. Bovet learned to work with laboratory animals and collaborated with Pasteur Institute chemists on a variety of problems, including hypnotics, the chemotherapy of malaria, local anesthetics, and antiseptics. Nitti had interrupted medical studies in his native Italy to join his father in political exile from fascism. Completing his medical studies in Paris with a thesis on use of autovaccines in treatment of bronchial asthma, he entered the Pasteur Institute on a fellowship to continue his research and stayed on in the vaccine service.[10]

At first, Bovet and Nitti were unable to reproduce Domagk's results. Animal trials carried out with the Pasteur Institute's good collection of bacterial cultures were negative. The cultures were not sufficiently virulent, and Prontosil was without effect. Success came with a fresh culture from a human streptococcal infection, obtained through a friend at the Hôtel-Dieu. The new culture killed mice with the necessary efficiency, and infected mice treated with Prontosil survived. After three months of trials, the collaborators were confident that they had replicated Domagk's animal model and that they could now proceed to screen new compounds.[11]

By June 1935, conditions were in place for Fourneau's service to proceed with the synthesis and screening of new compounds. The chemical work was done by Jacques and ThérèseTréfouël, who had before them the model of Fritz Mietzsch and Joseph Klarer's patent application for Prontosil. By July 13, the Tréfouëls had produced the first azo dye other than Prontosil, and on July 25 Fourneau wrote to Blaise that he had in hand a compound labeled 1095F that surpassed Prontosil in activity.

Now the pace quickened as the work became routinized. Between July and early November, the Tréfouëls synthesized forty-four azo derivatives, of which eighteen were sulfonamides. Bovet and Nitti conducted animal trials on some eighty compounds, and Bovet tested each for toxicity after the example of Domagk's February 1935 paper. The urgency of the work was underlined by positive clinical reports on Prontosil and its French homologue, Rubiazol, that arrived in the summer and early fall from both French and German clinicians.[12]

Prontosil and its copy, Rubiazol, were dyes, and so were many of the compounds synthesized and tested in Fourneau's service between July and November. The Pasteur Institute team saw little reason to depart from a research path that was accessible, clearly marked, and rich in possibilities. That they did so was the result of a discovery that came upon them suddenly and unexpectedly on November 6–8.

The story has been told in detail by Bovet. On the morning of November 6, Bovet and Nitti began with forty mice. Dividing them into groups of four, they gave each an intraperitoneal injection of the same dose of a highly virulent culture of streptococcus. They left one group untreated and gave a second group what they judged to be a curative dose of a Prontosil clone. The remaining eight groups were to be treated with oral doses of new compounds. Only seven such compounds were available, however, leaving an extra group of mice. Bovet recalled that "I thought, why not simply try p-aminophenylsulfonamide, the molecule common to all the compounds being tested?" The large brown glass flask from Vitry containing the intermediate stood before him on the table. He quickly prepared the solution and administered it to the last four mice.

Checking their animals the next day, Bovet and Nitti found the controls dead as expected, while those mice treated with the Prontosil clone were still alive. Only one of the seven new compounds prepared by the Tréfouëls showed activity, confirming an earlier observation. Arriving finally at the last cage containing the four mice treated with the intermediate, Nitti and Bovet were surprised to find its occupants in good condition. Bovet recalled that his and Nitti's first response was disappointment, since the activity of the intermediate seemed to render all the work to prepare and test dyes of the previous four months "suddenly and completely useless." The let-down was short-lived. "A moment of reflection," Bovet wrote, "was sufficient for us to appreciate the results before us. The last V [indicating survival] was not yet written [on the laboratory record] before Nitti and I were convinced that the future belonged to 'colorless products'. From this moment on the patents of the German chemists would be without value."[13]

Bovet and Nitti conducted more trials of the intermediate the following week, on larger numbers of animals, with positive results. Once *p*-
aminobenzenesulfonamide's powers had been demonstrated empirically,
explanations for them were soon in coming. The Pasteur Institute team noted
analogies in the structure of *p*-aminobenzenesulfonamide (hereafter PABS) and
two other chemotherapeutic agents, atoxyl and stibamine. Perhaps the more complex dye molecules of which PABS was a constituent were broken down in the animal organism, releasing the intermediate to act on its own. If so, all of the French
and German laboratory and clinical investigators preparing and testing different
compounds over the past several months had, unknowingly, merely confirmed the
efficacy of a single simpler substance. There was general recognition on
Fourneau's service that a real breakthrough had occurred. Jacques Tréfouël saw
an explanation for what to him had been a puzzling similarity in therapeutic action of very different compounds. Bovet found himself overcome with emotion
when he observed even animals infected intravenously recover after treatment
with PABS. Fourneau began immediately to plan studies of derivatives belonging
to neighboring chemical series.[14]

Once they had confirmed the action of PABS, its role as the common factor
in the activity of a variety of azo dyes seemed obvious to the Pasteur Institute
workers, and the experiments that revealed that role were open to anyone. To ensure priority in the discovery, they sought the quickest vehicle of publication. For
French researchers in the life sciences, the path of choice was a short note in the

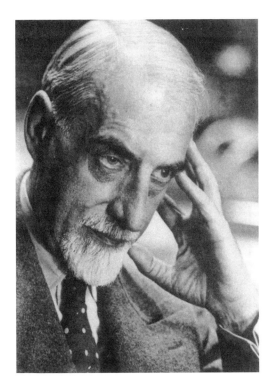

Figure 6.1. Ernest Fourneau
(1872–1949) c. 1930 (© Institut
Pasteur, reprinted with permission).

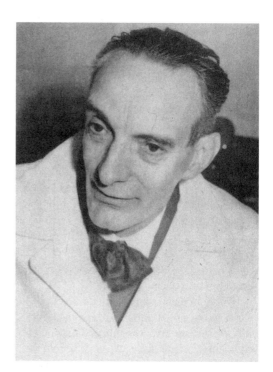

Figure 6.2. Daniel Bovet (1907–1992) in his laboratory c. 1955. Swiss by origin, Bovet worked at the Pasteur Institute in Paris from 1924 to 1947. In 1957 he received the Nobel Prize in Physiology or Medicine for his work on antiallergenics and synthetic curares (© Institut Pasteur, reprinted with permission).

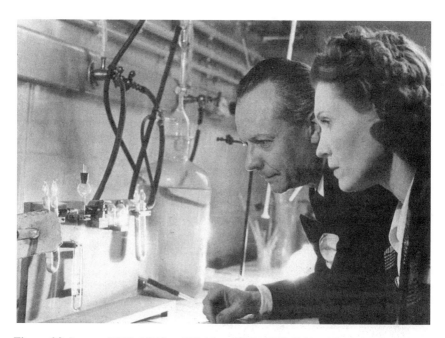

Figure 6.3. Jacques (1897–1977) and Thérèse (1892–1978) Tréfouël in their laboratory of therapeutic chemistry at the Pasteur Institute, Paris, c. 1945 (© Institut Pasteur, reprinted with permission).

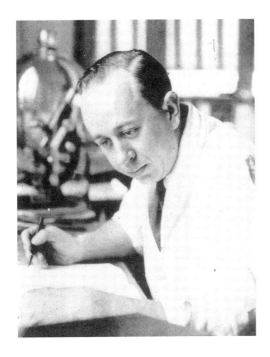

Figure 6.4. Frédéric Nitti (1905–1947) in his laboratory at the Pasteur Institute, Paris, c. 1945 (© Institut Pasteur, reprinted with permission).

Comptes Rendus des Séances de la Société de Biologie. The Société de biologie, founded in 1848 and counting among its early presidents Pierre Rayer, Claude Bernard, and Paul Bert, continued to thrive in the 1930s in a dual role as testing site for candidates for the Académie de médecine and Académie des sciences and as receptacle for a large scientific correspondence. Since 1929, it had published three volumes of *Comptes Rendus* a year. In 1935 alone, these volumes comprised 4,756 pages and some 2,000 notes or short communications. Not known for selectivity—no editorial committee reviewed its notes for content, and it was sometimes referred to with affectionate humor as the *"Comptes des mille et une nuits"* (in a play on *Contes des mille et une nuits, Tales of the Thousand and One Nights*)—the *Comptes Rendus* did have the virtue of efficiency, its weekly installments appearing like clockwork. Neither Nitti nor Bovet was a member of the Société, but both knew the secretary and had published other notes in the *Comptes Rendus* during 1935. The Pasteur Institute team's note was read to the Société on November 23, 1935, and printed on November 28.[15]

The published note is remarkable in several respects. Although the discovery of the therapeutic efficacy of PABS was made in Fourneau's service, and the collaborators referred to the compound as 1162F in his honor, Fourneau declined to include his name as co-author. Bovet surmised that his chief did so either to advance the careers of his younger colleagues or as a gesture of respect to Hörlein and the Elberfeld scientific staff whose prestige might be damaged by the publication. Because notes in the *Comptes Rendus* were held to strict limits of length, the Pasteur Institute team, facing a week's delay in publication, withheld from the text the protocol of their initial experimental finding. Most striking, in light of Bovet's later narrative of events, is the rational reconstruction that the note imposes on the discovery. The note first reports that the Pasteur Institute team had found that derivatives of Prontosil differing in their physical and chemical properties had an analogous antistreptococcal power. It then continues,

> in order for such different compounds to act in an almost identical manner, is it not because they undergo in the organism a series of modifications of which the first result will be the cutting of the double bond with formation of aminophenylsulfonamide? This hypothesis led us to study the activity of the hydrochloride of P-aminophenylsulfonamide or 1162F.

In the published note, therefore, the chance conjunction of an extra set of mice and Bovet's casual, impromptu decision to try the intermediate that stood before him on the table is effaced in favor of an experiment proceeding from prior reasoning and a clearly framed hypothesis.[16]

Assuming that Bovet's later reconstruction was accurate, why did the Pasteur Institute team represent their discovery in 1935 in a way that diverged from the actual sequence of events? A clue may be found in Bovet's remark that once PABS's activity was confirmed, its role as common source of the activity of a variety of azo dyes seemed obvious. So obvious, we may surmise, that retrospective explanation was easily converted into prior hypothesis when the time came to present the discovery to the medical and scientific communities. The *Comptes Rendus* note of November 1935 appears to be a case not of willful misrepresentation but of the priority frequently ceded to logical order over historical reconstruction in scientific publications.[17]

The November 1935 note's masking of the element of chance involved in the discovery of PABS's activity, and the representation of the discovery in hypotheticodeductive terms, may help to account for later speculations such as those of bacteriologist Ronald Hare that attributed a similar discovery to the Elberfeld group. If the reasoning was so clear to the French, so the argument would go, it must have been equally clear to the Germans, who suppressed it only to protect their profits from Prontosil. Bovet's revelation that the reasoning was not obvious to the Pasteur Institute team until after it had made its chance discovery thus undermines the Hare thesis and provides additional reason to suppose that the Elberfeld team had not come to the same conclusions independently.[18]

Given the importance attached to their discovery by the Pasteur Institute team, and the role that it did eventually have as starting point for a new generation of sulfa drugs, the reception of the discovery in France is surprising and at first sight, baffling. Within the Pasteur Institute itself, response to the discovery outside of Fourneau's own service ranged from indifference to hostility. No other head of service expressed curiosity or desired a part in the follow-up research. What was worse, the finding appears to have created displeasure on the part of the institute's directors. In a letter of March 23, 1936, to director Louis Martin, Fourneau wondered what the institute expected from his laboratory and whether the council clearly perceived the importance of chemotherapy:

It appears that you are very unhappy with what has just happened for antistreptococcal products, but I admit that I do not understand at all the
reasons for your unhappiness. We can only be very proud to confirm that
in a domain where the Germans are past masters, in which they dispose
of a considerable number of workers and of raw materials in, so to speak
infinite quantities, the French have been able to create for themselves a
personal place.[19]

Two reasons may be suggested for this unfriendly reception. One has to do
with the threat posed by PABS, and by bacterial chemotherapy generally, for
older biological products on which the Pasteur Institute relied for a part of its financial support. Since the time of Pasteur the institute had derived prestige and
income from the development and manufacture of vaccines and serums. By early
1936, Prontosil/Rubiazol had already begun to render antistreptococcal serums
obsolete, and the prospect that other serums, for meningococcal and pneumococcal infections, dysentery, and plague, would suffer similar fates was clearly dis-
cernible. Bovet recalled that he and Jacques Tréfouël had jokingly accused
themselves of cutting off the branch on which they sat. It is unlikely that the institute's executives found the idea so amusing. Competition for resources within the
institute may have been another ground for the cool response of the other services. Fourneau pushed for an expansion of his unit in light of the increased importance of the chemotherapy of infectious disease. His requests were finally
approved by the institute council in November 1938, three years after the PABS
discovery, possibly over the resistance of other researchers who resented the already well-supported section of therapeutic chemistry.[20]

Meanwhile, PABS fared no better in the hands of French manufacturers.
Rhône-Poulenc, which might have been expected to move 1162F quickly to clinical trials and to market, instead sought a closely related derivative that could be
patented. The result was the synthesis in early 1936 by Rhône-Poulenc chemists
of *n*-benzylsulfonamide. After bacteriological and toxicological tests by company
employees Mayer and Halpern and clinical trials by H. Bloch-Michel, M. Conte,
and P. Durel, the new compound was marketed in March 1936 by the *Société
parisienne d'expansion chimique* (Spécia) under the trade name Septazine. Bovet
and his colleagues were not impressed. Septazine was almost entirely insoluble—
a "plaster," in Bovet's and Nitti's terms—and was only moderately effective in
Pasteur Institute animal trials; it had no demonstrated clinical advantage over
PABS. PABS was kept off the French market until the spring of 1937, well after it
had been made available to doctors and patients in Germany and Britain in 1936,
and even after its introduction in the United States earlier in 1937. Bovet could
only conclude that Rhône-Poulenc and Spécia did not want competition for their
specialty in the French market.[21]

Finally, in March 1937, F. Albert-Buisson, the new managing director of
Rhône-Poulenc, visited Fourneau's unit and was persuaded of the importance of
PABS. In May 1937, eighteen months after discovery of its therapeutic action at
the Pasteur Institute, 1162F (by now called sulfanilamide in the United States)
went on the French market under the trade name Septaplix, manufactured by the

new pharmaceutical company Théraplix, created by Albert-Buisson and Rhône-Poulenc. It was an immediate success.[22]

The same month witnessed the opening of the *Exposition internationales des arts et des techniques* in Paris. The exposition's displays illustrating the material progress of civilization were housed in a new *Palais de la découverte* (Palace of Discovery) exhibition. Among the booths was one devoted to therapeutic chemistry, in the care of Fourneau, Lecomte de Noüy, and Jacques Tréfouël. Bovet recalled with pride that here "for the first time in history," the most recent results with "synthetic bactericides," the sulfonamides, were presented on large panels alongside the more familiar research on antiparasitic medicines. Jean Perrin, who had conceived the idea for the *Palais de la découverte*, wrote after its opening that in spite of wars, economic crisis, and other troubles,

> the development of civilization becomes more and more rapid, thanks to techniques that are ever more supple and effective, in domains more and more extensive. The exposition . . . expresses our legitimate pride in the material progress that we owe to [those techniques]. Almost all have appeared in the last century, developing or applying inventions . . . which seem to have realized or surpassed the desires expressed in our old fairy tales.

Thirty-seven million people attended the exposition, of whom 2,250,000 entered the *Palais de la découverte*. On the last day, November 25, the organizers awarded a large number of prizes, including a gold medal to Domagk. Bovet recalled that when Perrin spoke of "the domination of matter," and of "the techniques already victorious over smallpox, diphtheria, typhus, and perhaps soon all diseases," he and his colleagues in Fourneau's service almost imagined that Perrin was speaking for them. Perhaps they also shared Perrin's sense that "suddenly, by a sort of glory, we have entered into a new age."[23]

"Something Which May Save a Human Life"

The new age was also arriving across the English Channel, but at a more deliberate pace. On March 18, 1935, Henry H. Dale, the director of Britain's National Institute for Medical Research in London, wrote to F.H.K. Green, secretary of the Medical Research Council's Therapeutic Trials Committee (TTC) regarding Prontosil. Dale informed Green that Leonard Colebrook, a London physician well known to both of them, was interested in trying the new preparation, that Dale had written to Hörlein to request a supply, and that Hörlein had readily agreed to provide one through Bayer's London office. Colebrook wrote separately to Green the next day reporting his communication with Dale and expressing his willingness to undertake "some preliminary investigations" if the TTC wished him to do so.[24]

The immediate occasion of this exchange was Domagk's publication of the previous month. Dale had long been aware of the existence of Prontosil, however, and indeed may have been the first non-German medical researcher to learn of it.

Over two years earlier, in January 1933, Dale had given a lecture to the Medical Academy of Düsseldorf. Dale's invitation to speak had come in part from Werner Schulemann, a medical doctor and chemist of the Elberfeld research establishment, and among Dale's audience were other I.G. Farben staff from Elberfeld and Leverkusen. After speaking on January 9, Dale stopped in Elberfeld the next day on his way back to London, met the research staff, and visited the laboratories. Late in his life, Dale recalled few details of the visit, with one exception: his encounter with Domagk. Dale had the impression that Domagk's colleagues, "whom I was primarily visiting, had not yet taken him quite seriously." Dale remembered that "they said to me, in effect, that they thought it would be rather kind of me if I would say how d'you do to *Kollege* Domagk, who had rather a bee in his bonnet about a discovery he thought he had made, of a chemotherapeutic agent for bacterial infections." Dale obliged his hosts, visited Domagk, "and found him, at the time, an almost painfully modest and apologetic personality." At the time Domagk seemed hesitant about his results and had no immediate intention to publish. Dale was puzzled by this reticence in the face of what appeared to be straightforward evidence, but ascribed it to the skepticism then widespread among bacteriologists regarding the possibilities of bacterial chemotherapy, and felt obliged not to speak of Domagk's findings pending publication.[25]

Dale's brief encounter with Domagk in 1933 may have made him more receptive to news of Prontosil, and he later claimed that it was at his initiative that Colebrook was induced to test the new drug. Dale also later asserted that Colebrook, as a loyal follower of Almroth Wright's doctrine that bacterial chemotherapy would prove impossible, had at first resisted the idea of testing Prontosil. Neither claim has been verified from contemporary correspondence. What is certain is that Colebrook viewed the German publications of February 1935 as "from the scientific point of view . . . quite inadequate to justify a large scale human experiment" and that he therefore intended first to carry out *in vitro* and animal tests. On March 20, Green replied to Colebrook on behalf of the TTC, promising to bring the matter before the committee as soon as a formal application had been received from Bayer Products, and responding sympathetically to Colebrook's request to be the only British physician to test Prontosil through the TTC for the time being.[26]

In turning to the TTC, Dale and Colebrook were following what had become, by the mid-1930s, standard procedure for the testing of new drugs in Britain. Established in 1931 at the urging of the Association of British Chemical Manufacturers, the TTC was the Medical Research Council's response to a situation in which the need of the British pharmaceutical industry for clinical tests of new preparations was thwarted by the fears of physicians that any association with industry, but especially subsidized clinical trials, would compromise their reputations for scientific impartiality. Commercial or academic laboratories submitted new medicines to the TTC along with information on chemical composition and animal tests that supported the requests for clinical trials. The TTC then made arrangements with one or, usually, more than one clinician to carry out the tests. The TTC reviewed clinicians' evidence and conclusions. If results were negative, the committee returned a report to the manufacturer, usually without publication.

If favorable, the report was published in the medical press under the clinician's name as "Report to the Medical Research Council's Therapeutic Trails Committee." Green, the TTC's secretary, was on the permanent staff of the Medical Research Council, and its membership included distinguished representatives of the medical and medical research communities. Dale himself served as first chair, and later as member. Between 1931 and the beginning of the war in 1939, several important drugs entered medical practice through reports to the TTC, including in addition to Prontosil and sulfanilamide, calciferol for rickets, digoxin for auricular fibrillation, and stilbestrol for menstrual disorders. The success of the TTC in legitimizing clinical trials of commercial preparations contributed to its demise during the war. Doctors and pharmaceutical companies were now better able to make arrangements with one another directly, and physicians could publish on their own responsibility without need for a TTC stamp of approval.[27]

On April 1, 1935, George H. Morrison, of Bayer Products in London, wrote to Green expressing the company's wish to submit Prontosil to the TTC for trial. Green replied on April 3, encouraging the submission and asking for details on Prontosil. Bayer Products was slow to respond but, after further prompting by Green, sent a four-page summary of information on chemistry, animal experiments, pharmacology, toxicity, mode of administration, dosage, and the results of German animal trials on Prontosil. In early May, Green wrote to T.R. Elliott, a professor at University College Hospital Medical School in London and chair of the TTC, to ask if the committee would accept Prontosil and its sister compound, still called Streptozon S, for trials. Elliott readily agreed, noting that he was aware of the papers published by Domagk and others in the *Deutsche Medizinische Wochenschrift* in February and that "the work in Germany is not a sudden sky rocket but has been burning steadily for some time." Elliott was only irritated by Colebrook's request to restrict the first trials to his own unit at Queen Charlotte's Hospital and insisted that this limitation to a single investigator not become a precedent for the TTC. After more consultation with Colebrook, Green wrote to Bayer Products on May 11 to inform them that Prontosil and Streptozon S had been approved for trial and requesting 500 tablets of Prontosil and 500 cc of Steptozon S. Colebrook thought that these quantities would be enough for experimental work and treatment of twenty or thirty cases.[28]

Supplies were slow in reaching Colebrook. On May 13, Bayer Products reported a "hitch" in obtaining the needed quantities, and the rest of May, June, and early July passed with no delivery. In the meantime, other physicians approached the TTC to request Prontosil for clinical trials. One of these was C.H. Browning of the Pathology Department at Glasgow University, who had a long-standing interest in chemotherapy and whose work was supported by another committee of the Medical Research Council. Inexplicably, Bayer Products was able to supply Browning, with the TTC's permission, in mid-June, while Colebrook continued to wait. Other physicians were informed by Green that the TTC could not supply them with Prontosil while preliminary trials were in progress but that they could approach Bayer Products directly (and without TTC sanction) for samples if they wished. Finally, on July 18, after prompting by Green, Bayer Products sent Colebrook supplies of Prontosil and Streptozon S, although not quite in the quantities he had requested.[29]

Colebrook began animal trials of Prontosil in July, and these continued quietly through August and September. In the meantime, Bayer Products sent Green a five-page letter clarifying the forms and dosages in which Prontosil and Streptozon S would be supplied. This letter emphasized that the company intended henceforth to supply Prontosil only in tablet form, and that Streptozon S (later called Prontosil Soluble) in 2.5 percent solution would be the sole liquid form for injection. A postscript to the same letter revealed that by August 15 Bayer Products had sent supplies of Prontosil or Streptozon S to at least three British physicians in addition to Colebrook and Browning. Green continued to receive inquiries from individual doctors, either directly or through Bayer Products. These, and Green's response to them, make it clear both that Green was willing to approve limited usage of the new medicines outside the framework of the TTC investigation and that Bayer Products was committed to work through the TTC in spite of the delays in marketing this entailed.[30]

On October 3, 1935, Hörlein delivered a lecture titled "The Chemotherapy of Infectious Diseases Caused by Protozoa and Bacteria" at the Royal Society of Medicine in London. Addressed to the society's section of tropical diseases and parasitology, the lecture drew a contrast between the many successes of the chemotherapy of protozoal diseases and the relative failure of bacterial chemotherapy. Hörlein attributed the difference to the more highly differentiated structure of protozoan parasites, which offered more points of attack to chemotherapeutic agents. He devoted more than half the lecture to the piroplasmoses, infectious diseases caused by protozoa of various species afflicting large numbers of domestic animals that brought serious economic losses in tropical, subtropical, and temperate zones. Hörlein claimed that a new compound, developed by I.G. Farben and recently introduced under the trade name Acaprin, was clearly superior to medicines used previously against piroplasmoses, including trypan blue and trypaflavine. More surprising for his audience, given the contrast with which he began, was his description of Prontosil and Prontosil Soluble, the latter identical to what the TTC was testing as Streptozon S. Hörlein recounted Domagk's, Mietzsch's, and Klarer's early finding that Prontosil and other azo compounds containing sulfonamide were effective against streptococcal infections in mice. Drawing heavily on the February 1935 publications by Domagk and others in the German medical press, he described the results of animal experiments, and the pathological, toxicological, and clinical findings on the new compounds. Hörlein concluded that "a breach had been created in the ramparts of bacterial diseases."[31]

In the discussion that followed Hörlein's talk, it came out that G.A.H. Buttle, a medical doctor working at the Wellcome Research Laboratories, had been conducting his own tests of Prontosil on experimental infections in mice. Whereas Domagk had seen all his test mice recover, Buttle, using different strains of streptococci, had succeeded only in delaying the death of his animals. Buttle acknowledged that the divergence of results might be grounded in differences of laboratory technique, and he thought he had confirmed that Prontosil had at least some degree of therapeutic activity. In response to a question from L.P. Garrod, Hörlein emphasized that the limits of the clinical value of Prontosil would have to be established by more investigation and practice. Despite these notes of hesitation, the section president, P.H. Manson-Bahr, "voiced the impression of all present that a contribution to chemotherapeutics had been made by Professor Hörlein and his co-workers which might indeed prove to be monumental."[32]

Whatever the ultimate import of his message, Hörlein's talk sparked immediate interest among British physicians who heard of it directly or indirectly. One of the first reactions came from A.H. Douthwaite, a Harley Street doctor who wrote to the TTC the next day asking for a supply of Prontosil to treat cases of arthritis associated with streptococcal infections. As he usually did in response to similar inquiries, Green replied granting the TTC's permission for Douthwaite to obtain Prontosil directly from Bayer Products for use in his own cases. The response to Hörlein's talk evidently prompted a sense of urgency, for on October 17 Green wrote to Colebrook mentioning the requests from clinicians and remarking that "I should be glad to learn as soon as possible about the results of your test of Prontosil and Streptozon S."[33]

Colebrook, not yet convinced of the monumentality of Hörlein's revelations, replied with a bucket of cold water. "Up to date my experiments with mice give no support whatever to German claims," he wrote, "and since their clinical reports seem to me to be quite worthless I have not felt justified in giving it to patients." He was given pause, he said, only by talk with a man at Wellcome (Buttle was meant) who had observed some prolongation of life in infected mice treated with Prontosil. Although these results did not fully support German claims, Colebrook remarked, they were suggestive enough to justify a few more tests. Colebrook advised Green that "I think you will do nothing but good by checking the optimism and hopefulness of inquiries meanwhile." Green obliged, and his replies to doctors during the balance of October and until late November included a warning that TTC experimental tests had so far failed to confirm published claims by German investigators. Skepticism was reinforced by Browning's report from Glasgow October 28 that his mice trials had so far failed to show any high therapeutic efficacy for Prontosil. In what may have been the nadir of Prontosil's reception in Britain, Green wrote to Dale within a month after Hörlein's Royal Society of Medicine talk that "I think it is rather unlikely that the Committee will decide to arrange for any large-scale trials of this substance."[34]

If Colebrook would not be stampeded, neither would he succumb to a pessimism reinforced by past failures. In mid-November, he wrote to Green apologizing for the delay in his report but making it clear that he intended to push on to definite conclusions. A week later, he visited Green with the news that his recent experiments were more encouraging than those he had done earlier. Colebrook now felt that Prontosil had some protective power against streptococcal infections, was of very low toxicity to animals, and appeared to increase the organism's resistance to infection. He was now prepared, with the approval of the TTC and of the Medical Committee of Queen Charlotte's Hospital, to move ahead to trials in patients. When Green informed him that Elliott of University College Hospital was interested in trying Prontosil in cases of infective arthritis, Colebrook responded that there was an a priori case for doing so as "a shot in the dark." Acting with his customary efficiency, Green telephoned both Elliott and

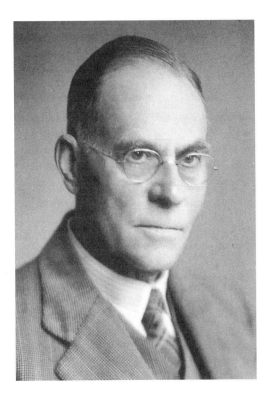

Figure 6.5. Leonard Colebrook
(1883–1967) in 1946 (© The Godfrey Argent Studio, reprinted with
permission).

Bayer Products the same day, arranging for Elliott to receive supplies of Prontosil
and Streptozon S.[35]

Colebrook's slightly more optimistic view is reflected in Green's responses
to continuing inquiries about Prontosil from practicing physicians through late
November, December, and January. Caution still prevailed, but phrases such as
"so far failed to confirm" German claims or "almost entirely discouraging" were
replaced by "laboratory tests of [Prontosil's] action are at present being made . . .
in an attempt to confirm the German claims for its efficacy." As weeks passed with
no firm results, however, Green became uneasy. In early January 1936, he wrote
to both Browning and Colebrook asking about the status of their tests with Prontosil. Both replied that there was still no clear basis for its clinical use. A shortage
of suitable cases at Queen Charlotte's Hospital had prevented Colebrook from
undertaking even a handful of clinical trials. Colebrook's mouse experiments had
shown some effect of Prontosil against highly virulent strains of streptococci in
mice but little or no effect against strains isolated from human infections. "It
seems to me, therefore," Colebrook wrote to Green, "unlikely that we shall get
any good results in human cases, but since its mode of action is quite obscure,
there is a possibility, and I am going to try it, but I am afraid it will take several
months before one can formulate any opinion owing to the high spontaneous recovery rate in these cases."[36]

By early February, Colebrook had no more than six patients under treatment
with Prontosil, and Green was seeking ways to expand the clinical trials. In a let-

ter to Dale he proposed asking W.R. Snodgrass, a Glasgow physician in charge of
400 hospital beds, to undertake clinical tests of Prontosil in streptococcol infections other than puerperal fever, in particular, chronic infections associated with
arthritis. Dale endorsed the idea and warned of new pressures on the TTC:

> The position as I see it is that some enthusiasm, carefully stoked by the
> I.G. [Farben], is beginning to glow in the German literature on this sub-
> stance, and that, if we keep it hanging too long without some definite re-
> port for or against it, there is danger of a clamour from medical men in
> England, that they cannot get hold of this wonder-working remedy, be-
> cause the M.R.C. are holding it back.

Dale cautioned that "that is a danger which we always have to watch, when taking
on the investigation of something which is already supposed to have good continental credentials." The TTC should not rush to judgment, Dale concluded, but
should expand its clinical trials of Prontosil.[37]

Dale's warning was timely. On February 1, the first notice of Prontosil appeared in *Lancet*. The single unsigned paragraph described the claims of German investigators, their so far only partial confirmation by British researchers,
and the recent more favorable findings of Levaditi and Vaisman in France. Noting that Prontosil's mode of action remained obscure, the author underlined the
need for more clinical studies. Despite its sober tone, this notice held out to
hard-pressed physicians the possibility of a drug treatment for streptococcal infections. The message was taken up and amplified the same month when Hörlein's talk of the previous October was printed in the *Proceedings of the Royal
Society of Medicine*.[38]

On February 24, T.W.P. Thompson of Bayer Products wrote to Green to ask
about the status of the TTC report on Prontosil. Thompson remarked that since
publication of the *Lancet* note and of Hörlein's talk, the company had received
many inquiries. He added that those doctors who already had been supplied with
Prontosil by permission of the TTC had "rather extraordinary ideas" about its indications, which he attributed to lack of authoritative information in the British
medical press. The onus for this state of affairs, Thompson implied, was on the
TTC. Green responded with a telephone call to Colebrook, who informed him
that the clinical results were good so far and that he would send Green an abstract
of his results by February 28 and a more detailed report the following week.
Green also called Thompson to arrange to meet later when he had Colebrook's results in hand.[39]

Colebrook's five-page report summarized his findings on trials with thirty-
four mice and seven human cases. Results were mixed for both mice and people
but gave enough indication of the positive action of Prontosil to warrant its continued testing and even its routine use in all but the mildest cases "until we have
enough data to allow a critical comparison with untreated cases." Although the
numbers were small, they also sufficed to alter Colebrook's outlook on the now
not so new medicine. In his covering letter to Green, he remarked that "it seems
as if we may be at the beginning of an important new chapter in chemotherapy."
He also suggested that "in view of the very scrappy data given by German and

French papers," it might be desirable to publish a short paper after a few more human cases and animal experiments had been accumulated. Colebrook's findings were taken into account by the TTC in its meeting of February 28, 1936, and used to justify expansion of clinical trails to other sites and kinds of streptococcal infections.[40]

If the TTC was picking up its pace, the activity was not visible to the outside world. Dale's prediction of a "clamour" from British physicians may have seemed about to come true in early March when Green received a letter from F.W. Eurich, a consulting physician to the Royal Infirmary in Bradford. Eurich said he often had cases of streptococcal sepsis to treat, had heard Hörlein's Royal Society of Medicine talk, and read reports on Prontosil in the German medical press. Bayer Products was prepared to supply him, he said, but only with TTC permission. Eurich's frustration was plain. "It is, I confess, very galling to feel that there is something which may save a human life when everything else fails and to find impediments to a speedy application of what may be a remedy."[41] How much of Eurich's frustration was shared by other physicians who politely applied to the TTC, or by those who held back from even this step, is unknown. What is clear is that the TTC now adopted a change in policy. On March 7, Green met with Thompson of Bayer Products and brought him up-to-date on Colebrook's work and on TTC plans to extend clinical trials. Green informed Thompson that, in view of the large numbers of inquiries about Prontosil now coming in from physicians, it would be in order for Bayer to respond directly, without consulting the TTC. For his part, Thompson undertook to supply British physicians with Prontosil at a nominal charge on condition that they did not publish their results until the TTC's investigation was completed.[42]

In March and April, the TTC pushed ahead with efforts to expand clinical trials of Prontosil and Prontosil Soluble to conditions other than puerperal fever and to investigators other than Colebrook. Green wrote to Browning in Edinburgh asking him to assist Snodgrass in his trials of Prontosil in cases of arthritis thought to be related to streptococcal infections. Green also arranged with Bayer Products to send supplies of both medicines to A.W.M. Ellis of London Hospital, who would test them in selected cases of arthritis, and to Sir David Wilkie of the Department of Surgery of the University of Edinburgh, who would try them in acute hemolytic streptococcal infections encountered in surgery. Another member of the TTC, Edward Mellanby, called upon J.H. Brincker of the London County Council to arrange for clinical trails of the Prontosils in cases of scarlet fever and measles, on the idea that their use might prevent middle ear infections and bronchopneumonia in these diseases. Brincker obliged, making possible tests in at least two fever hospitals under direction of the council. None of these investigators returned substantial findings before June 1936, although a preliminary report from one of the London County Hospital studies concluded that Prontosil had no marked effect on scarlet fever except to reduce complications.[43]

Meanwhile, Bayer Products responded with alacrity to the TTC's requests for supplies and on March 16 submitted a formal four-page application to the committee on behalf of Prontosil and Streptozon S. Thompson informed Green on April 3 that the company was "receiving enquiries about Prontosil from a great many doctors and hospitals." He recommended that the TTC arrange with medical journals not to publish on Prontosil in advance of the TTC's report, fearing that "unless some such precaution is taken, it is not unlikely that some enthusiastic user may publish his experiences with this new preparation." Green took the advice and telephoned *Lancet* and *British Medical Journal* the next morning to make the arrangements.[44]

The extension of clinical trials and increasing interest in Prontosil in the British medical community were welcome to Bayer Products but also found the company unprepared in at least one respect. Thompson admitted to Green in late March that Bayer had only German packaging for Prontosil, and in early April the company was not able to respond immediately to a request for English translations of German medical reports on Prontosil. By April 21, Thompson had in hand a seven-page leaflet on Prontosil and Prontosil Soluble (the name Streptozon S had been dropped by this time), which he described as "the only printed literature available in English." The leaflet, prepared at Elberfeld, echoed claims made for the medicines in the German medical press and was therefore considerably more positive than the TTC was prepared to be at the time, and about a wider range of infections.[45]

The *Lancet* publications in February and the increasing interest in Prontosil among British physicians, some of whom were beginning to use the new medicine, placed added pressure on Colebrook and the TTC to produce an official report. Not only was there a danger, as the months passed, that a freelance investigator would preempt the TTC report by publishing independently, but there was also the hazard, as Thompson worried, that physicians lacking official guidance would misuse Prontosil. Finally, as Dale warned, there was a danger that the TTC would be perceived by the British medical community as actually blocking the introduction of a new and useful drug.

On April 7, Colebrook informed Green that he was starting to write a short paper on Prontosil but that he would have to be guarded about its therapeutic value. On May 15, Colebrook hand delivered the typescript to Green, telling him that he had arranged for publication in *Lancet* if the committee approved the report. Mellanby and A.J. Clark (also a member of the TTC) read and approved the manuscript the same afternoon. The same day, Green received a call from the *Lancet* editorial offices with the news that Colebrook's paper would be published at the earliest possible date and that *Lancet* had also received a paper from Wellcome Laboratories "on chemotherapeutic tests of substances related to Prontosil." Would the TTC object to publishing the two papers together? The Wellcome paper, by Buttle and his colleagues, was known to Colebrook, who had supplied Buttle with streptococcal cultures. Green readily agreed to simultaneous publication. Finally, Thompson of Bayer Products came by to read Colebrook's paper and declared himself pleased. Green informed Thompson, on Mellanby's authority, that "as the publication of Colebrook's report would doubtless lead to a great demand for *Prontosil* from practicing physicians . . . the firm would be at liberty, so far as we were concerned, to put *Prontosil* on the market on an ordinary commercial basis once the report had appeared."[46]

At least two other TTC members, Dale and Elliott, read the report before it was formally approved for publication on May 26. Dale read the manuscript "with very great interest" and was troubled only with what he perceived to be an insufficiently clear distinction between Prontosil and Prontosil Soluble. Elliott approved publication but found the manuscript not well written and unlikely to "do much more than to incite some other investigators to try the substance." Elliott's reservations evidently were not shared by the rest of the committee. Green wrote to Colebrook on May 26, assuring him that "we look forward keenly to publication of the report, and anticipate that the results will create something of a stir." Co-authored with Meave Kenny, Colebrook's colleague at Queen Charlotte's Hospital, the paper appeared on June 6 under the title "Treatment of human puerperal infections, and of experimental infections in mice, with Prontosil." It was further described as "a preliminary report to the Therapeutic Trials Committee of the Medical Research Council."[47]

Colebrook and Kenny began their long-awaited report by recalling the striking results reported in Domagk's first paper. Domagk's single animal experiment had not been followed up by other reports of animal trials in the German literature, they pointed out. Moreover, animal trials carried out in France by Levaditi and Vaisman and by Bovet and Nitti had demonstrated curative effects of Prontosil that varied depending on the culture used and that were not consistently as strong as those reported by Domagk. German reports of clinical use of Prontosil in puerperal fever, erysipelas, and other conditions were uniformly favorable, the authors noted. Unfortunately, Colebrook and Kenny asserted, "their evidential value must be regarded as small," since the German authors did not sufficiently allow for the tendency to spontaneous cure of the infections in question, and since the bacteriological and clinical data supplied were nearly always "scanty." For example, the German literature did not always specify whether all the cases studied were infected by hemolytic streptococci, whether cocci were present in the blood before treatment, or whether in the cases studied a clinical condition such as peritonitis was present or not. Colebrook and Kenny conceded that the German clinical reports had shown Prontosil to be well tolerated by humans and had established effective dosage levels. To go beyond this, they felt, new animal and human trials were needed.[48]

In the initial trials carried out at Queen Charlotte's Hospital, Colebrook and Kenny infected mice with strains of streptococci freshly isolated from human puerperal infections. They injected cultures previously known to be 10–100 times the minimum lethal dose into the peritoneum, and then after one and one-half to two hours administered a single dose of Prontosil or Prontosil Soluble by stomach tube or subcutaneous injection. In some trials, they gave a series of doses at one and one-half, five, twenty-four, forty-eight, seventy-two, and so forth, hours after infection. Although they varied the dosage and used six different strains of streptococci, the results were uniformly disappointing. Some treated animals survived longer than untreated controls, but there were very few survivals, and "the experiments were regarded as negative, failing to confirm Domagk's claim."[49]

Colebrook had learned from Buttle of Wellcome Laboratories, whom he had previously supplied with a streptococcal strain isolated from a case of puerperal fever, that Buttle had had better success with this strain modified by passage through a series of twenty-three mice. The passage had sharply increased the virulence of this strain, called "Williams," for mice and had at the same time made mice infected with it more susceptible to treatment by Prontosil. Taking a cue from Buttle's work, Colebrook and Kenny had created their own highly virulent passage strain, called "Richards," and "with this strain we began at once to get striking curative results in mice." They displayed results of the "Richards" strain trials for thirty-five mice, an unspecified fraction of the total number studied, in two tables indicating quantities of cultures administered, size and intervals of dosages of Prontosil Soluble given, numbers of untreated controls, and numbers of deaths in each successive twenty-four-hour period after infection. The authors commented that the results "seem to indicate quite clearly that the administration of the drug does exert some curative effect upon infections by those hemolytic streptococci in the mouse, which normally terminate in peritonitis and septicemia."[50]

Colebrook and Kenny extended the animal phase of the investigation in three directions. To test the prophylactic action of Prontosil, they injected 50 mg of the medicine subcutaneously in mice, and then after four days infected the mice with streptococcal culture. The results, presented in a third table, indicated some protective action by Prontosil. Responding to the Pasteur Institute team's discovery of the efficacy of PABS, they tested this compound (supplied by chemist Harold King of the National Institute of Medical Research) in mice infected with the "Richards" streptococcal strain, with positive results displayed in a fourth table. Finally, the authors raised the question "upon what does the antistreptococcal influence of Prontosil depend?" Laboratory tests of serum, whole blood, and leukocytes from infected animals yielded no positive answers to this question. Colebrook and Kenny considered a number of possibilities but could only conclude with the negative finding that "at present it appears very unlikely that the cocci are actually destroyed, either by the drug itself or by some compound formed from it in the animal body."[51]

Surveying the results of animal trials, Colebrook and Kenny found that they gave at best ambiguous support to the idea that Prontosil might be effective against infections in humans. The results had been positive but had become so only after modification of the streptococcal strain away from its condition in the human subject. Nevertheless, since the import of high mouse virulence was unclear, and the German clinical reports on Prontosil uniformly favorable, Colebrook had decided to undertake treatment of a group of puerperal fever cases. All were patients in the isolation block of Queen Charlotte's Hospital. The fifth table of the article summarized the treatment record for thirty-eight patients, including age, pathological condition, blood culture (positive or negative), day of puerperium (since childbirth), Prontosil dosage in grams (by injection, orally, and total), number of days administered, result (recovery or death), and remarks. At first, Colebrook and Kenny had treated only the most severe cases, comprising ten of those included in the table. For the past several weeks, however, they had treated every case of infection with hemolytic streptococci, adding twenty-eight to the table. With the exception of two individuals, none of these patients had received any medication other than Prontosil or Prontosil Soluble. Colebrook and Kenny had followed the example of recent German authors and had given relatively large doses, at first 20 cc of a 2.5 percent solution of Prontosil Soluble (0.5 grams) injected intravenously or intramuscularly and six 0.3 g Prontosil tablets by mouth per day. Later they increased the amount given by injection for some patients to 40 cc, 60 cc, or 90 cc per day. Observing the sometimes severe malaise and nausea occasioned by intravenous injections, they decided to restrict this mode of administration to the first dose.[52]

Colebrook and Kenny began their evaluation of the clinical trial by throwing out forty-five percent of the data, or seventeen cases (cases 17–33 of the table). This was done, they explained, because "all of them would, in all probability, have recovered without the treatment—and perhaps as quickly." In general, they pointed out, it was extremely difficult to interpret signs and symptoms in puerperal infections caused by hemolytic streptococci: "at every point it is a matter of fine judgment, instructed by long experience." Of the remaining twenty-one cases, sixteen, or forty-two percent (cases 1–16 of the table) of the total, did appear to provide useful information. All presented serious symptoms of septic infection. For Colebrook and Kenny, all were cases that, "in the light of our previous experience over several years, surprised us by the prompt clinical improvement and remission of fever following the first few doses of Prontosil."[53] Three of these, cases 10, 14, and 16, the authors found to be "of specially great evidential value." In all three, the authors believed that the infection had spread to the abdominal as well as the pelvic peritoneal cavity, and in case 14 they found streptococci in the bloodstream, an especially serious sign. After beginning treatment with large doses of Prontosil and Prontosil Soluble, the physicians observed rapid improvement in all three cases. Given Colebrook's long experience with puerperal fever and relentlessly sober, cautious, and critical view of therapeutics, the language of the entries in table 5 is instructive. For case 10: "General peritonitis . . . Desperately ill. After massive doses of Prontosil signs of peritonitis rapidly abated. A very striking result." For case 14: "Early generalizing peritonitis with septicemia . . . Very ill on admission; T. 104°, P. 140, rising; diarrhea. Spectacular remission of symptoms and signs within 24 hours. Steady improvement followed." And for case 16: "Acute generalising peritonitis . . . Ill nourished woman, very ill. Spectacular and rapid abatement of signs of peritonitis." Considering the seriousness of their condition and that all three women were older than thirty, Colebrook and Kenny thought it very unlikely that any of them would have made a spontaneous recovery.[54]

The last five cases of the group of thirty-eight were more problematic. For the two of those who recovered, Colebrook and Kenny suspected that Prontosil may have hindered rather than assisted the recovery. The remaining three, the only deaths of the series, all presented with very severe preexisting infections. In one case, and possibly in a second one, the infections were complicated by thrombophlebitis. In two of the fatal cases, the physicians did not administer the heavy doses that were apparently successful in cases 10, 14, and 16, leaving some doubt as to what the result might have been if that measure had been taken. The last patient died in spite of massive doses of the medicines.[55]

Three deaths in thirty-eight cases yielded a mortality of eight percent, a figure that Colebrook and Kenny found to compare favorably with that for the thirty-eight cases preceding these (23.7 percent), and the average rate for the years 1931–1934 (twenty-two percent). While they felt bound to caution that such a small series of cases could not predict future results, Colebrook and Kenny were persuaded that "the very low death-rate, taken together with the spectacular remission of fever and symptoms observed in so many of the cases, does suggest that the drug has exerted a beneficial effect." They found that these benefits came at minimal cost in toxic or other untoward effects. Among these were faintness and nausea following intravenous injection, a reddish or terra cotta coloring of the skin with heavy dosages, mild irritation of the urinary tract, and most curiously, cyanosis associated with sulfahemoglobinemia in a few cases. They concluded that "the clinical results, together with the mouse protection experiments, support the view that further clinical trial is amply justified, and that there is more hope of controlling these streptococcal infections by the early administration of this or some related chemotherapeutic agent than by any other means at present available."[56]

Comparison of the Colebrook and Kenny paper with early German clinical reports on Prontosil that accompanied or followed Domagk's first publication reveals both similarities and differences. Like the German authors, the British physicians gave close attention to the particulars of individual cases. Like them, too, their initial skepticism was at least partially overcome by striking positive results in a few cases. Like the German doctors, Colebrook and Kenny saw difficulties in distinguishing the effects of Prontosil from those of the body's own healing powers or of other therapeutic measures but nevertheless were prepared to be guardedly optimistic about the new medicine's prospects. What set their paper apart from the German work was the systematic gathering, organization, and presentation of data. Without losing sight of the particularity of each case, Colebrook and Kenny created a standardized format, best exemplified in table 5, that greatly facilitated comparison and analysis. Years of experience with puerperal fever under comparable conditions allowed the British doctors to speak with confidence, and with some precision, about mortality rates before and after Prontosil. Finally, Colebrook and Kenny, unlike the German clinical writers on Prontosil but like the Pasteur Institute team, had made a serious effort to replicate Domagk's animal trials of Prontosil, with mixed results that added a further note of caution to their conclusion.

Animal trials also figured prominently in the paper by Buttle, W.H. Gray, and Dora Stephenson that immediately followed Colebrook and Kenny's article in the June 6 issue of *Lancet* and that explored the action of PABS (later called sulfanilamide) on streptococcal and other types of infection. The work was done at the Wellcome Physiological Research Laboratories in Beckenham, Kent, and at the Wellcome Chemical Laboratories in London. Buttle and his co-authors reviewed the German literature, including Domagk's early papers on Prontosil and Hörlein's Royal Society of Medicine talk. They gave special emphasis to the French work, however, citing the partial confirmation of Domagk's results by Levaditi and Vaisman, and by Nitti and Bovet, and especially the Pasteur Institute's finding that PABS had an antistreptococcal action comparable to that of Prontosil.[57]

Buttle, Gray, and Stephenson had confirmed the Pasteur Institute team's results and had extended the French researchers' work by testing the action of PABS at different dosages, against streptococcal cultures of different quantities, and at different treatment times after infection. They had also used six different strains of streptococci, four of which they obtained from cases of human puerperal sepsis via Colebrook, who they thanked for the strains and for serological typing, and all of which had been made more virulent by repeated passage through mice.[58]

In addition to their testing of PABS and comparison of its action to that of Prontosil, Buttle and his colleagues moved beyond the narrow focus of Colebrook's investigation in two directions. First, they took on infections other than streptococcal ones. In preliminary experiments on mice, they had found that PABS had a favorable effect against meningococcal infections but little or no action against those involving staphylococci or pneumococci. They had also tried PABS against the nonbacterial infections *Trypanosoma equiperdum* in mice and malaria in canaries, without effect. Second, they had begun to seek out chemical variants of Prontosil and PABS, noting in the paper that "the success obtained with these simply constituted compounds naturally directed attention to the study of others more or less closely related to them, with the object of obtaining a clue to the chemical structure requisite for the development of this form of bactericidal activity." The authors had tested more than thirty compounds, in addition to PABS, for antistreptococcal activity. These were subdivided on the basis of the kinds of modifications to PABS they represented. In one set an amino group of PABS was modified or replaced, in a second the sulfonamide group in the molecule was modified, while in a third elements other than carbon were substituted in the benzene nucleus. Other tested compounds were *p*-toluenesulfonamide derivatives, sulfuric acids, or naphthalene derivatives. In only one case, a compound called *p*-aminobenzenesulfonanilide, in which $-C_6H_5$ had been substituted for one of the hydrogens in the sulfonamide group, did one of its relatives show an antibacterial action comparable to PABS.[59]

Lancet followed the two papers with an editorial that captured both the hope and the caution of the new publications. Echoing Hörlein's Royal Society of Medicine lecture, the editorial recalled a past littered with failures. "The history of attempted chemotherapy in bacterial infections is so discouraging that any indisputable success in this direction is almost totally unexpected," the author began, adding that "nothing has been more uncertain or perhaps more frankly disappointing than the effect on such a condition as streptococcal septicemia of administering all manner of supposedly bactericidal compounds." Against this background, the first reports from Germany on the success of Prontosil were "startling," the editorial continued, and scarcely to be credited on the basis of experiments on mice and "a number of rather uncritical but highly enthusiastic clinical reports of its effect in acute streptococcal infections in man." Now that English workers had "fully satisfied themselves of the validity of these claims on the experimental side, and reached a significant if not conclusive stage in clinical trials," the importance of the discovery was more evident. The key point to grasp, in the author's view, was that unlike older antiseptic substances that were bactericidal and acted only locally, Prontosil was probably not directly bactericidal and acted when introduced at sites distant from the site of infection. "This at any rate is something quite new," the editorial emphasized, since "it is the first time that any drug has been shown to have a specific and regular effect on an acute bacterial infection when administered by the mouth." Caution was still necessary, the author noted. The action of Prontosil was still limited to infections due to *Streptococcus pyogenes*. Clinical trials were needed on streptococcal infections other than puerperal fever. And the mode of action of Prontosil was still almost entirely unknown. All this admitted, there was no question that Prontosil was "obviously a therapeutic advance and possibly the prelude to others."[60]

The upbeat conclusions of the *Lancet* papers and editorial were echoed in the *Times* of London, whose medical correspondent said of the two papers that "the results which they describe are so good as to deserve widespread attention." The article also repeated the cautions expressed in the *Lancet* publications but made it clear to readers that a new kind of medicine was on the scene.[61]

Some British physicians were already using Prontosil before the June papers appeared in *Lancet*. Others were probably drawn to do so by Colebrook and Kenny's favorable conclusions. Glimpses of practice gained from the medical press suggest that physicians were seriously interested but less than dazzled. A meeting of the British Medical Association's Section of Public Medicine, reported in *Lancet* in August, for example, focused on the hemolytic streptococcus, with special reference to scarlet fever. Discussion ranged over several topics including geographical distribution of streptococcal diseases, sources of infection, preventive measures, and the effectiveness (or lack thereof) of antistreptococcal serums. Two discussants mentioned Prontosil. B.A. Peters of Bristol said that he was trying Prontosil in cases of erysipelas, with encouraging results. While treatment with Prontosil had been effective in most cases, he said, he doubted whether the results had been any better than those obtained by treatment with the symmetrical ureas, a relatively obscure alternative therapy for erysipelas. H.J. Parish of Beckenham reviewed the use and limitations of antistreptococcal serums, adding that "if the initial promise of the Prontosil group of chemicals were fulfilled chemotherapy might replace serotherapy to some extent in many streptococcal infections." At the October meeting in Dublin of the Royal Academy of Medicine in Ireland, members of the Academy's Section of Obstetrics traded impressions of treatments of puerperal fever. Prontosil occupied a place, though a peripheral one, among other therapies, including antistreptococcal and antiscarlatinal serums, intrauterine glycerine, local antiseptics, and surgery. Discussants were also much occupied with matters other than therapeutics, including the source of infection (was it usually the patient, or the patient's environment including nurses?), preventive measures, the need for routine bacterial cultures of nurses and patients, the advantages of large or small wards, and so on.[62]

Meanwhile, the TTC continued to encourage broader clinical investigation of Prontosil. On June 5, Green wrote to Snodgrass in Glasgow urging him to continue the trials already under way and to extend them to include cases of erysipelas and, referring to Buttle's *Lancet* paper, menigococcal infections. Snodgrass, who found the clinical evidence in Colebrook and Kenny's paper "only suggestive, but not convincing," was amenable. By early July, he was able to report promising results in treatment of both erysipelas and other streptococcal infections with Prontosil but still warned that "stricter evaluation is necessary." By September, he had increased the number of cases and had used Prontosil in treatment of surgical streptococcal and staphylococcal infections, chronic infectious arthritis, chronic sinus infection, cholecystitis, bacterial endocarditis, and erysipelas, all without decisive evidence that Prontosil made a significant difference in the outcome. Snodgrass had read translations of German physicians' reports on use of Prontosil in erysipelas and was critical of their methods, especially the lack of controls and exclusive reliance on clinical judgment. He was persuaded to continue by the striking outcomes of a few severe cases in which recovery coincided with the use of Prontosil but warned that "a long time must elapse and many cases must be treated before a final decision is reached."[63]

On July 18, Green received a report from J.S. Anderson of the London County Hospital Public Health Department on use of Prontosil and Prontosil Soluble in measles and scarlet fever. Anderson had found that use of Prontosil appeared to reduce the incidence of complications in measles due to secondary invading organisms, mostly streptococci, including otitis media, pneumonia, osteomyelitis, and cellulitis. Complications including tonsillitis, otitis media, and rheumatism also appeared to be reduced in cases of scarlet fever in which relatively high dosages of Prontosil were given. Anderson asked permission of the TTC to publish his findings, but the committee, Brincker of the London County Council, and Colebrook thought the numbers of cases (fifty-six of measles, forty-three of scarlet fever) too low and controls inadequate. Anderson agreed to extend his investigation.[64]

As Prontosil became commercially available in the wake of Colebrook and Kenny's *Lancet* paper, cost of treatment emerged as an issue for the first time. Colebrook wrote to Green in July complaining that at the current prices set by Bayer Products, the average cost of treatment for each patient would be £3 or £4. He worried that the "monstrously high" price would discourage adequate dosage and that "the drug may fall into disrepute in consequence." At Colebrook's urging, Green took the matter up with Thompson at Bayer Products, who in turn raised the question with his directors. Thompson explained that the company had not anticipated the high dosages recommended by Colebrook, and he pointed to discounts available for bulk purposes.[65]

The cost of Prontosil would soon be rendered less significant by the ascent of its constituent molecule, PABS. Even as he complained of Prontosil's price, Colebrook announced to Green that he intended to switch to the intermediate in clinical trials as soon as he felt his animal trials were sufficient. That would not be until October, when Colebrook and Kenny sent the manuscript of their second paper on Prontosil to the TTC. In the meantime, Colebrook and other British clinical investigators were preempted by Bayer Products, which released PABS to the British market in September under the trade name Prontosil Album. The new preparation was quietly introduced in the Bayer Products publication *Clinical Excerpts*, in such a way as to underline its continuity with Prontosil. "The indications, dosage, and therapeutic effects of this substance are exactly similar to those of the original product," the journal noted, adding that besides being simpler and cheaper "animal experimental, and clinical trials on the continent have testified to its value, and it is believed that in practice it will gradually replace the original tablet [Prontosil]," while Prontosil Soluble would remain for treatment by injection. By October, Bayer Products was routinely sending out Prontosil Album in response to requests for Prontosil, unless doctors specified "red Prontosil."[66]

The shift by Bayer Products to Prontosil Album prompted some hesitation on the part of physicians still testing Prontosil in the clinic. Green, who received the manuscript of Colebrook and Kenny's second paper on Prontosil in early October, urged his correspondents to continue trials of the older compound for the time being, while holding out the possibility of a changeover to "the sulfonamide" (Prontosil Album) in the not-too-distant future. Ripley Oddie of Bayer Products informed Green in early November that the company would be glad to supply clinical investigators with Prontosil and Prontosil Soluble, "although most of the business in these products is now being transferred to the sulfonamide preparation." Green wrote that he thought Bayer Products "may have been somewhat premature" in switching to the colorless compound, "of which clinical tests in this country are only now beginning!" Oddie, in reply, explained that the company was responding not only to published experimental and clinical work in Germany but also to a demand "which had already been making itself felt." Bayer Products, he wrote, felt "that we should, as the firm responsible for the opening up of this new aspect of chemotherapy," be able to supply the "complete range of products." In other words, Bayer Products now feared being left behind in the market. With Prontosil Album even more than with Prontosil and Prontosil Soluble, the diffusion of the new drug into practice was outpacing the TTC's slow and deliberate trials procedure.[67]

Green circulated Colebrook and Kenny's second paper on Prontosil to members of the TTC in October, and it was published in *Lancet* on December 5. The authors had added twenty-six new cases to the thirty-eight reported in June, and ventured new summary remarks on their experience. All but one of the twenty-six patients had been diagnosed with puerperal fever and infection by hemolytic streptococci. Apart from treatment with Prontosil, all patients had received minimal treatment, which was standard general care. None had died. Colebrook and Kenny judged that in twelve cases the patients would "almost certainly" have recovered without Prontosil. In the remaining fourteen more severe cases, rapid and complete recovery made it "seem probable that the treatment assisted recovery." In the most severe cases, the authors deemed the role of Prontosil "more than probable." They gave details of the two most serious cases:

> Mrs. F. 1-para; admitted on fifth day of puerperium, with temperature of
> 103°F and pulse of 140 rising to 150, signs and symptoms of generalised

peritonitis, and a positive blood culture. (This combination has almost invariably in our experience proved fatal.) After three days' treatment her temperature and pulse-rate became persistently normal, and all signs of peritonitis disappeared.

Mrs. S. 1-para; developed fever to 105°F on third day, and on admission was very gravely ill. Blood culture gave a growth of more than 5,000 colonies per c.cm. on the first two days, and over 3,000 on the third day, most, if not all, of the colonies being hemolytic streptococci. . . . On the fourth day of treatment a blood culture was sterile and the temperature fell to normal . . . She was discharged in good health 21 days after admission to hospital and has suffered no relapse.

Of the second case, Colebrook and Kenny remarked that "in view of the fact that blood cultures yielding such a large number of hemolytic streptococci (equivalent to something like 30 millions in the whole blood stream) have never previously been observed by us except in the terminal stages of a fatal infection, this patient's prompt recovery was astonishing." They included a chart of this case to show "a typical scheme of dosage," in which the dramatic turn of the patient's condition is graphically plain.[68]

In their commentary on all sixty-four cases, Colebrook and Kenny emphasized the "sudden and remarkable fall in the death rate" in cases of puerperal fever caused by hemolytic streptococci. They also noted that the tendency of puerperal infections to spread to the cellular tissues of the parametrium and to the pelvic walls had been "conspicuously absent" in Prontosil-treated cases, a circumstance reflected in the prompt fall and stabilization of temperature and in

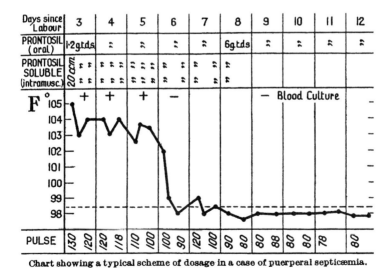

Chart showing a typical scheme of dosage in a case of puerperal septicæmia.

Figure 6.6. Patient chart from Leonard Colebrook and Meave Kenny, "Treatment with Prontosil of puerperal infections due to hemolytic streptococci," *Lancet* 2 (1936): 1319–1322.

shorter average hospital stays. Finally, they reported that none of the sixty-four patients had had to be readmitted, and all had been found to be in good health in follow-up visits. All of this had been achieved without significant toxic effects.[69]

Several problems remained for future research, Colebrook and Kenny conceded. Dosage levels, the relative value of oral and parenteral administration, the possible effects of Prontosil on other than hemolytic streptococci, and the relative efficacy of Prontosil and "the sulfonamide" were still to be determined. Nevertheless, they found that their investigation made it "difficult to resist the conclusion that the remarkable improvement in the clinical results had been chiefly due to the introduction of the treatment with Prontosil," a conclusion "strongly supported by the analogous and unmistakable curative effects obtained in experimental animals."[70]

In their December 5 paper, Colebrook and Kenny announced that in the next few months they would treat a new series of patients with PABS (Prontosil Album). They reported that "the sulfonamide," as they also called the simpler compound, had given better results than Prontosil in animal trials and also conferred "a much greater bactericidal power on the blood." These remarks were based in part on collaborative work that Colebrook had done with Buttle of Wellcome Laboratories and R.A.Q. O'Meara of the Bernhard Baron Memorial Research Laboratories at Queen Charlotte's Hospital, which appeared in *Lancet* immediately following Colebrook and Kenny's paper.[71]

Colebrook, Buttle, and O'Meara had taken as starting point "a number of new facts which have recently come to light," by which they referred especially to the Pasteur Institute team's suggestion that PABS was formed *in vivo* after administration of Prontosil and was the therapeutically effective part of the medicine. To test this idea, they had added Prontosil or PABS to bacterial cultures and to blood serum or whole blood inoculated with hemolytic streptococci. They gauged the bactericidal or bacteriostatic effects of the compounds both when they were added to blood *in vitro* and when they were administered to infected or uninfected human subjects from whom blood samples were then taken. They found that administration of either compound to humans gave the blood or serum a powerful bacteriostatic action against hemolytic streptococci but that only PABS showed a comparable action *in vitro*. These results, joined to those of British biochemist A.T. Fuller showing that the simpler compound was produced by reduction of Prontosil in the body, tended to confirm the Pasteur Institute team's conjecture.[72]

The same issue of *Lancet* also carried an editorial underlining the importance of the new findings. By confirming and extending their original conclusions, the editorialist asserted, Colebrook and Kenny had left no room for doubt that Prontosil worked. In their studies of Prontosil and "sulphonamide," he wrote, Colebrook, Buttle, and O'Meara had completely reversed the earlier view that "the disinfection of the bloodstream in septicemia is by nature a complete impossibility." Now "only the most rigid sceptic" could deny the efficacy of the new compounds, the writer stated, concluding that "it has become an imperative duty to employ them not only in puerperal fever, but also in other severe forms of streptococcal infection." It was only a small step beyond the language of the *Lancet* papers and editorial when *Clinical Excerpts* described Prontosil later the same month as "what may well prove to be one of the most remarkable medical discoveries of this century."[73]

"A Medical Miracle"

Remarkable discovery or not, Prontosil and its offspring, PABS, were still unknown to most physicians in the United States. For many months, the strenuous activity surrounding Prontosil and its relatives in German, French, and British laboratories and clinics found no echo across the Atlantic. Not until September 1936, over a year and a half after Domagk's first publication, did a notice of Prontosil appear in the *Journal of the American Medical Association* (*JAMA*). Even then, the report came in the form of abstracts of Colebrook's and Buttle's first papers in *Lancet*. Most American physicians learned of the new drugs only in December 1936, when the president's son, Franklin D. Roosevelt, Jr., was cured of a life-threatening streptococcal infection by Prontylin (a Winthrop Chemical Company trade name for PABS) and Prontosil Soluble, amid great publicity. From then on, the curve of recognition of Prontosil and related compounds by the American medical community rose steeply, as did the research attention the new medicines received.[74]

That the president's son could be treated was, however, due to earlier initiatives taken by a handful of American medical researchers. Perrin Long and Eleanor Bliss, both of Johns Hopkins, attended the Second International Congress of Microbiology in London in July 1936. There they heard Colebrook summarize his work on Prontosil. Long immediately grasped the importance of Colebrook's findings. He wrote to Johns Hopkins to ask that they request supplies of Prontosil and Prontosil Soluble, and to E.I. Dupont de Nemours and Company to ask that its laboratories prepare PABS. On their return, Long and Bliss began animal trials. In early September, Long treated his first patient, a seven-year-old girl suffering from erysipelas, with PABS. The successful outcome in this case persuaded Long to continue clinical trials. Colleagues at Johns Hopkins were drawn into the effort. In October, pharmacologist Eli Kennerly Marshall, Jr., began studies of PABS, tracing its absorption and excretion in the body and devising colorimetric methods for estimating its concentration in the blood. A few other American physicians, learning of the medicines, began to use them to treat patients. In November, Long and Bliss gave a preliminary report to a meeting of the Southern Medical Association, urging that clinical tests be vigorously pursued. In December, just before news broke of FDR Jr.'s cure, Long treated his first case of streptococcal meningitis with PABS. The patient recovered from a disease that until then had a nearly 100 percent mortality.[75]

In January 1937, Long and Bliss published their first paper on the new compounds, describing *in vitro* and animal experiments and summarizing in tabular form nineteen clinical cases. Citing a now extensive list of papers from the German, French, and British literature, they went on to largely confirm the findings

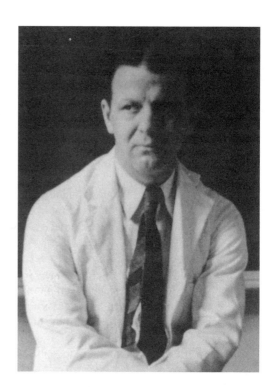

Figure 6.7. Perrin H. Long
(1899–1965) (reprinted courtesy
of Alan Mason Chesney Medical
Archives of The Johns Hopkins
Medical Institutions).

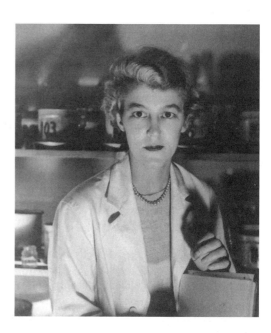

Figure 6.8. Eleanor A. Bliss
(1899–1987) (*Harper's Bazaar*).

of the British researchers. Even so, they could not withhold a note of caution, warning that "it is always necessary in testing new therapeutic agents to adopt a skeptical attitude toward the results obtained," since "too often have early brilliant therapeutic successes eventually proved to be due to chance or to optimism of the reporter." Skepticism was yielding to what now seemed unambiguous experimental evidence, however, and they were prepared to conclude that "the careful clinical use of para-amino-benzene-sulfonamide and its derivatives in the treatment of human beings ill with infections due to beta-hemolytic streptococci is warranted." *JAMA* agreed, summarizing in an editorial the results of research from Domagk through Long and Bliss and calling for more and better controlled clinical trials.[76]

The field was now open to American medical researchers. Between January and June 1937, reports of experimental and clinical trials of the new medicines began to flow into the American medical press. Prontosil and PABS were tried in several kinds of bacterial infections, including streptococcal and meningococcal meningitis, gonorrhea, and pneumococcal type III infections, with results ranging from somewhat favorable to strikingly successful. At least two publications were authored by Long's and Bliss's colleagues at Johns Hopkins. From the Brady Urological Institute, origin of the earlier vogue for mercurachrome, came a promising report on use of PABS (by now called sulfanilamide) in treatment of gonorrhea. On Long's advice, John E. Dees and J.A.C. Colston had treated nineteen patients without prior animal trials, a measure reflecting not only the difficulty of infecting laboratory animals with the gonococcus but also Long's growing confidence in the efficacy and safety of the medicine. Marshall presented the first results of his research, begun the previous October, on absorption and excretion of PABS and of methods of determining its concentrations in the blood and urine. Starting with PABS, Marshall produced an azo compound that, when coupled to dimethyl-1-naphthylamine, yielded a purple-red dye that could be readily estimated by colorimetric comparison. By opening the way to more exact knowledge of blood concentrations of the medicine over time, Marshall provided a new basis for both therapeutics and mode of action studies.[77]

In April, the American Medical Association's Council on Pharmacy and Chemistry announced the adoption of "sulfanilamide" as the official generic name for PABS. Although at the time the council was still considering the compound for inclusion in its list of New and Nonofficial Remedies, it was moved to act by the proliferation of proprietary names for the same substance. The council would have preferred a shorter name but accepted "sulfanilamide" because it expressed the compound's composition and was said to be already in use abroad. By comparison with the chemical nomenclature, the new term still came out as a measure of economy.[78]

In May, the council issued its official report on "Sulfanilamide and Related Compounds." The report listed thirteen British and American companies now manufacturing sulfanilamide, under eight different names, including the official generic one. The proprietary names, and manufacturers, were Prontylin (Winthrop Chemical Company), Prontosil Album (Bayer), Stramid (Alba Chemical Company), Streptocide (Evans Sons Lescher & Webb, Ltd., London), Colsulanyde (Crookes Laboratories, London), Sulfamidyl (Abbott Laboratories), and Sulphonamid P (Burroughs,

Wellcome & Co.). The six other firms already involved in manufacture of the medicine were Calco Chemical Co. Inc., Lederle Laboratories Inc., Eli Lilly and Company Inc., Merck & Co. Inc., Parke Davis & Company, and E.R. Squibb & Sons. The report summarized the "rapidly increasing evidence that Sulfanilamide and its derivatives are useful therapeutic agents in the treatment of infections with beta-hemolytic streptococci, both local and generalized," endorsed their use in such cases, and added sulfanilamide to its list of New and Nonofficial Remedies. Perhaps sensing a rising tide of enthusiasm among practitioners and the public, the council added a word of caution. Toxic effects of the drug were not yet fully known, the report noted, and it "should not be used indiscriminately. It is not a panacea."[79]

The warning was timely. Enthusiasm for the new medicines was beginning to break through the customary restraint of professional medical and scientific language. Reporting on the impressive showing made by Prontosil and sulfanilamide at the Atlantic City meeting of the American Medical Association in June, a writer for the journal *Science*, Jane Stafford, described Prontosil in glowing terms as "the new chemical remedy that has already saved thousands of lives and promises to conquer four of mankind's major germ enemies." Stafford had gained the impression from physicians' discussions at the meeting that both sulfanilamide and Prontosil were effective treatments for all manner of diseases caused by streptococci, pneumococci, meningococci, and gonococci. She had the assurance of Morris Fishbein, editor of *JAMA*, that "hundreds of similar cases were now ready for publication in the *Journal*." [80]

In this effusiveness, the popular press had taken an early lead. Already, when reporting on the FDR Jr. case in December 1936, *Time* magazine had referred to Prontosil as possibly "the medical discovery of the decade." By April 1937, *Colliers* magazine was deploying the full language of superlatives. "A scientist in Germany, tinkering with molecules, produced a red dye. Immediately, patients scheduled to die from streptococcus infection began to get well. Here is the dramatic story of a modern miracle." So began J.D. Ratcliff's article "Magic Dye" in *Colliers* for April 3, 1937. Ratcliff skillfully spotlighted one of Long and Bliss's early cases, a five-year-old girl pulled back from the brink of death from septicemia by treatment with Prontosil. He went on to recount for his readers the dangers of streptococcal infections, mentioning the death of Calvin Coolidge's son from such an illness and the saving of FDR Jr., the initial discoveries at Elberfeld, their confirmation by Colebrook and Kenny, and the French researchers' findings on PABS. Casting aside the careful hedging and reservations of the research literature, Ratcliff hailed Prontosil as "a brilliant new chapter in medical history—possibly the most brilliant of our day" and as "wonder-working," commenting on one case that "you would have to turn to Biblical literature to duplicate a miracle like that."[81]

Some popular representations of the new medicines were more restrained. Writing in the *Baltimore Sun* in June 1937, Arthur Musgrave gave a strongly positive but careful, detailed, and cautious account of Long and Bliss's successful use of PABS in treatment of spinal meningitis due to streptococci. Musgrave credited Long and Bliss with introduction of the compound in the United States and described dramatic cures of a disease that had previously had a nearly 100 percent mortality in Baltimore hospitals. Perhaps because he was directly in touch with Long, however, Musgrave did not exaggerate the drug's powers, noting that its effectiveness against meningococcal, gonococcal, and pneumococcal infections was under study but not yet demonstrated. Still, he was willing to write of "the unparalleled workings of the compound" against streptococcal infections. And in the title and headings of his article, Musgrave mixed the increasingly common metaphors of military victory ("medical science conquers a foe") and divine powers ("a medical miracle"). At least in the minds of some Americans, the age of miracle drugs had arrived.[82]

The Paths Converge

By the spring of 1937, sulfanilamide was on the market in France, Britain, and the United States. Its clinical use under specified conditions had been endorsed by medical researchers in all three countries. Although Prontosil and Prontosil Soluble were still available, they were being displaced in both research and practice by their constituent compound. The search was on, especially in industrial laboratories, for a new generation of antibacterial agents, derivatives of sulfanilamide. Although many differences persisted in the biomedical worlds of the three countries, on these few points a degree of convergence had occurred.

The paths of this convergence differed markedly. The differences are revealing of national differences in the way new medical knowledge was generated, diffused, and assimilated and suggest a number of comparisons. First, there is the question of how new medical knowledge gets across national boundaries. In all three of these cases, the crossing was initially effected by medical researchers who themselves had crossed the boundaries in question (Fourneau had trained in Germany, Dale had visited Elberfeld, Long and Bliss met Colebrook in London). In the cases of Fourneau and Dale, the prior experience in Germany led to a continuous monitoring of German research on chemotherapy. Lack of such contact by American researchers in chemotherapy may have been a factor in the delayed response to Prontosil in the United States.

To differing degrees, yet to be fully explored, the crossing of borders was aided by the competition and emulation inherent in the relationship between the French, British, and American pharmaceutical industries and German industry. French industry responded rapidly to the I.G. Farben patent application. British industry initiated work on sulfanilamide and its derivatives in Britain, apparently independently of the Medical Research Council. Long and Bliss were supported in part by the Chemical Foundation, an American organization set up with an eye to competition with German industry. Early research on Prontosil and sulfanilamide was facilitated by institutionalized connections between medical researchers and the pharmaceutical industry. Fourneau's service of therapeutic chemistry at the Pasteur Institute was closely linked to Rhône-Poulenc. In Britain, the Medical Research Council mediated between industry and clinical researchers, while in the United States the links were less centralized and often less formal.[83]

Patents played a mixed role. Information on Prontosil first reached France in the form of the I.G. Farben patent application and, once there, became the basis of a French industry copy, Rubiazol. That French industry was willing and able to ignore patents on German pharmaceutical products was a source of some bitterness for I.G. Farben. As early as 1915, Fourneau had argued that French law permitted manufacture of products covered by German patents, whether or not a chemical process different from the one patented was used, and that it would be foolish for French manufacturers to forgo the opportunity. German patents and trademarks had been seized during the war, and after the war stiff restrictions on German imports had been imposed. Hörlein had complained in 1926, not restricting his remarks to France, that "in the pharmaceutical field a circumstance prevails that is not all that different from that of the robber knights of the Middle Ages." In 1935, he returned to the same theme, citing as "classic example" of the successful theft of intellectual property rights the French copying of Prontosil, "a discovery that was the result of work carried out with tenacity for years and with the expenditure of extensive material means, and of great intellectual energy."[84]

German patents appear to have been respected in Britain and the United States. By the fall of 1936, however, the movement toward testing and use of the nonpatentable PABS freed researchers, practitioners, and companies from any such restraints. Paradoxically, introduction of sulfanilamide was delayed longest in France, where a related alternative displaced it until the spring of 1937.

In two of the three cases, professional meetings played significant roles in carrying knowledge of Prontosil across national boundaries. Hörlein's talk at the Royal Society of Medicine in October 1935 (printed in *Lancet* in February 1936) brought first news of Prontosil to many British physicians. And Long and Bliss's encounter with Colebrook at the Second International Congress of Microbiology sparked the first American research on the new medicines.

Professional medical journals appear to have been effective in diffusing knowledge of Prontosil and sulfanilamide within national boundaries once that knowledge was in possession of advanced medical researchers. They appear to have been less effective as vehicles for the cross-national transmission of knowledge. Fourneau and other French researchers made use of early German publications by Domagk and others, but only after learning of Prontosil through a patent application. Dale had first learned of the compound that became Prontosil in a visit to Elberfeld. It is striking that *JAMA* printed nothing on Prontosil or sulfanilamide until September 1936, despite the presence in Berlin of a *JAMA* correspondent reporting regularly on German medical news, and regular *JAMA* abstracts (in English) of papers in German medical journals. A possible explanation, yet to be confirmed, is that Fishbein, the *JAMA* editor, had been embarrassed by overly hasty publication of news of new drugs in previous years and now erred on the side of excessive caution. In contrast, American newspapers and magazines appear to have played a significant role in alerting many physicians and the public to the new medicines, in the first instance by granting wide publicity to a single celebrity case.

Perceptions of one national research community by another, and the related problem of differing national standards for the laboratory and clinical evaluation of new drugs, also played roles in the reception of Prontosil and sulfanilamide. In

France, a copy of Prontosil went on the market just five days after the first reports of animal trials were published, and two months before publication of the first French clinical studies, a fact that could reflect either a casual attitude toward clinical trials or, more likely, confidence in earlier published German clinical reports. In Britain, in contrast, the Medical Research Council's Therapeutic Trials Committee discounted German publications and insisted on meticulous and time-consuming laboratory and clinical trials before approving Prontosil for commercial sale. Colebrook, who restricted his study to one disease in which he had years of clinical research experience, and who went to considerable trouble to organize and present his data systematically, set an especially high standard. Some American researchers may have initially discounted German reports on Prontosil because they emerged from Germany under the Hitler regime. Once engaged with the new medicine, American researchers seem to have given special weight to prior British studies, but conducted their own laboratory and clinical trials anyway.[85]

Finally, skepticism regarding the very possibility of bacterial chemotherapy undoubtedly played a role in all three countries (as it did also in Germany), but to different degrees. It was least evident in France, where response to the news from Germany was immediate and positive. Even in France, however, the prior existence of skepticism may be reflected in the absence of an active research program in bacterial chemotherapy at the Pasteur Institute before March 1935. It was pronounced in Britain, where Colebrook, for example, had been imbued with his teacher Wright's doctrine that bacterial chemotherapy was an impossibility and had seen other chemicals come and go through long years of research on puerperal fever. And it may well be the single most important reason for the delayed American response to Prontosil, which occurred against a background of failure of mercurachrome and numerous other compounds from the 1910s to the early 1930s.[86] One of the remarkable things about this story is that the skepticism about bacterial chemotherapy, so pervasive in early 1935, was everywhere dissipated by the spring of 1937. Ehrlich's prediction of the achievement of such a chemotherapy, long unfulfilled, had at last taken on substance.

CHAPTER 7

M&B 693

Late in 1943, at the height of the Second World War, Winston Churchill visited the Middle East for conferences with Britain's allies. He met Chiang Kai-shek in Cairo, then flew to Teheran to talk with Stalin, and finally returned to Cairo for a meeting with President Roosevelt. Exhausted from work and travel, he boarded an airplane at 1 A.M. on December 11 for a flight to Tunisia, where he was to stay at Dwight Eisenhower's villa near Carthage. Off course, the plane made an unscheduled stop forty miles from its destination. Churchill sat on his luggage on the runway in a cold wind for an hour before completing his journey. Later that day Churchill had a pain in his throat and a bad headache. The next day he had a fever of 101°F. Lord Moran, Churchill's personal physician, called in nurses and a pathologist from Cairo. A portable X-ray machine was brought from Tunis. X-rays showed a shadow on Churchill's lung, which the doctors diagnosed as pneumonia. Moran immediately put Churchill on one of the recently developed sulfa drugs manufactured by the British company May & Baker, a drug familiarly known as M&B. Churchill began to have heart trouble.[1]

Alarmed and fearing the worst for his 69-year-old patient, Moran called in leading specialists from the Mediterranean theater. From Cairo came Brigadier D. Evan Bedford, a prominent heart specialist, and from Italy Lt. Colonel G.A.H. Buttle, who as a civilian researcher before the war had conducted some of the earliest animal trials of sulfonamides in Britain and who was now regarded as an expert on the administration of M&B. Churchill's condition continued to deteriorate. His lungs became congested. He had heart fibrillations. A planned side trip to Italy to visit the troops was canceled, and Churchill's stay at Carthage was extended indefinitely. Then, much to the relief of everyone around him, he began to improve. By Christmas Day, he was feeling better and working. On December 27, he flew to

Marrakesh to continue his convalescence, during which he worked on plans for the Anzio invasion, the Normandy invasion, and other, lesser operations. From Marrakesh he flew to Gibraltar in mid-January, and from there sailed for England, arriving on January 17, 1944.[2]

No one, not Churchill himself, not his doctors, not the press or the public who anxiously followed the Prime Minister's illness and recovery, doubted that he had been brought back from the brink of death by the new medicine, that is, by M&B. After arriving in Marrakesh, Churchill issued a bulletin that was immediately printed in the British newspapers that said in part

> This admirable M&B, from which I did not suffer any inconvenience, was used at the earliest moment; and after a week's fever the intruders were repulsed. I hope all our battles will be equally well conducted. . . . The M&B, which I may also call Moran and Bedford [Churchill could not resist the joke on his physicians' names], did the work most effectively. There is no doubt that pneumonia is a very different illness from what it was before this marvellous drug was discovered.[3]

All very good. But what was "M&B"? Martin Gilbert's otherwise exhaustive biography of Churchill is not more specific, nor is Richard Lovell's biography of Lord Moran. A compound called M&B 760 (chemical name sulfathiazole) may have been used. One of the specialists attending Churchill, a Lt. Colonel R.J.V. Pulvertaft, had participated in research on penicillin with the British Middle East forces. But the presumption of most doctors, the press, and the public was that the drug that had saved Churchill's life was M&B 693, or sulfapyridine.[4]

Thanks to Churchill's recovery enjoying its most brilliant moment in the public eye, M&B 693 was a "miracle drug" that had not existed six years earlier. And even as it was reported that Churchill had taken it, M&B 693 was being displaced by newer, more effective or less toxic medicines, first other sulfas such as M&B 760, later by penicillin. M&B 693, in fact, was one of a flood of sulfonamide compounds that appeared from the late 1930s to the late 1940s. It was but one instance of a spreading revolution in the therapeutics of bacterial infections set in motion by the introduction of the first sulfa drugs, Prontosil and sulfanilamide, in 1935. With the way shown by Prontosil and sulfanilamide, pharmaceutical companies in several countries had joined an intensive search for new derivatives to treat a widening spectrum of bacterial diseases with lower risks to the patient.[5]

By 1945, a decade after the entry of Prontosil into medical practice, more than 5,000 compounds had been synthesized, and some small fraction of these had gone on the market. Chemotherapies were available for many infections previously untreatable, or treated only with great difficulty, including puerperal fever, erysipelas, septicemia, urinary tract infections, gonorrhea, bacillary dysentery, and bacterial pneumonia. At the end of the war, penicillin was beginning to displace the sulfa drugs as the medicine of choice in bacterial infections, but for most of World War II it was the sulfa drugs that carried the main therapeutic burden, on both sides.[6]

The first sulfas, Prontosil and sulfanilamide, were effective mainly against streptococcal infections. M&B 693 burst on the medical scene in 1938 as the first effective chemotherapy for bacterial pneumonia, a major scourge counted by William Osler among the "captains of the men of death." A study of case fatalities in pneumonia published in the *American Journal of Public Health* in 1943 showed a drop in mortality from more than twenty percent in the period 1935–1937 to less than four percent between 1939 and June 1942. The same study estimated that by 1943 M&B 693 and other sulfa drugs were saving at least 25,000 lives a year in the working population of the United States alone. Churchill was only the most celebrated beneficiary of the new medicines.[7]

M&B 693 enjoyed about five years in the limelight as a miracle drug. In the brevity of its career, it exemplified the fate of other medicines in the fast-changing domain of bacterial chemotherapy, where patents were often rendered superfluous by the pace of obsolescence. It may be representative of the new generation of sulfa drugs in other respects, and not least in the way it was discovered.

M&B 693 emerged from an industrial research effort in which a deliberately constructed system of methodical trial and error was complemented by serendipity. It was greeted by the medical community with measured but genuine enthusiasm and was appropriated by the popular press in ways that frequently exaggerated, misrepresented, or distorted its significance. Viewed in retrospect by participants and observers, the discovery of M&B 693 became subject to competing interpretations, most of which, nevertheless, presupposed that the discovery could be isolated to a single point in time and that credit could be assigned to one or two individuals.

As in Churchill's case, the greatest impact of sulfapyridine came in treatment of pneumonia. On the whole, British physicians and researchers received sulfapyridine with enthusiasm, although the headlong rush to introduce it into medical practice also prompted warnings about the drug's potential toxicity, especially if misused.

In the United States, medical researchers at first greeted sulfapyridine with caution, but by the spring of 1939 American physicians had embraced the new medicine. A prior history of therapeutic reform conditioned early reaction to sulfapyridine, and it became a focus of government efforts to formulate regulatory policy in accordance with the federal Food, Drug, and Cosmetic Act of 1938.

The Industrial Invention of Sulfapyridine

In principle, the Pasteur Institute discovery in 1935 that sulfanilamide was the therapeutically effective part of Prontosil opened the way for a new program of chemotherapeutic research based on substitution for the hydrogen atoms in the sulfanilamide molecule. In practice, it seems that it was not immediately obvious to industrial researchers which direction to take, and response was slower than one might think in retrospect. One complication was that it took a while for researchers and doctors to be convinced that Prontosil itself worked, and still longer for them to recognize that sulfanilamide was Prontosil's equal. This was especially true in Britain and the United States.[8]

At the laboratories of May & Baker, at Dagenham outside London, interest in the sulfa drugs did not surface until January 1936, when George Newbery, one of the company's small staff of research chemists, synthesized Prontosil. Even then, a crash program of sulfonamides research was not in the works, still less one that took as starting point the Pasteur Institute finding published two months earlier. Company chemists made a few azo compounds, evidently with the thought of extending the Prontosil model. At research director Arthur J. Ewins's instigation, they also synthesized a number of stilbene compounds. Stilbene derivatives, with their aromatic groups linked by a double bond between two carbon atoms, were important in the dye industry, and their structural analogy to azo dyes may have prompted Ewins's interest in their possible therapeutic activity. At the same time, however, company chemists were working on compounds without direct relation to the sulfonamides, including cyano compounds and oil-soluble arsenicals.[9]

Arthur James Ewins, who was fifty-four years old in 1936, already had thirty-six years of experience in pharmaceutical and chemotherapeutic research, including twenty years as director of research at May & Baker. The son of a railroad signalman, he had begun his career in 1899 by proceeding directly from secondary school to a post as research apprentice and technical assistant at the newly created Wellcome Physiological Research Laboratories. In at the ground floor of the then novel pharmaceutical research establishment, Ewins had the good fortune to work for and with a succession of exceptionally talented senior colleagues, including Edward Mellanby, George Barger, and Henry Hallett Dale. From Barger he gained a practical and theoretical knowledge of organic chemistry, and most of Ewins's early publications were co-authored with his mentor. Among the projects on which Ewins worked with Barger was research on ergot, its specific alkaloids, and the active amines found in its extracts. When Barger left Wellcome in 1909, Ewins, who had meanwhile earned a chemistry degree at the University of London, was appointed to a staff position in chemistry by Dale, who by then was director of the laboratories. With Dale, Ewins continued the work on ergot extracts, assisting with Dale's early studies of histamines and participating in the isolation of acetylcholine. In July 1914, just before the outbreak of war in Europe, Ewins moved with Dale from the Wellcome Laboratories to the Department of Biochemistry and Pharmacology in Britain's new National Institute of Medical Research.[10]

When the war began, Britain's supply of medicines from Germany was suddenly cut off. Wartime increase in the incidence of venereal disease made the disappearance of Neosalvarsan (neoarsphenamine) an especially serious problem. Dale and Ewins worked closely with British pharmaceutical firms to develop methods for manufacture and quality control of Neosalvarsan substitutes. Ewins took on the main responsibility for the project, and this brought him into contact with Robert Blenkinsop of May & Baker. Impressed with Ewins's ability to handle chemotherapeutic problems, Blenkinsop offered him a position, with the opportunity to build up a new research division at the company. It was an offer Ewins could not refuse, and he left the National Institute for Medical Research for industry in 1916.[11]

Neosalvarsan was an organic arsenical. So, too, was tryparsamide, a sleeping sickness remedy developed by the American researchers Michael Heidelberger and Walter A. Jacobs as part of their wartime program to seek specific chemotherapies for trypanosomal and spirochetal infections. While still with Dale, Ewins developed a new method for estimation of arsenic in organic compounds. He took this method, and a permanent interest in medicines for tropical diseases, with him to May & Baker. Among the few papers published under his own name after joining the company were three that appeared in 1927 and 1928 on organic arsenicals, and May & Baker researchers were still investigating compounds of this type when they took up Prontosil in early 1936.[12]

With a handful of chemists and staff, and relatively modest resources by comparison with I.G. Farben, Ewins was able to create a research group in which a commitment to long-term development of chemotherapies took precedence over short-term economies and in which morale was high. According to Dale and H.J. Barker, the latter of whom worked closely with Ewins at May & Baker, part of the key to Ewins's success was his readiness to give subordinates a sufficient degree of freedom to work out their own ideas. Personally kindly and modest, he was also generous in allowing those under his direction to take credit for the work of the laboratory, a quality that did not prevent him from acquiring a high reputation among other researchers and among physicians interested in chemotherapy. In Dale's view, Ewins lacked the sort of mind that strove to theoretically comprehend a problem or that opened up "really new scientific territory." What he did have, according to Dale, was "an exceptional promptitude in recognizing possibilities of practical developments from new discoveries made elsewhere," a characteristic that suited him well for industrial research and that was brought into play in May & Baker's response to Prontosil and sulfanilamide.[13]

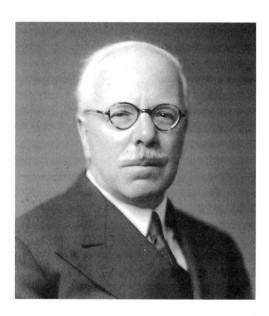

Figure 7.1. Arthur James Ewins (1882–1957) in 1946 (© The Godfrey Argent Studio, reprinted with permission).

It was only in May 1936 that Newbery turned to making derivatives of sulfanilamide. Two explanations may be suggested for this shift. One is that Newbery was asked to do so by his superior, Ewins, who was in turn asked to initiate research on sulfanilamide derivatives by his superior, Nicholas Grillet. Grillet was general manager of the French chemical firm Rhône-Poulenc. In 1927, one of the parent companies of Rhône-Poulenc, Établissements Poulenc Frères, had bought a controlling interest in May & Baker, and this was retained after the merger that gave rise to Rhône-Poulenc in 1928. Grillet, a manager who understood research problems, therefore presumably had the authority to direct Ewins to initiate a new line of research. That he did so was later asserted by Jacques Billon, another manager at Rhône-Poulenc. Billon wrote that Grillet ordered Ewins at May & Baker, and Edmond Blaise, the scientific director of Rhône-Poulenc, to divide up the work in the search for derivatives of sulfanilamide. Rhône-Poulenc was to concentrate on derivatives substituted in the N^4 position on the benzene ring, that is, the amino group. May & Baker was to concentrate on derivatives substituted in the N^1 position, that is, the sulfonamide group.[14]

The case for a Rhône-Poulenc intervention is strengthened by the circumstance that the French company had launched its first sulfanilamide derivative in April. This was benzylsulfonamide, introduced to the French market under the trade name Septazine. Rhône-Poulenc asked May & Baker to market the same compound in Britain as Proseptazine. Lacking in-house facilities for animal trials, Ewins turned to Lionel Whitby, a pathologist at Middlesex Hospital in London, to conduct tests of Proseptazine on experimental infections in mice. Whitby's laboratory findings on Proseptazine, and subsequent trials of the compound by clinicians, were not impressive. Nevertheless, Proseptazine provided an occasion both for May & Baker work on sulfanilamide derivatives and for the company's initial connection with Lionel Whitby.[15]

A second explanation for the May & Baker research staff's shift of attention to sulfanilamide derivatives points to sources closer to home. In the spring of 1936, Buttle, a researcher at Wellcome Laboratories in London, was following up on the Pasteur Institute discovery by testing the therapeutic efficacy of sulfanilamide and its derivatives in animal trials. Buttle also had arrangements with Leonard Colebrook to conduct clinical trials of his compounds. Word of Buttle's success with sulfanilamide itself and with one derivative may have reached May & Baker staff even before he published his first results in June 1936.[16]

Either or both explanations may be correct, although the Billon story is placed in some doubt by the circumstance that May & Baker chemists did not confine themselves to preparation of N^1-substituted derivatives but also made N^4-substituted ones. In any case, one day in the spring of 1936, Ewins met with two of his chemists, Newbery and Montague Phillips, and agreed on a program for synthesis of various derivatives of sulfanilamide. No written record of the plan survives, but according to recollections of at least one chemist who was working in the laboratory at the time, the idea was to look for water-soluble compounds. This would make sense, because one drawback of sulfanilamide as a medicine was that it was relatively insoluble. Part of the aim was apparently to increase the basic quality of the molecule so that it would form neutral salts with an inorganic acid.[17]

The first sulfanilamide derivative was entered in the laboratory test book in May 1936. Thereafter, the program was pursued, sporadically, through the rest of 1936 and the first ten months of 1937. Whitby conducted trials of the new compounds on experimental infections in mice. Some fifty sulfonamide compounds were made, many of them by Newbery, who was simultaneously engaged in other projects.[18]

By the time he began collaborating with May & Baker chemists, Whitby had already established a reputation as an outstanding pathologist. The son of a West County glove maker, he was headed for Cambridge on a scholarship when war broke out in 1914. He immediately joined the army, was decorated for bravery, and rose to the rank of major before losing a leg to a severe wound in 1918. After leaving the army, he studied medicine at Cambridge, and then moved to Middlesex Hospital in London, where he was appointed assistant pathologist in 1923.[19]

Whitby's choice of pathology as a specialty was at least partly determined by the limited mobility imposed by his wooden leg, but the field proved compatible with his interests and talents. By the time he took his medical degree in 1927, he was doing research and writing on pernicious anemia and on the organisms causing empyema (pus in a body cavity). His strong commitment to the connection of laboratory research and clinical practice found expression in a series of textbooks summarizing the current state of knowledge in concise, readable, and practical form. *Medical Bacteriology* first appeared in 1928, followed by *The Laboratory in Surgical Practice* in 1931 and *Disorders of the Blood* in 1935. His growing reputation in

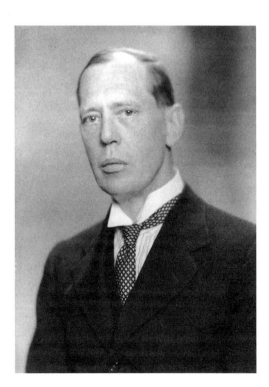

Figure 7.2. Sir Lionel E. H. Whitby (1895–1956) in 1947 (National Portrait Gallery, London, reprinted with permission).

these years resulted in his inclusion in the medical team treating King George V during his illness in 1929.[20]

Whitby undertook the work on sulfonamides eagerly but in the midst of numerous other responsibilities. In the mid-1930s, he supervised the routine bacteriology and blood counts of Middlesex Hospital, gave an annual course of lectures and practical classes, ran an extensive private practice, and prepared new editions of his *Medical Bacteriology*. Students and colleagues later recalled him at work in his laboratory on the second floor of the Bland-Sutton Institute, seated at the end of a long bench in a worn white coat, surrounded by manuscripts in preparation and, as the sulfonamides trials began, boxes of white mice.[21]

One day in October 1937, someone in Ewins's laboratory, possibly Newbery himself, noticed an old bottle sitting on the shelf. It turned out to be a sample of the base aminopyridine, prepared by a chemist named Eric Baines back in 1930 for another chemist who had since left the company. The sample had been moved from Wandsworth to Dagenham when the company relocated in 1934 and had stood on the shelf collecting dust ever since. Looking back two and a half decades later, company chemists, including Baines, agreed that it would have been very unlikely that this compound would have been prepared for use in the sulfanilamide derivatives program. But since it was there, "at the front of the third shelf on the left hand side of the cupboard," as another chemist, L.E. Hart, recalled, it was used. "Well, you know what would happen very much in those days," Baines remarked to company colleagues in 1961, "you would set out to try and make something, and you would find something on the shelf, and you would try it."[22]

On October 29, 1937, a laboratory assistant named Alexander, probably on the direction of Newbery, condensed the aminopyridine with acetanilide sulfonyl chloride. The result was a compound called acetyl sulfapyridine. Ordinarily in preparing sulfanilamide derivatives, the acetyl group would be removed with hydrochloric acid. Memories of laboratory workers differ on whether this was actually attempted. If it was, it failed, yielding merely sulfanilic acid. What is certain is that four days later, on November 2, Phillips successfully removed the acetyl using the unconventional sodium hydroxide, yielding sulfapyridine. The new compound was duly entered in the test book as T693.[23]

At this stage, it must be emphasized, T693 was nothing special, just another compound to be sent on to Whitby for animal trials. Chemists who were present in the May & Baker laboratories at the time or shortly thereafter recalled that when the first sample of T693 was sent to Whitby he was away from his laboratory, perhaps on holiday. Moreover, his laboratory was temporarily out of streptococcus-infected mice, the standard subjects for tests with sulfonamide compounds. In this situation, Whitby's assistant, acting on a hunch, decided to try T693 on mice with pneumococcal infections. Contrary to expectation, the first results were positive. So, too, were trials in mice with streptococcal, meningococcal, staphylococcal, and gonococcal infections.[24]

At some time in November or early December 1937, Ewins sent a sample of T693 to Richard Wien, a researcher at the Pharmacological Society in London, for toxicity tests. The report came back on December 23. It must have been favorable, for Ewins wrote to Wien a few days later thanking him and remarking that "this product becomes more and more interesting." "Interesting" was also the word used by Whitby to describe his first impressions of T693 to Ewins. In the meantime, one or more healthy members of the company research staff had swallowed T693 without ill effect.[25]

It is clear that by late December the May & Baker research team was beginning to focus its attention on T693 and that hopes were on the rise for the new compound. Still, it was by no means clear to them yet exactly what they were dealing with, either biologically or chemically. One incident is revealing. A sample of sulfapyridine prepared after the first one supplied by Phillips was found to have a melting point 7–8°C higher than Phillips's sample. Hart recalled that there was a big flap, and "we were virtually told that we hadn't made the right material." But then they found that Phillips, "in his inimitable way," had not done a thorough job in determining the melting point. The chemists were also concerned that later samples of sulfapyridine, not prepared with what one chemist called the "scruffy," impure sample of aminopyridine used by Phillips, although less toxic, would turn out to be therapeutically inactive. Fortunately, Whitby found that this was not the case.[26]

In January 1938, May & Baker production chemists, under technical manager R.W.E. Stickings, began working on the first larger batch of T693. Ron Welford, who was delegated much of the work, recalled that the first production equipment was improvised from whatever things were available around the works. For example, since the chemists lacked a vacuum still for distillation of aminopyridine, Welford carried out the distillation in one- or two-liter flasks in the semitechnical laboratory next to the research lab. "After much struggling," Welford remembered, "just over a kilogram of T693 emerged sometime in February." It came out "a glorious pink color." Unfortunately, it was supposed to be white. Stickings intervened, and further operations produced a liquid closer to the proper color and largely free of acetic acid. The chemists called this kilogram or so of T693 "Batch 1."[27]

By mid-February 1938, Ewins was convinced of the low toxicity of the compound and was talking of clinical trials. Sometime in March, a decision was made to give T693 to a human patient. The man selected was a Norfolk farm laborer thought to be near death from lobar pneumonia. Treated with T693 from Batch 1, his condition improved, and he went on to a full recovery.[28]

If there was any more doubt in the minds of Ewins and his staff, this cure must have ended it. The production chemists were asked to raise their output to the maximum that was feasible. From January to October 1938, they struggled with inadequate equipment, intermediates of low quality or insufficient quantity, and kinks in the production processes. In smoothing out the latter, they were helped by Rhône-Poulenc, which now entered the program to develop T693.

Both the difficulties faced by the chemists and the nature of the support provided by Rhône-Poulenc are illustrated by the development of one stage of the production process, the making of sodamide ($NaNH_2$). Sodamide was a key ingredient in the manufacture of M&B 693 since it was reacted with pyridine to yield 2-aminopyridine, which in turn was reacted with p-aminobenzenesulfonamide to form the immediate precursor of M&B 693.

At the time, in early 1938, sodamide was a laboratory chemical available only in small quantities. May & Baker's sole source was British Drug Houses Ltd. (BDH), a company that specialized in the production of laboratory chemicals. Sodamide was made by reacting ammonia gas with sodium according to the equation $2Na + 2NH_3 \rightarrow 2NaNH_2 + H_2$.

The reaction is straightforward but had to be carried out above the melting point of sodamide. Sodamide, moreover, is a dangerous substance that readily forms peroxides, which are explosive. May & Baker chemists thought that BDH had run the molten sodamide onto trays, cooled it, and then coarsely broken up the resulting solid. May & Baker received it from BDH in 500 g chunks that had to be roughly ground in a mortar and pestle before use.[29]

The challenge faced by May & Baker chemists was to design a plant in which sodamide could be safely manufactured in much larger quantities. The substance had to be obtained as a solid product of small particle size for reaction with pyridine, a reaction that took place in a solvent, toluene, in which sodamide had a negligible solubility. First efforts in the research laboratory resulted in a serious accident. Blockage of a pipe ejected molten sodium from the reaction, severely burning a chemist on the hands and face. May & Baker staff persisted and by the summer of 1938 had succeeded in constructing a small plant. Its centerpiece was a fifty-liter mild (i.e., relatively malleable) steel gas-heated vessel into which gaseous ammonia and nitrogen were fed through a distributor pipe. The vessel was charged with about twenty kilograms of sodium and heated to 400°C. At the same time, chemists fed in nitrogen gas, to maintain an inert atmosphere, and ammonia from a weighed cylinder to start the reaction. Exhaust gases—ammonia, hydrogen, and nitrogen (before the start of the reaction)—were fed to a water scrubber to remove the ammonia and to a gas meter to measure the hydrogen. When no more hydrogen was evolved, chemists took the reaction to be complete. They then inserted a dip pipe into the molten sodamide and blew it out onto a mild steel tray using nitrogen pressure.[30]

Once the sodamide had cooled below its melting point of 220°C and solidified, workers broke it up coarsely with a hammer and chisel. They then took the chunks and crushed them, a little at a time, between sheets of brown paper using a two-kilogram flat iron weight, producing a very coarse powder. Welford, who was closely involved, later reflected on the dangers of this stage of the work with some sense of disbelief. "Although we had no serious mishaps with this plant," he recalled, "minor fires and explosions were a daily occurrence." Another complication in the early development work derived from the paraffin wax coating on the sodium used for the reaction. The wax solidified in the pipework, and workers had to strip the pipes, heat them to melt the wax, flush them with water, and allow them to dry. "These operations resulted in a minor display of pyrotechnics," Welford recalled, "due to traces of sodium and sodium peroxide." Later, May & Baker was able to obtain supplies of sodium uncoated with wax.[31]

In the fall of 1938, this process was markedly improved as a result of information obtained from Rhône-Poulenc. The main innovation involved replacement of the original mild steel vessel by one fitted with a *raclant* (scraping) agitator. This was a device that was closely fitted to the bottom and sides of the containing vessel and that subjected any solid contained in the vessel to a shearing and grinding action. Working with information from the Rhône-Poulenc research chemist who had developed the process, May & Baker staff quickly designed and built a thirty-liter mild steel *raclant* vessel. This was charged with sodium and heated with a gas ring. After the sodium had melted, chemists passed ammonia gas down the hollow shaft of the agitator. After the reaction was complete, they allowed the sodamide to cool slowly. As it did so, it was ground to a coarse, crystalline, free-flowing powder by the agitator. This "extremely elegant solution," in Welford's words, was an immediate success. May & Baker engineers promptly designed a 100-liter *raclant* vessel, which was equally successful. The sodamide problem was solved.[32]

A footnote to this story reported by Jack Hodgson reveals that intracorporate communication was not always so efficient. Rhône-Poulenc had invented the *raclant* process and had used it extensively in the large-scale manufacture of acetic anhydride at their factory at St. Fons outside Lyon. St. Fons was also the site for Rhône-Poulenc's manufacture of sodamide and the sulfonamides. When the Rhône-Poulenc factory at Vitry outside Paris began to use sodamide in the manufacture of antihistamines, it developed its own process to make sodamide, evidently without knowledge of the *raclant* process used at St. Fons. A May & Baker employee visiting Vitry was horrified to find workers using a non-*raclant* process and using a pneumatic hammer to break the sodamide into lumps to be fed into a grinder. The upshot was that the Vitry plant wrote to May & Baker for details of the *raclant* process, which May & Baker had obtained from St. Fons. Apparently in this case, the distance from St. Fons to Vitry exceeded that from St. Fons to Dagenham.[33]

In March 1938, while the chemists were wrestling with sodamide and other problems, May & Baker made arrangements with physicians at Dudley Road Hospital in Birmingham to treat patients admitted for pneumonia with T693 over several months.[34]

Meanwhile, Whitby continued his animal trials of T693, publishing his first results in *Lancet* at the end of May. His conclusions were forthright and unequivocal: "These experiments represent the one striking success in the chemotherapy of pneumococcal infections in an assessment of no less than 64 related sulphanilamide compounds [all obtained from May & Baker]," he wrote. Not only did M&B 693 (as Whitby now referred to it) possess "great chemotherapeutic activity against pneumococci of several types," but it was also as effective as sulfanilamide against hemolytic streptococcal and meningococcal infections, and apparently of low toxicity.[35]

Publication of the first clinical trial followed five weeks later in *Lancet*. Between March and June 1938, G.M. Evans and Wilfrid F. Gaisford, physicians at Dudley Road Hospital in Birmingham, treated with M&B 693 about 100 patients suffering from lobar pneumonia; 100 other patients admitted with lobar pneumonia during the same period were given the conventional nonspecific treatment by other physicians. In the control group, the mortality was twenty-seven percent, a figure very close to the case mortality rate for lobar pneumonia in the same hospital in the preceding year and a half. In the treated group, the rate was eight percent.

Gaisford and Evans called this "a striking fall in mortality" and hoped that others would confirm their findings.[36]

Whitby continued his animal tests, and the company made arrangements for further clinical trials. In the eyes of May & Baker executives, however, enough was already known to justify making the new compound generally available to doctors. In October 1938, M&B 693 went on the British market under the trade name Dagenan. Great pressure was placed on the company's production team, which put its first plant in operation in October. By the end of the year, May & Baker had licensed Merck to make and distribute sulfapyridine in the United States, which it did in time for the pneumonia outbreak that winter.[37]

Treatment of Pneumonia before Chemotherapy

When M&B 693 came on the medical scene, pneumonia was still among the most common and most deadly of diseases caused by bacteria, claiming tens of thousands of lives each year in Britain and the United States alone. Not for nothing had Osler dubbed it "Captain of the Men of Death" in the 1901 edition of his textbook of medicine. It is hard to improve on Harry F. Dowling's description of the typical course of pneumonia as observed by the clinician:

> Lobar pneumonia, the most characteristic form of this disease, usually begins dramatically with a chill or sharp pain in the chest. Cough is an early symptom, and the sputum is likely to be pink, red, or otherwise dis-colored by the presence of blood. Following the chill, the temperature rises as high as 104–105°F and, in the absence of specific therapy, re-mains high for several days. During this time the patient is miserable. He breathes rapidly and coughs frequently; each breath and each cough may cause a sharp pain in the chest, resulting from inflammation of the pleu-ral covering of the lung. With the high fever goes a flushed face, hot, dry skin, and mental dullness that sometimes proceeds to delirium. After five to ten days, sometimes more, the fever subsides, either rapidly or over the course of two or three days. Complications are frequent; especially serious are meningitis, endocarditis, or inflammation of the inner lining of the heart, and empyema, or pus in the pleural cavity. The other variety of pneumonia, bronchopneumonia, affects one or more localized areas in the lungs rather than entire lobes and occurs particularly in elderly persons or as a complication of other diseases. Although its onset is less dramatic and its symptoms less pronounced, it is just as likely to be fatal as lobar pneumonia.[38]

By 1938, physicians believed that they had a full causal picture of the disease but decades of research had yielded therapeutic measures of only limited utility. The pneumococcus bacterium was first recognized in 1881 and in the following years gradually came to be seen as the pathogen primarily responsible for pneu-monia, although other kinds of bacteria could also be involved. Attempts to in-duce immunity to pneumococcal pneumonia began in the 1890s, and physicians used vaccines for prevention with uncertain results at least through the 1920s. Vaccines were also occasionally used on a hit-and-miss basis as treatments for pneumonia, but this practice never established either a theoretical or an experimental justification.[39]

In 1897, researchers at the Pasteur Institute in Paris recognized that there was more than one kind of pneumococcus, and by 1913 other workers in Germany and the United States had divided all pneumococci into type I, type II, type III, and a miscellaneous set named group IV. By 1932, medical researchers recognized thirty-two types of pneumococcus, among which types I, II, and III were generally the most fatal.[40]

Typing of pneumococci opened the way for preparation of antipneumococcal serums according to the principles of passive immunization defined by Emil von Behring in the 1890s. Serums were prepared by removing blood from animals infected with a specific bacterium and separating the blood's fluid component from the cells contained in it. The fluid, or serum, contained antibodies produced by the animal in response to the infection. When administered to a human infected by the same type of bacterium, the antibody-containing serum assisted the patient in resisting the infection.

One of the first to venture into this territory was Rufus Cole, the first director of the hospital attached to the Rockefeller Institute for Medical Research in New York. When the hospital opened in 1910, Cole decided to devote most attention to pneumonia as "the most serious acute disease with which physicians have to deal." Cole's research group took the lead in typing efforts and in 1913 reported treatment of patients with type I and type II serums. For the next two decades, Cole and other researchers, with the assistance of commercial firms including the U.S. company Lederle Laboratories, labored to improve the quality of antipneumococcal serums and methods of diagnosis and administration.[41]

Despite these efforts, progress was slow. By the mid-1930s, an effective serum was available only for use against the type I pneumococcus, which was responsible for about thirty percent of all pneumonia cases. Even for type I serum, treatment was hedged with difficulties. To be most effective, diagnosis and treatment had to be done as quickly as possible. The physician had to be trained in typing techniques, and results had to be correctly interpreted. Whitby participated in a study of pneumococcal pneumonia published in 1935 that identified three possible sources of error: (1) a case might be diagnosed as pneumococcal pneumonia but later develop a streptococcal complication; (2) a case might be diagnosed from a sputum sample as due to one pneumococcal type and later be determined to be due to a different type; or (3) the pneumonic process might be found to be due to more than one type in a single patient. Even if typing was done correctly, the doctor needed to be trained to administer the appropriate serum and had to have the necessary equipment on hand. Adverse reactions due to hypersensitivity might occur and could be severe or fatal. Finally, the expense of serum therapy discouraged its widespread use.[42]

Whatever the problems and difficulties, serum therapy could have its rewards. Recounting his days as an intern at the Boston City Hospital in the 1930s, Lewis Thomas recalled that serum treatment "could turn out a technological *tour de force*, the only genuine cure within an intern's grasp. . . . When it worked, it worked within an hour or two. Down came the temperature, and the patient, who might have been moribund a few hours earlier, would now be sleeping in good health." In a typical city hospital in the United States, pneumonia mortality rates dropped from around thirty percent for patients receiving no specific treatment to around seventeen percent for those given serum. To meet problems of cost and administration, state programs began to be set up, starting with Massachusetts in 1931. In 1939, the federal government began to provide support for these programs.[43]

In contrast, the search for an effective chemotherapy for pneumonia was littered with failures. Whole bile or sodium salts of bile acids, soaps, coal tar dyes, metals and metallic salts, epinephrine, camphor, formaldehyde sulfoxylate, potassium permanganate, and other agents had all been tried without success. Most promising were the quinine derivatives such as optochin (ethylhydrocupreine) first introduced by Joseph Morgenroth and his associates in the 1910s. But even these had proved too toxic at effective dosages for routine therapeutic use.[44]

Other failed or at best problematic therapeutic measures sometimes undertaken in pneumonia included morphine, oxygen therapy, sodium chloride replacement, digitalis, quinine, alcohol, diathermy (heating of the lungs above the temperature of the rest of body), and artificial pneumothorax (deliberate collapse of the affected lung to rest it, relieve pain, and promote healing). Of more assured value, though lacking dramatic effect, were rest and reassurance.[45]

On the eve of the introduction of sulfapyridine, then, leading medical researchers in Britain and the United States recognized serum treatment, especially of type I pneumonia, as the only proven specific therapy available. Beset with difficulties as it was, even serum therapy had yet to dissipate "the doubts which linger in many a medical mind," as Benjamin White pointed out in his 1938 textbook, and its widespread application was just being consolidated by the establishment of state programs in the United States. Against a background of previous failures, both White and Cole wrote hopefully but vaguely of the promise of chemotherapy.[46]

Reception by Physicians

In this context, it is hardly surprising that M&B 693 was enthusiastically embraced by many physicians, and increasingly also by the public, which began to hear of "miracle cures" by the wonderful new drug. Between the summer of 1938, when May & Baker began to distribute M&B 693 to selected clinicians, and June 1939, by which time the new drug had been on the market for eight months, use of M&B 693 in treatment of pneumonia expanded dramatically. It began to be studied and used in treatment of other bacterial infections, including, most notably, gonorrhea and cerebrospinal meningitis. Already in August 1938, a *British Medical Journal* editorial included M&B 693 in a review of the "specific rapid curative effect" on gonorrhea exercised by the sulfonamides, an effect "so striking as to make older forms of treatment appear by comparison almost futile." Clinical investigations, followed by favorable reports, continued through the next eight months. Surveying the accumulated evidence in April 1939, a group from the Aberdeen Public Health Service concluded that M&B 693 "has proved the most effective therapeutic agent yet introduced in the treatment of gonorrhea."[47]

In June 1939, W.J. Roche and C.J. McSweeney, two physicians at the Cork Street Hospital in Dublin, reported on their experience with use of M&B 693 in treatment of cerebrospinal meningitis. In patients two years old or younger, the "classical" mortality for this disease was more than seventy-five percent, a figure not much improved upon by serum therapy. Roche and McSweeney wrote that combined use of serum and sulfanilamide had reduced mortality in this group to fifty-seven percent. Starting in October 1938, they had replaced sulfanilamide with M&B 693 and had subsequently recorded a mortality of sixteen percent. At Dudley Road Hospital in Birmingham, site of the earliest clinical trial of M&B 693, use of the new medicine became routine in treatment of pneumonia in August 1938. Under the new regimen, mortality dropped to six and one-half percent, compared to twenty-two to twenty-three percent for 1936 and 1937 and for the patients not treated with M&B 693 in 1938.[48]

Doctors had reason for enthusiasm, but in the eyes of some researchers and practitioners the headlong rush to embrace M&B 693 and other sulfa drugs could be precipitous and even dangerous. Some of the earliest warning notes with regard to M&B 693 came in connection with its use in treatment of gonorrhea. The same August 1938 editorial in the *British Medical Journal* that welcomed the addition of M&B 693 to existing chemotherapies cautioned that "it is still by no means certain, however, which of the available compounds is the most effective, or how it should be used." The availability of sulfa drugs over the counter combined with the tendency of gonorrhea patients to self-medicate drew a sharp response from the journal:

No more potent drugs than these have ever been placed in the hands of ambulant patients, and none whose self-administration is fraught with more disadvantage and danger have been available for sale without prescription. It is very necessary that patients instructed to take them should be impressed with the absolute necessity for following directions exactly, and it is even more necessary that indiscriminate sale should be prohibited.[49]

In November 1938, Whitby welcomed the impending prohibition of direct sale of sulfanilamide to the lay public and noted that this medicine had been "used by an experimentally minded profession for many diseases concerning which little or no controlled experimental work is available or possible." Similarly, Whitby pointed out that "the complete field of activity is as yet unexplored, and it would be hasty to claim too much before M&B 693 has passed that proper phase of clinical assessment which it undoubtedly deserves."[50]

The same kinds of reservations were brought forward again in a March 1939 discussion in the Royal Society of Medicine on the treatment of pneumonia. Maurice Davidson conceded the value of M&B 693 but felt moved "to make some protest against the indiscriminate use of this and other preparations of the sulphanilamide group." Davidson maintained that "apart from the fact that wholesale administration of such drugs in various febrile conditions, without a certain diagnosis and without scientific control, was wrong in principle, . . . a risk might be entailed of damage to vital organs of the body." In particular, he suggested that "it seemed likely a priori that a drug sufficiently potent to deal effectively with a virulent organism must be capable of damaging possibly the renal epithelium or even the myocardium."[51]

In reply, H.L. Tidy, the Section of Medicine's president, acknowledged the force of Davidson's criticism and extended it: "The 'wild use' of these drugs in general practice was," he thought, "largely due to the travelers [detail men, sales representatives of pharmaceutical companies] who went round visiting doctors." Most cases, Tidy believed, "were now receiving sulphonamide preparations in one form or another," and "they were undoubtedly given uselessly, and there were likely to be cases in which they were to some extent harmful." Finally, Tidy conceded, there was the possibility that these medicines might produce serious aftereffects. All this admitted, Tidy pointed out that passage of time had not confirmed long-term damage. The same point was made by Whitby, who remarked that although "there must have been tons of these drugs [sulfonamides] used (or abused) by now," nevertheless "there had been no widely advertised coroner's inquests."[52]

In the context of a generally positive evaluation of the use of M&B 693 in gonorrhea, the Aberdeen Public Health Service team remarked:

> That M & B 693 is a remarkable drug cannot be questioned. What may be, and probably will be, debated for some time is how best to employ it: early during gonorrhea or later on in the disease; in short intensive courses, single or multiple, or by more prolonged, easy-going methods; with or without urethral lavage, or perhaps with or in alteration with some other forms of adjuvant treatment yet to be devised; how long it should be given to apparently resistant cases before trying some other method of treatment, and so on.[53]

In the case of gonorrhea alone, assessment of M&B 693 was only beginning.

One problem in need of clarification was the relation of established serum therapies to the new chemotherapy. The issue surfaced in the March 1939 discussion of recent advances in the treatment of pneumonia in the Royal Society of Medicine. G.J. Langley, who had pursued clinical research on serum treatments of pneumonia for the preceding five years, regarded M&B 693 as possibly promising but also as something that could potentially complicate diagnosis and serum treatment. Referring to the "high grade of efficiency" attained in state serum treatment programs in the United States, he called for similar statistical scrutiny of M&B 693. That events were already proceeding in a different direction was indicated by Gaisford's remarks in the same discussion. Gaisford stated that, following clinical trials at Dudley Road Hospital in Birmingham in the spring and early summer of 1938, use of M&B 693 had been made routine in treatment of pneumonia beginning in August. A similar conversion was described in June 1939 by Roche and McSweeney of Dublin's Cork Street Hospital, who since 1937 had overseen the changeover from serum therapy to combined serum therapy and M&B 693 in cases of cerebrospinal meningitis in young children. Such experience appears to have been sufficient to convince practitioners in advance of evidence from rigorous statistical studies.[54]

While M&B 693 was beginning to replace serum treatments for pneumonia and other acute infectious diseases through the middle of 1939, question marks continued to hang over the new medicine. Alexander Fleming raised the issue of potential acquired resistance to the drug by pathogenic bacteria. More immediately pressing was the matter of toxicity. In November 1938, Whitby judged animal trials to have shown M&B 693 to be "extremely non-toxic" and that limited clinical trials had shown no toxic effects in humans apart from the relatively mild ones of cyanosis, nausea, and occasional vomiting. Doctors in Edinburgh trying M&B 693 in 102 cases of gonorrhea reported in December 1938 that, along with a high percentage of apparent cures, they observed mild toxic effects, including headache, nausea, dizziness, skin eruption, lassitude, and cyanosis in less than a third of the cases, and that these symptoms responded to reduction of dosage. Similarly, the Aberdeen Public Health Service team studying treatment of gonorrhea with M&B 693 described only minor toxic reactions that subsided rapidly on withdrawal of the drug.[55]

In the midst of this cautious optimism on the part of British researchers, a cloud appeared in the form of a preliminary report on sulfapyridine—the generic name assigned to M&B 693 in the United States—by Council on Pharmacy and Chemistry of the American Medical Association (AMA). A *British Medical Journal* editorial in late March 1939 summarized the AMA report as asserting that

> there is sufficient evidence of [sulfapyridine's] value in pneumonia to warrant further trials under controlled conditions, but not to justify general use or the abandonment of serum treatment; that such trials should also embrace staphylococcal and Friedländer's bacillus infections; and that there is no evidence of the superiority of the drug over sulphanilamide for treating infections by haemolytic streptococci, meningococci, gonococci, or *Cl. welchii.*

While the *British Medical Journal* editorial faulted the Americans for being unduly cautious and predicted a full recognition of the value of sulfapyridine in pneumonia in the United States, it conceded the need for careful observations on a more extensive scale than heretofore. The editorial admitted the full force of the AMA report's claim that pharmacological investigation of sulfapyridine had been neglected, and in particular that Eli Kennerly Marshall, Jr.'s experimental findings had demonstrated wide variation in the absorption of the drug from the alimentary tract. The editorial also asserted that Marshall's findings on toxicity using the highly soluble sodium salt of the compound "must be held to supersede English results, which are undoubtedly vitiated by failure to take into account the factor of incomplete absorption." In March 1939, the Medical Research Council's Therapeutic Trials Committee concluded that more clinical study of M&B 693 was needed.[56]

American criticisms of M&B 693 came as no surprise to Ewins, who had begun consulting with pharmacologist Wien as early as January 1939 on how to respond to Marshall's published remarks. Nevertheless, he and others closely involved in the research must have been stung by the editorial rebuke in the British medical press. In the Royal Society of Medicine discussion on pneumonia just three days after publication of the *British Medical Journal* editorial, Whitby, without referring explicitly to American attacks, reported that he was doing, and advocated doing, more of the kind of coordinated laboratory and clinical studies of M&B 693, taking into account absorption efficiency and so on, that Marshall had called for.[57]

In a letter to the *British Medical Journal* just two weeks after the appearance of its editorial, Ewins conceded that much remained to be learned about the fate of M&B 693 in the body but faulted Marshall for his reliance on the highly soluble sodium salt of the compound in his assessment of toxicity. It was precisely the sparing solubility of the original drug that was its own safeguard, Ewins maintained. Ewins also responded sharply to the Americans on the comparison of M&B 693 and sulfanilamide, arguing that since M&B 693 had a wider range of activity, it should be the preferred medicine "for empirical use in clinically probable acute coccal infections," that is, in cases in which a rapid bacteriological diagnosis was not possible.[58]

Ewins's letter drew its own response from Paul Gross and Frank B. Cooper, investigators at the Western Pennsylvania Hospital. Gross and Cooper rejected Ewins's claim that animal experiments had shown M&B 693 to be harmless, pointing to their own on rats that demonstrated the formation of urinary calculi with partial or complete urinary obstruction, resulting in hematuria or even death. The animal results deserved serious attention, they insisted, since clinical observation of hematuria following treatment with M&B 693 had already been reported.[59]

Setting a Pattern for Regulation

In the United States, the reception of sulfapyridine was enmeshed from the beginning with government efforts to formulate regulatory policy in line with recent passage of the federal Food, Drug, and Cosmetic Act of 1938. Indeed, how the U.S. Food and Drug Administration (FDA) handled sulfapyridine, the first important new drug to be considered under the 1938 Act, set the pattern for the FDA's subsequent regulation of new drugs until 1950.[60]

As far as medicinal drugs were concerned, the 1938 Food, Drug, and Cosmetic Act resulted from a conjunction of longstanding efforts by therapeutic reformers within the medical and scientific community, the political environment of the New Deal, and a fatal calamity in the autumn of 1937 that dramatized the need for stricter controls on new drugs.

Desire for therapeutic reform, including reform of drug therapy, existed in the American medical community in the nineteenth century. Only in 1905, however, did the AMA create the Council on Pharmacy and Chemistry (CPC) that would attempt to regulate medicinal drugs and their promotions. Composed largely of academics involved in pharmaceutical research, the CPC represented specialists and educators rather than ordinary practicing physicians. It published a column in the *Journal of the American Medical Association* (*JAMA*) in which it made known its judgments on products submitted by manufacturers. It reviewed each drug for chemical composition, validity of therapeutic claims, and advertising. Each year, it published its New and Nonofficial Remedies, in which approved drugs were listed.[61]

In its evaluations of medicinal drugs, the CPC relied on chemical analysis, animal experimentation, and clinical investigations. The last of these proved to be the most problematic. Often, it was not possible to get competent clinical study of a drug by qualified investigators. In practice, the CPC often relied instead on the opinions of a few investigators it deemed able. A more serious constraint on realization of CPC goals was the difficulty faced by the experimental ideal where it counted most, in the practices of physicians. Faced with overriding pressures to attract and retain patients, most physicians followed their own inclinations regarding drug therapy, whether or not these were in line with CPC judgments. Nevertheless, reformers' optimism persisted, sustained by the support of an academic elite, a firm association in their minds between science and morality, and distrust of the influence of commercial interests on medicine.[62]

Beginning in the late 1920s, therapeutic reform took another direction. In the context of a widespread emphasis on cooperative research in the United States during and after World War I, studies were undertaken that enlisted the joint efforts of specialists at institutions across the nation, or of practitioners within a state. Advocates of cooperative studies touted the advantages of considering large numbers of patients, of joining the judgments of veteran investigators, and of standardizing methods of selecting and treating patients and for analyzing outcomes. Despite those apparent advantages, however, cooperative clinical studies were beset with problems, including uneven success in mobilizing stable financial support, lack of or failure to devise adequate organizational forms and practices, and persistent gaps between researchers and the great majority of practicing physicians.[63]

Field studies of serum treatment for lobar pneumonia supported by the Commonwealth Fund between 1938 and 1940 exemplify some of the problems. The aim of these investigations was to determine whether, in spite of the difficulties and costs of serum therapy for pneumonia, it would be worthwhile for state governments to manufacture and distribute serum to doctors, especially general practitioners, and whether general practitioners could be induced to use serum therapy. Results of two major programs, one run by the Massachusetts Department of Public Health and the other administered by the New York State Medical Society, were mixed. But the net effect in both cases was that most physicians did not adopt serum therapy for pneumonia. Serum treatment remained predominantly the domain of the hospital-based urban practitioners. Most other physicians feared not only toxic reactions to serum treatment but also damage to their relationships with their patients if they recommended the costly treatment and it failed. As in the case of the Cooperative Clinical Group study of syphilis, the Commonwealth Fund field studies of serum treatment for pneumonia foundered on failure to close the gap between elite therapeutic reformers and the majority of practitioners.[64]

Nearly coincident in time with early efforts at therapeutic reform was the passage of legislation establishing the first federal regulation of drugs. The Biologics Control Act of 1902 directed the Public Health Service's Hygienic Laboratory to oversee "biologics," that is, pharmaceutical products derived from living organisms, including serums and vaccines. The Pure Food and Drug Act of 1906 authorized regulators in the Department of Agriculture to take action against medicines judged to be adulterated or misbranded. In practice, both acts were of limited effect. Hygienic Laboratory officials could move decisively when able to make judgments on the basis of laboratory findings, but were reluctant to intercede if it was the clinical value of a product alone that was in question. Those enforcing the Pure Food and Drug Act could take action against a product only after it was on the market, had no authority over advertising, and were severely hampered in court cases by the need to prove fraudulent intent on the part of those they prosecuted.[65]

The inadequacy of the 1906 law was long keenly felt by those responsible for enforcing it, but until the coming of Franklin D. Roosevelt's administration in 1933, no serious revision of the law was ever considered by Congress. Roosevelt's new Assistant Secretary of Agriculture, Rexford G. Tugwell, backed a stronger drug law, and New York Senator Royal S. Copeland was persuaded to sponsor the measure. First introduced in 1933, the bill went through several versions, as the medicinal drug industry lobbied to reduce the powers invested in regulators while consumer groups attacked even the original version as too weak, and administration officials struggled to ensure that something useful, if not ideal, made its way into law.[66]

Passage of a stronger replacement for the 1906 law was delayed by several circumstances. Tugwell was perceived by many as a socialistically inclined wild man. Roosevelt's support for food and drug reform, though real, was not vigorous and tended to be overshadowed by other priorities. That part of industry opposing a strong bill lobbied more effectively than did consumer groups supporting one. Newspapers and national magazines felt pressure from advertisers of foods, drugs, and cosmetics, putting a damper on muckraking zeal. An attempt to pass a bill in 1936 died in part due to conflict over whether the FDA or the Federal Trade Commission (FTC) should have control over food, drug, and cosmetic advertising. In the midst of economic depression and more dramatic federal programs, Americans were not easily excited by drug reform.[67]

Not until 1938 did the House of Representatives again vote on a comprehensive food and drug bill. In the meantime, three of the obstacles to a new law had been reduced or eliminated. Tugwell had resigned as Assistant Secretary of Agriculture to take a job in private industry. The FDA–FTC dispute was settled in favor of the FTC. And public interest in drug reform was inflamed by a fatal incident with a new product introduced in the fall of 1937 that dramatically exposed the weakness of the 1906 law.[68]

By mid-1937, Americans had embraced sulfanilamide. As if to make up for delayed recognition of the drug's powers, demand soared, reinforced by reports that sulfanilamide could cure gonorrhea. At least 100 companies marketed proprietary brands of sulfanilamide, all in solid form. Rewards beckoned for the company that could find a way to put the relatively insoluble compound into liquid form for those patients, especially children, who had difficulty taking the solid medicine. A chemist employed by the S.E. Massengill Company of Bristol, Tennessee, thought that he had found the desired solvent. Harold Cole Watkins mixed his solvent with sulfanilamide, water, and several substances added for flavor, scent, and color, and the company marketed the resulting product, dubbed Elixir Sulfanilamide, on September 4, 1937.[69]

On October 11, the AMA in Chicago received telegrams from physicians in Tulsa, Oklahoma, reporting deaths of six patients who had taken Elixir Sulfanilamide. The AMA replied that no solution of sulfanilamide had been approved by the CPC. From the S.E. Massengill Company, the AMA learned that the solvent was diethylene glycol. Tests in the AMA's chemical laboratory quickly confirmed the compound's identity, and animal experiments confirmed its toxicity. Reports of deaths from Elixir Sulfanilamide in St. Louis indicated that the problem was not confined to Tulsa. On October 18, the editor of *JAMA* issued a warning to the public over radio and newspaper.[70]

Word of the fatalities in Tulsa first reached the FDA on October 14. An FDA agent reached Tulsa the next day and on October 16 confirmed the deaths. The FDA immediately ordered seizure of all outstanding shipments of Elixir Sulfanilamide and started a massive effort, coordinated with state and local officials, to recover all of the remaining preparation. Most of the FDA's field force of 239 inspectors and chemists took part, tracking Elixir Sulfanilamide through dealers, wholesalers, retailers, druggists, and doctors, and ultimately to the patients themselves. When they made their final accounting, officials found that of the 240 gallons manufactured, eleven gallons and six pints had been dispensed by prescription or over the counter, and that of this amount, about half was consumed and caused the 107 deaths that eventually resulted.[71]

Death from Elixir Sulfanilamide poisoning was not quick or easy. The Secretary of Agriculture reported that "the victims of the 'elixir' were ill from about seven to twenty-one days. They suffered intense pain. All exhibited very much the same symptoms: stoppage of urine, severe abdominal pain, nausea and vomiting, and stupor; convulsions preceded death in some cases." Many of the victims were children.[72]

When questioned by federal agents, the Massengill chemist Watkins disclosed that his working formula for Elixir Sulfanilamide was as follows:

Sulfanilamide	58 pounds
Elixir flavor	1 gallon
Raspberry extract	1 pint
Saccharin soluble	1 pound
Amaranth solution 1/16	1 pints
Caramel	2 fluid ounces
Diethylene glycol	60 gallons
Water, q.s.	80 gallons

Watkins stated that he thought that glycols were well known not to be toxic. Glycols as a class were widely used for commercial purposes, for example, as antifreezes, to lower the freezing point of dynamite, and as solvents. Diethylene glycol was not ideal as an antifreeze, since it could dissolve a car's paint on contact. It was used as a humectant for tobacco and other products.[73]

What Watkins did not know but should have known was that for several years the FDA had advised against the use of glycol solvents in foods, that the principal manufacturer of diethylene glycol discouraged its use in food or drugs, and that the toxicity of diethylene glycol had been reported in medical journals. Watkins had done no toxicity tests of his own, an omission that was, unfortunately, routine. One exasperated FDA agent reported that "the most amazing thing about the company was the total lack of testing facilities. Apparently they just throw drugs together, and if they don't explode they are placed on sale."[74]

As the deaths mounted through October and November, so too did fear and anger. One of the more focused responses came from the leadership of the AMA. Even before diethylene glycol was confirmed to be the toxic agent, a *JAMA* editorial characterized Elixir Sulfanilamide as "a preparation not standardized by any reliable agency, semisecret in composition and apparently hastily rushed into the market to meet an overenthusiastic reception of a new remedy." By October 30, *JAMA* was calling the unfolding events "the most unfortunate incident in the pharmaceutical industry within the last decade" and was looking to Congress for more comprehensive and effective legislation.[75]

A week later, on November 6, *JAMA* editorialized in even stronger terms, distributing blame among manufacturers, detail men, pharmacists, and physicians. The writer conceded that the FDA could not be faulted, since "under our present laws . . . [the FDA] is as inefficiently armed as a hunter pursuing a tiger with a fly swatter." Manufacturers were most culpable, *JAMA* asserted, for their willingness to put on the market "semisecret preparations, untested as to either toxicity, potency, or therapeutic value." Second in line, the editorial continued, were those physicians who ignored repeated warnings—those of the AMA's CPC were meant—against the use of such preparations. The editorialist concluded bitterly that "surely there has been no blacker picture of the inadequacy of our present food and drug laws or the lack of common scientific decency in drug manufacture than that illustrated by this tragic disaster" and warned of future disasters if laws were not strengthened.[76]

On December 11, in the same issue that printed the Secretary of Agriculture's report on Elixir Sulfanilamide, *JAMA* backed the report's recommendations for stronger drug control laws. These included prohibition of drugs shown to be dangerous when used as recommended by the manufacturer, licensing of new drugs after they had been proved safe for use, a requirement that drug labels have directions for use and warnings about misuse, and a prohibition of secret remedies by a requirement that labels "disclose fully the composition of drugs."[77]

High public interest and the sense of urgency now felt by many in the medical establishment were not sufficient to push through new legislation. Several months of lobbying and compromises, resolution of the FDA–FTC dispute on regulation of advertising, and clarification of the process of court appeal in relation to FDA regulations were necessary before Congress could pass the new law. When it was enacted on June 25, 1938, however, the Federal Food, Drug, and

Cosmetic Act contained a provision for the safety of new drugs that responded directly to the dangers thrown into sharp relief by the Elixir Sulfanilamide disaster. Under Section 505 of the law, manufacturers were required to demonstrate to the FDA the safety of any new drug offered for sale in interstate commerce. Applications for new drugs had to include samples, full information on composition and manufacture, specimen of labeling, and reports of investigations made to assess safety.[78]

In developing its procedures and practices for implementation of the new law, the FDA drew heavily on the methods for evaluation of medicinal drugs developed by therapeutic reformers over several decades, including laboratory screening, clinical investigation, and use of expert consultants. In the first eighteen months of the law, the FDA received almost 1,700 new drug applications. Most were not problematic, given the preliminary screening and informational requirements of the law. Difficulties arose in the cases of medicines of known therapeutic efficacy that could be dangerous if used inappropriately. A prime example of the latter category was sulfanilamide, the potential toxicity of which was well known before the Food, Drug, and Cosmetic Act went into effect. In the summer and fall of 1938, the FDA and drug manufacturers worked out principles for the labeling of sulfanilamide that would go far toward preventing its "indiscriminate use by the lay public."[79]

The new law went into effect in June 1938 just as the first reports of M&B 693 were beginning to appear in the British medical and popular press. Sulfapyridine—the generic name was favored in the United States—was an obvious candidate for FDA review. The first application for sulfapyridine, from Merck, reached administration officials on October 7, 1938. Acting partly on the advice of Perrin H. Long at Johns Hopkins, the FDA asked Merck for more data. By December, officials were satisfied with animal toxicological results but regarded existing clinical data as insufficient to determine mode of administration and other conditions under which sulfapyridine would produce toxic effects such as nausea and vomiting.[80]

Despite these uncertainties, some researchers, including early skeptics Perrin Long and Marshall, had concluded by the end of December that sulfapyridine should be released to the medical profession. Through January and February, the FDA consulted with clinical investigators working with sulfapyridine. Some, including the AMA's CPC and *JAMA* editor Morris Fishbein, thought that the drug should be held back pending further clinical investigation. Others thought that enough evidence of benefit was already available and that patterns of toxicity would take a long time to establish. Support for sulfapyridine in the popular press and the urgencies of the winter pneumonia season created additional pressure for release. On March 9, 1939, the FDA notified the six companies by then awaiting its decision that it would not reject their applications. Approval came with the stipulation that labeling and advertising be designed to make clear the necessity for physician supervision and that manufacturers make physicians aware of sulfapyridine's toxicity and its management.[81]

Sulfapyridine set the initial pattern for FDA review and oversight of problematic new drugs under the 1938 law. The administration would confine itself to determining that a new drug was safe when used appropriately. It would not attempt to regulate physicians' practice. It would rely on manufacturers for extensive information on laboratory and clinical testing, on the medical research community for independent assessment of a new drug's value, and on practicing physicians to regulate their own use of the drug in practice.[82]

"There Seemed to Be No End to Its Uses"

In the United States, the divergence between cautious researchers and enthusiastic physicians and patients was, if anything, more pronounced than it was in Britain. A reading of *JAMA* from February to May 1939 leaves the impression that the use of sulfapyridine by American physicians quickly outran the measured pace that the CPC or cautious investigators such as Long would have preferred to follow. In publishing a special report summarizing opinions on sulfapyridine that it had collected from physicians with some experience with the drug in May 1939, the AMA conceded that it did so "in the absence of clinical reports giving detailed information on the drug in the treatment of pneumonia, and because of its importance in present day therapy in pneumonia." While admitting the usefulness of sulfapyridine, the May special report cautioned physicians about the many uncertainties that remained with regard to toxicity and the circumstances in which continued use of serum therapy might be called for. But these warnings came in the context of rapidly expanding use. Despite the CPC's hesitations, the floodgates had been opened. By May 1939, *JAMA* was overwhelmed with papers submitted by physicians wanting to report their experiences with sulfapyridine.[83]

By November 1939, eighteen months after Whitby's first publication, sulfapyridine had been used to treat thousands of cases of pneumonia in many countries. An article in the *British Medical Journal* reviewing the literature concluded that "it is now established that sulfapyridine is a most effective agent against infections by pneumococci of all types" and "an outstanding medical advance." The article stated that the relative value of sulfapyridine in most other bacterial infections compared to other sulfonamides remained to be determined but noted that it was already shown to be the most effective of the sulfas against gonorrhea.[84]

From the time that Whitby did his first mouse trials of T693 in 1938 to Churchill's cure in 1943, sulfapyridine was tried in the treatment of many kinds of human bacterial infections. The *British Medical Journal* reported trials in meningitis of several varieties (pneumococcal, staphylococcal, meningococcal), Pfeiffer's bacillus (*Haemophilus influenzae* type b), in pneumococcal peritonitis, in human anthrax, in bacterial endocarditis, in gas gangrene, in cerebrospinal fever, in acute bacillary dysentery, in suppurative otitis media, and in corneal ulcers. Tests of M&B 693 in gonorrhea had begun by the summer of 1938, and by June 1941 sulfapyridine treatment of gonorrhea was routine in the British army. As one harried production chemist who had rushed to meet the early demand recalled, "there seemed to be no end to its uses." [85]

A product of industrial invention, sulfapyridine was an early representative of the generation of sulfa drugs that followed on the introduction of Prontosil and

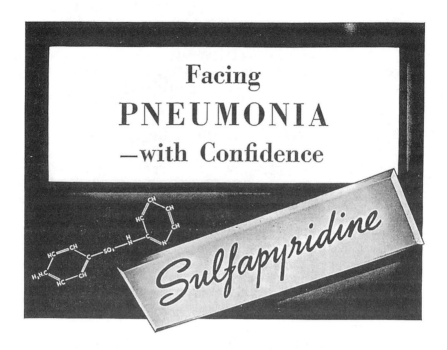

THIS year the physician has been able to view pneumonia with a degree of confidence that was impossible in the past. The striking therapeutic results obtained with sulfapyridine in pneumococcic pneumonia have profoundly altered the prognosis in this disease.

An analysis of more than 3,000 cases of typed pneumococcic pneumonia treated with sulfapyridine during the winter of 1938-39 showed the following case fatality rates:

Total No. of Cases	3,005
Gross Fatality	6.0%
No. of Bacteriemic Cases	240
Fatality	23.3%
No. of Non-bacteriemic Cases	2,765
Fatality	4.5%

During the pneumonia season of 1939-40 this clinical experience was duplicated in a large number of cases. A statistical review† of 9,162 cases revealed that the fatality rate in pneumonia patients treated with sulfapyridine was less than half that obtained with previous methods of treatment.

With wider dissemination of knowledge concerning this remarkable drug and its more widespread use, it is to be expected that the fatality rate from pneumococcic pneumonia throughout the nation will be reduced to a new low level during the current pneumonia season.

†Faller, C. P., Quickel, K. E., and Smith, C. W., Penn. M. J. 43:789-800, March, 1940

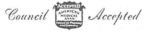

Council **Accepted**

Figure 7.3. Merck advertisement that appeared in *Journal of the American Medical Association* and other American medical journals in 1941 (reprinted courtesy of the Merck Archives).

sulfanilamide. Greeted with some caution by medical researchers, especially in the United States, where the views of therapeutic reformers were influential and where new drug legislation had been recently introduced, it was enthusiastically embraced by most physicians and patients. That this could be so was due in part to the warm reception it received beyond the circles of medical research and practice.

CHAPTER 8

Acclaim and Expansion

Behind the rising demand for M&B 693 in Britain lay not only favorable medical reports but also publicity in newspapers, magazines, and other media that began early and that loudly proclaimed the virtues of the new medicine. A sampling of British newspapers and magazines, particularly in the twenty months following publication of the first clinical trial in June 1938, conveys some sense of what the public was told about the meaning of the discovery, its import for the future of medicine, and the hows and whys of innovation in medical research. Also visible in the press accounts are the extent to which representation of the discovery for a lay audience incorporated reservations or cautions voiced by medical researchers, the likely role of popular demand in speeding the marketing of the new drug, the rapid diffusion of use of the new drug to distant sites including Africa, and the prominent role perceived for M&B 693 in the early war effort.[1]

The success of sulfapyridine that was reflected in, and reinforced by, its reception in the popular press also gave a powerful impetus to the expansion of research and development efforts in the international pharmaceutical industry. This expansion was under way before World War II, was accelerated by the war, and continued in the postwar decades. Its beginnings are visible in the histories of May & Baker in Britain and of Merck and Sharp & Dohme in the United States.

M&B 693 in the British Press

The tenor of the media reception is partly captured in a few headlines. "Germs Disarmed by a New Drug—Success Claimed in Treatment of Pneumonia," proclaimed the *Yorkshire Evening Post* in a June 1938 report on early clinical trials. Already in July 1938 *Everybody's* began a story on M&B 693 with the heading "Disease You Need No Longer Dread—New Drug Conquers Deadly Germ." First reports of meningitis cures by M&B 693 in September 1938 prompted a fresh burst of press coverage. "Dread Disease Cured by New Drug—Pneumococcal Meningitis Need No Longer Be Fatal," from the *Glasgow Herald*, was typical.[2]

Newspapers brought forward details of individual cases, often with dramatic effect. Under the headline " 'Miracle' Drug Saves Life of W'ton Girl—Mother Wishes It Had Been Discovered Before," the *Midland Counties Express* told the story of seven-year-old Betty Walters. Brought to the Royal Hospital in Wolverhampton on July 13, 1938, desperately ill with pneumococcal meningitis, Betty was given M&B 693 supplied to doctors by May & Baker. Her full recovery stunned even her parents, who had lost two other children to meningitis. "I thought that little Betty was going to be the third of my children to be stricken down in the same way," her mother told reporters. "We were told we had little to hope for. Consequently, I was amazed to hear first that Betty might live, then that she would live, and finally that she would be completely cured. I can hardly believe it, but when I saw Betty at last she was looking as fit as she has ever looked. When she was finally cured of the meningitis she looked marvelous." With the text came a picture of a smiling Betty beaming out at the reader from her hospital ward.[3]

Many press reports pointed beyond the success of the new drug and its dramatic cures to the wider implications of these events for the future. Referring to M&B 693 as a "spectacular but solid therapeutic achievement," the *Times* concluded that "chemotherapy is coming of age, and its benefits extend now to tropical as well as to temperate climates. Thus the dream of Paul Ehrlich, the great pioneer in this field whose labours shed such luster on science in Germany, is being realized." The *Yorkshire Evening Post* along with other papers took note of M&B 693's apparent ability to strip the protective capsules from pneumococci and inferred that this discovery "opens up an entirely new field of work the tilling of which is likely to occupy research workers during many years." In a similar spirit, the *Lancashire Daily Post* thought it "likely that many other allies [to M&B 693] will be unearthed and soon a great new defensive force will be built up. The spirits of Lister and Pasteur and Koch must be overjoyed these days; there is every good reason why they should."[4]

M&B 693 provided the occasion for predictions of a glorious future. Under the headline "Freedom from Disease in Fifty Years' Time?" the *Birmingham Gazette* reported remarks made by Sir Edward Mellanby, Secretary of the Medical Research Council, at a university luncheon. "In 50 years' time the new Hospitals Centre would be put to uses quite other than those intended today," went the reporter's paraphrase. "It might, of course, be full of motor accident cases or of aged people whiling away the quiet end of their days. On the other hand, it might be used only for teaching. But it certainly would have other purposes 50 years hence," Mellanby was reported to say, "for the rate of progress in medicine was becoming extraordinarily rapid. The disabling of people in early life from child diseases was going to disappear." In a similar vein, a writer for the *Daily Express* ventured that "this is chemotherapy. The future will undoubtedly see a number of other new drugs added to the existing specific substances we already possess. It is along those lines that, one day, man will hold in his hand the key to the mystery of infection." In January 1939, the *Daily Express* speculated that thanks to M&B 693 "pneumonia may be going the way of smallpox and diabetes. The drug may be adding one more to the list of diseases of which men need no longer live in dread." About the same time, the *Sunday Dispatch* drew its readers' attention with the headline "Miracle Drugs Start 'a New Era'," announcing in bold type that "a new group of drugs which cure in a few days patients suffering from such diseases as pneumonia, scarlet fever, puerperal fever, erysipelas, and septicaemia is revolutionizing medical science. The method is known as chemotherapy and is totally different from the old system of antiseptics and serums."[5]

In March 1939, the *Bristol Evening Post* reported claims by Charles F. McKhann, a professor at Harvard Medical School, that thanks to sulfapyridine "people just won't die from pneumonia any more" and that measles and whooping cough would lose their dangers because the pneumonia often associated with them was no longer a threat. *Reynolds News* quoted prominent physicians as saying of M&B 693 that "in some cases it works like a charm" and that "this drug is the biggest discovery of our generation" and drew the conclusion that "its discovery opens the door to further discoveries and research, and is a stepping-stone towards other medical progress." "How Science Advances—Drugs That Conquer Death" headed an article by "a doctor" in the *Doncaster Gazette* that summarized recent achievements of chemotherapy. Recalling the heavy toll taken by streptococcal and pneumococcal diseases, the writer affirmed that "yet today, most of them can be cured more quickly than the average cold in the head and there is every prospect that in a few years time death from these causes will have dwindled almost to the vanishing point." Further, "there seems little doubt that the time is not far distant when most of the diseases caused by microbes will be robbed of their terrors. If a substance has been found that will prevent one group of microbes from multiplying in the body, there seems no reason why other groups and families of these merciless killers should not be dealt with equally effectively." Even viruses would be brought within the purview of effective therapy, according to this physician. "Once we can study them and learn something of their habits," he continued, we may be able to prepare a chemical that will deal with them just as easily as 'M. and B. 693' deals with pneumonia."[6]

For such wonders, credit must be assigned. In some of the earliest reports, it went to Lionel Whitby, as in the *Evening Standard*'s flat statement in June 1938 that "Dr. Lionel Whitby, of the Bland Sutton Institute of Pathology at the Middlesex Hospital, has discovered a new drug for the treatment of pneumococcal infection." An attractive figure because of his distinguished military service in the 1914–1918 war and his position as a prominent London pathologist, Whitby became even more visible after the new war began, and now as Colonel Whitby, he took charge of the Army Blood Transfusion Service. At least one newspaper article told his life story in flattering terms, and another showcased the bacteriological laboratories of the Bland Sutton Institute.[7]

In parallel with the Whitby stories and apparently oblivious to them, other newspapers settled on May & Baker research director A.J. Ewins as the one responsible for the new medicine. Without citing Ewins by name, the *Manchester Guardian* referred in September 1938 to "the inventor" in the May & Baker research laboratories. Others were more forthright, as in the *Glasgow Sunday Post's* statement that "credit for the discovery of the new drug goes to Dr. Ewins and his assistants of the Dagenham (Essex) laboratories of Messrs. May & Baker, the manufacturing chemists." In some accounts, Ewins was made to step into the formulaic role of the heroic discoverer: he might be aided by others but would have to overcome difficulties; he was modest, perseverant, and dedicated to the welfare of humanity. "Holding up a test-tube to the light of a laboratory window overlooking the Thames at Dagenham, white-haired Dr. Arthur J. Ewins murmured: 'This is the 693rd attempt—I wonder if this is the one?' " So began a story in the *Sunday Chronicle*, which continued, "in the test tube was a white powder, the product of months of precise and painstaking experiment. Though he did not know it, the doctor's task was ended. He had perfected a compound which today is saving the lives of hundreds of victims of lobar pneumonia." The writer concluded, "and still the modest scientist goes daily to his work, unknown and unhonoured, refusing to take the credit he has earned for a discovery which, he would say, if he would speak of it at all, was due to teamwork in his laboratory. Discovery of M. and B. 693 would, to Dr. Ewins, be just a job of work."[8]

Like the *Sunday Chronicle*, other newspapers that credited Ewins usually took pains to account for the medicine's common name. "The new drug . . . is called 'M and B 693' because its inventor discovered it after 692 previous attempts to obtain a chemical compound of the precise molecular structure desired," explained the *Manchester Guardian*. A writer for the *Daily Herald* reported that "time after time the chemists thought they had discovered the secret. They were disappointed until the 693rd attempt proved right. Hence the name 'M and B 693.' " What the writers of such accounts failed to report, and were no doubt unaware of, was that most of the test book entries in the same numerical series had nothing to do with the specific research program that yielded sulfapyridine. The first sulfa drug prepared at May & Baker laboratories, in January 1936, was a copy of Prontosil bearing the test book number 576. All of the compounds from 1 to 575, and many of those from 577 to 692, were not directly related to the Prontosil- and sulfanilamide-inspired project. Whitby had received from May & Baker only sixty-some compounds for animal testing before his work on T693.[9]

The name proved tenacious, at least in Britain and its overseas connections. When May & Baker put sulfapyridine on the market in October 1938, the company made an effort to substitute its new trade name, Dagenan, a term derived from the location of the company in Dagenham. By this time, however, "M&B 693" was entrenched, and "Dagenan" was doomed to a furtive and obscure existence, except on May & Baker packaging. As one newspaper wrote, "the name of the drug tells something of the drama and romance of the discovery," something that was hard to give up. In 1944, the *Sunday Graphic* was still playing on this quality when it credited Ewins for the discovery and noted that "it was his 693rd experiment, it was made in May & Baker's laboratory, so he labeled it M&B 693, the name by which it is still best known to the public." In a muddled hybrid version of the Whitby and Ewins stories, the *Eastern Evening News* even reported that Whitby "spent nearly five years on 692 unsuccessful experiments before discovering the formula. In the process a small army of white mice died. Infected with pneumonia microbes, they were inoculated with one experimental formula after another, and 692 white mice succumbed to pneumonia. When the 693rd lived, a 'secret weapon' in the warfare against disease was discovered." If any further evidence of its charms were needed, the *Limerick Leader* pointed out that "the magic number will have an attraction for all superstitious people. Each of its digits is divisible by three, and the sum of the digits is divisible by nine."[10]

A variant of the Ewins story named Ewins and Montague Phillips (who had effected the last step in the synthesis of T693) as colleagues who had jointly produced the discovery. In at least one of these versions, Phillips was said to demur, assigning most of the credit to Ewins and other members of the May & Baker research staff: " 'We are only scientists doing our job' he said." In an interview with another newspaper in 1944, Phillips revealed the element of luck that had made possible the synthesis, in the shape of the nearly forgotten bottle on the laboratory shelf, thus injecting a rare demystifying note into the story. Many years later, in 1961, Phillips would bitterly attack May & Baker's version of the discovery, which presented it as a group effort led by Ewins, as a grave injustice to himself.[11]

Above the details of individual credits newspaper reports often flew the banner of national achievement. "From all over the world comes evidence that pneumonia is being mastered by the life-saving British drug 'M. and B. 693'," the *Daily Herald* told its readers. The *Sunday Sun* reported that "the story behind these little tablets is a fascinating one—it is a story of triumph for British research chemists." In a similar vein, a writer for *Reynolds News* claimed that "one of the most important and spectacular victories in man's age-old battle with disease has been won as the result of the discovery of a new drug, evolved and produced in this country." The *Manchester Evening Chronicle* told the story of M&B 693's development under the subheading "British discovery." National pride did not yet have to contend with the complication that May & Baker was French owned, a fact that was not available even to most of the company's employees.[12]

Whatever the variations and contradictions among the stories highlighting the role of Whitby, or Ewins, or Ewins and Phillips, all agreed in crediting laboratory research for the discovery of M&B 693. In most cases, this assignment of laurels to the laboratory was implicit, but occasionally it surfaced in more direct remarks. A physician writing for the *Lancashire Daily* noted that "the doctors who are investigating [M&B 693] are in collaboration with the bacteriologists, and after all it is the man in the laboratory with the microscope who is able most succinctly to determine the positive factors of any remedy." A writer for the *Picture Post* called M&B 693 "one of the most successful examples of the comparatively new science of chemotherapy" and noted that it was "based, like all modern miracles, on infinite patience in the chemical laboratory." Paraphrasing Mellanby, the *Sunday School Chronicle* reminded its readers that "while honouring the doctors we should not forget (as we generally do) to honour the research workers whose patient work has discovered such an important 'family' as the sulphonamides."[13]

Mellanby's reminder may have been prompted by other news reports that passed over Whitby, Ewins, and Phillips in order to credit or showcase others, often local clinicians or hospitals involved in early trials or use of M&B 693. "Big Birmingham discovery: 'M and B 63' [*sic*] drug for pneumonia," was the prominent subheading of a *Birmingham Gazette* article. The article quoted none other than Mellanby to the effect that "only a day or so ago there was announced one of the greatest discoveries of the time. It has come from Birmingham's own municipal hospital in Dudley-road." Mellanby was referring to the first clinical trial of M&B 693 in pneumonia, carried out by G.M. Evans and Wilfrid F. Gaisford. The effect of the article, however, was to convey the impression that the discovery had originated in Birmingham. In Wolverhampton, the *Daily Express* highlighted the efforts of two pathologists of the city's Royal Hospital in supplying "proof that even the most deadly types of pneumonia can be cured." Under the heading "pneumonia cure doctor works till 3 A.M.," a photograph showed doctors S.C. Dyke and G.C.K. Reid in their laboratory surrounded by microscopes and test tubes. The writer conceded that "if they could be induced to talk about what they have done they would probably ask for honours to be shared with a London doctor," referring to Whitby. Whitby and "chemists in laboratories in Ilford" earned a brief mention at the bottom of the article, but a large share of glory went to the local men, who had successfully treated several pneumonia patients with the new medicine.[14]

Other localities were not to be outdone. In an article that failed to differentiate clearly among Prontosil, sulfanilamide, and M&B 693 and that made no mention of Whitby or Ewins, the *Middlesex Independent* put forward Queen Charlotte's Hospital in London as the site of "a discovery of immense importance not only in times of peace, but more particularly in times of war." Prontosil had been discovered in Germany, the writer conceded, but "the Germans never discovered how to make it effective," a task left to Leonard Colebrook and his colleagues at Queen Charlotte's, who were reported to be working with Prontosil and its successors, including M&B 693. The *Manchester City News* reported the conclusion of a successful clinical trial of M&B 693 at a local hospital under the headline "Pneumonia Is Conquered: Crumpsall Hospital Verdict after Sensational Twelve-Months Test with 'Wonder Drug'." The writer credited Ewins with discovery of the medicine but devoted most of the article to local doctors' proof that pneumonia mortality could be reduced from thirty percent to 6.7 percent.[15]

In some cases, local pride was satisfied merely by the early successful treatment of a patient with the new medicine. "Saved by Miracle Drug—Swinden Man Owes Life to 'M&B 693' " ran a headline in the *Swinden Evening Advertiser*. Readers learned that the man, "who was saved from death at the 11th hour . . . was only the sixth man in the country to receive this drug." A writer for the *Croyden Advertiser* told his readers that "the new treatment of pneumonia by a drug known as M. and B. 693 should be of special interest to Croyden, since it is a cure that has been applied at Croyden General Hospital and used in his private work by at least one Croyden doctor." The reporter could not resist adding that "Croyden, in fact, appears to have adopted the cure before the successful application of the drug at the Royal Hospital, Wolverhampton, called attention to the matter" and concluded that "we may well feel proud that Croyden is in the front line in making use of this drug." The *Lewisham Borough News* found satisfaction in the successful treatment of a desperately ill local baby with M&B 693, "a new drug never before given to a new-born child."[16]

Not only was the site or agent of the discovery sometimes shifted in news reports to serve local interests, but the nature of the discovered entity occasionally proved elusive. Reporting on early trials of the new medicine in treatment of pneumonia, the *Daily Express* medical correspondent told readers that "proof of the success of the 'wonder drug,' sulphanilamide, in the most dreaded of all lung infections, has been obtained in Wolverhampton and Walsall." Sulfanilamide was also the drug credited with recent pneumonia cures at the Manchester Royal Infirmary by a newspaper in that city, and in all of Scotland by the *Glasgow Sunday Post*, which explained the name M&B 693 as "the short way of referring to sulfanilamide." *Pearson's Weekly* not only referred to M&B 693 as "a cryptic designation of sulphanilamide," but also described the medicine as "the discovery of German chemists experimenting with coal-tar dyes," a confusion of the new medicine with Prontosil. The same error was committed by a writer for the *Financial Times*, who reported that pneumonia "can now be warded off, or attacks greatly shortened, by injections of 'Prontosyl,' discovered by the chemists of the German Dye Trust and now known in this country as 'M. B. 693' [*sic*]." In what was perhaps the most bizarre incident in which M&B 693 was conflated with sulfanilamide, an Arkansas farmer was reported to have "cursed the drug which had saved his life." While "critically ill with pneumonia, he was given sulfanilamide," the *Daily Express* reported, "and while under its influence he confessed to half a dozen murders which he committed as a youth."[17]

More seriously, in the rush of elation and relief accompanying reports of cures by M&B 693, warnings were often ignored or brushed aside. Many news stories omitted mention of side effects or possible toxicity altogether. Others noted calls by physicians or laboratory researchers for more testing but in a context that tended to discount any hesitations. "Birmingham plea for caution in new drug 'cure' for pneumonia—'M. and B. 693' tablet research not yet complete," was the restrained headline of an *Evening Dispatch* article reporting on early clinical trials. The same article began, however, with the statement that "pneumonia may be conquered with a new drug, M. and B. 693," and ended by quoting Mellanby to the affect that this drug was "one of the greatest discoveries of the time, 'by which a considerable control has been achieved over that wild disease, that king of diseases, pneumonia'." An otherwise informative article in the *Lancashire Daily Post* reported that M&B 693 "can be taken without any ill effects and in comparatively small doses" and that "it is so mild and inoffensive that it does not even have much of a taste." The headline "Disease You Need No Longer Dread— New Drug Conquers Deadly Germ" set the tone for a confident and enthusiastic report on M&B 693 in *Everybody's*. The writer dutifully took note of researchers' continuing tests but expressed the opinion that "once the after-effects—or lack of them—have been duly observed, there seems little doubt that the drug will be put into regular use throughout the country" and concluded "it looks like a certain cure."[18]

Some of the most sober and balanced stories about M&B 693 failed to mention its possible harmful effects. The medical correspondent of the *Northern Whig* (Belfast) gave a historical account of the development of the sulfonamides in which he mentioned that Prontosil "was not without its dangers" and conceded that the mode of action of the sulfonamides was not yet clarified but mentioned only the curative properties of M&B 693. Offering practical health advice to the public, a physician writing for the *National Welfare* (Johannesburg) made it clear that M&B 693 was "not to be regarded as an absolute panacea" for pneumonia and should not be substituted for ordinary precautions such as personal hygiene or avoidance of overwork, fatigue, or excessive cold. The same writer made no mention of the hazards of the drug itself.[19]

On rare occasions, a negative note was sounded amidst the paeans of praise. British newspapers acknowledged the paradox when an American doctor known for his successful treatment of pneumonia with M&B 693 died of the disease himself in spite of receiving the same treatment. The availability of M&B 693 over the counter in its early months on the market prompted one doctor to issue a warning that "there is a grave danger that people who are suffering from any of these diseases, or relations and friends who wish to help them, may be induced to purchase the drug and have it administered independent of skilled medical supervision. This would be highly dangerous since the drug in unskilled hands may produce serious consequences." Similar warnings are to be found in the British press long after M&B 693 was classified as available by prescription only. In the wake of Churchill's cure in late 1943, the *Sunday Post* ran an article under the title "The Chemist Says 'No!'," noting that "many unauthorized people are asking for [M&B 693]" and advising that "some people react very badly to this drug or its allied compounds." Rarer still was the appearance in newspapers of descriptions of specific toxic effects associated with M&B 693 treatment. One such was a letter to the editor of the *Star*, signed by "M.D.," which pointed out that the drug, "if taken without proper safeguards, may cause an illness called sulphaemoglobinaemia, in which the patient's skin assumes a bluish colour and which is accompanied by severe nausea and vomiting and perhaps by loss of consciousness."[20]

Perhaps predictably, the most radical criticism of M&B 693 came from the antivivisectionist press. A writer for the *Antivivisection Journal* quoted a physician and a May & Baker executive on the toxic effects of M&B 693 and the need for caution in its evaluation and predicted that the new medicine would follow a cycle already established by its predecessors, Prontosil and sulfanilamide, of inflated claims, followed by disillusionment and recognition of hazards, and finally supercession by "some new wonder-working potion." Months later the same journal was still complaining of "the booming in the lay press of the new drug M&B 693" and, in criticizing evidence put forward on behalf of the new medicine, took the occasion to reject the whole research enterprise from which it emerged:

> For the whole case against modern medicine with its fallacious theories
> of specific causes and specific remedies, the fatal result of reliance on an-
> imal experiment, is based on the impossibility of knowing how any indi-
> vidual human being will react to disease under any given circumstances.

Standardised methods are both dangerous and misleading and their effects are quite incalculable.

In yet another attack, the *Antivivisection Journal* quoted a physician's letter to *Lancet* highlighting the toxicity of M&B 693 and other sulfa drugs and remarked with satisfaction that "it is not often that illusions are so soon shattered in respect of the playthings of the laboratory (launched as panaceas and whatnots by over zealous if gullible enthusiasts), as in the case of the sulphanilamides," adding mockingly, "What? So soon?"[21]

Whatever doubts or criticisms were voiced were swept aside by a wave of positive publicity that appears to have reached an early high point in September 1938 with the widespread and dramatic newspaper reports of the cure of seven-year-old Betty Walters of Wolverhampton of pneumococcal meningitis.[22] Even before the Walters case appeared in print, a question was raised in the House of Commons about the pace of research on M&B 693 and its restricted availability. After the Walters case broke, newspapers reassured their readers that production of the new medicine was being speeded up to meet the demand "from doctors and hospitals in all parts of the world."[23]

After working for months under rising pressure to develop its manufacturing processes and facilities, May & Baker announced in October 1938 that it could now make M&B 693 generally available to the medical profession. The new drug went on display at the London Medical Exhibition that month, featured prominently among thousands of items in the exhibition catalogue, including new surgeons' gloves, automatic shutoff valves for hospital oxygen pipelines, and the then novel and costly contact lens.[24]

One indication of the rapidity with which M&B 693's fame spread and the extent of its reach may be found in early reports from Britain's African colonial empire. As early as August 1938, May & Baker made supplies of the medicine available to colonial doctors for experimental purposes. Two of these, T. Farnsworth Anderson and R.M. Dowdeswell, working at the Native Hospital in Nairobi, Kenya, began using the drug in cases of pneumonia. Their report on 100 cases, which appeared in *Lancet* in February 1939, recorded sharp drops in mortality, length of fever, and time in hospital for treated patients in comparison with those not receiving M&B 693. Anderson later recalled that he found the results "dramatic" and "astonishing" and that the introduction of M&B 693 was the most exciting episode in his career. By June 1939, a British press report was calling the success of treatment of pneumonia with M&B 693 "the outstanding event of the year in Kenya's health records." The same report noted that the Masai were willing to sell cattle to obtain their own supplies of the drug.[25]

By the beginning of 1939, similar reports of effective treatment of pneumonia with M&B 693 were beginning to surface in British press reports on South Africa. Especially striking was the drop in mortality among the some 300,000 native workers in the Transvaal gold mines. In August 1939, one British paper reported that enthusiasm for the drug in South Africa was such that people had been "buying and using it indiscriminately," leading the South African Medical Association to ask for government restrictions on its sale. In the Sudan, where outbreaks of cerebrospinal meningitis had been a persistent problem in the 1930s, treatment of cases with M&B 693 resulted in a drop in mortality from between sixty-eight and eighty percent to around ten percent. News of these "astonishing" results began to reach British readers by April 1939.[26]

Soon after war broke out in September 1939, indications began to appear in press reports of the important role M&B 693 would play in the conflict. In October, the *News Chronicle*'s war correspondent, Philip Jordan, reported from "somewhere in France" that the British Expeditionary Force had already amassed nearly 300,000 units of M&B 693, "the magic drug that saves so many lives." In January 1940, advertisements solicited funds to supply M&B 693 to treat pneumonia among troops in Finland, and by February 230,000 tablets had been sent to this war zone alone.[27]

Churchill's cure, not once but twice in 1943 at the height of the war, confirmed M&B's status as a household word in Britain. The caption of a photograph that appeared in the *Glasgow Evening Times* was representative: "A nurse taking a tablet of M&B 693, the famous sulphonamide drug that has twice saved the life of Mr. Churchill. The drug is the one powerful specific against pneumonia, and has literally saved thousands of lives." M&B seemed to be everywhere, even at the circus, where the medicine was reported to have "pulled Nero, Royal circus lion, through pneumonia," and at the London Zoo, where Winnie the lioness was also treated with M&B 693 for pneumonia. For some reason, the initials invited humor, as Churchill's Moran and Bedford joke (chapter 7) was joined by others. A cartoon in the *Yorkshire Evening Post* showed a man with a visibly shiny nose in bed, attended by his wife and doctor. The wife remarked to the doctor "M&B? If that means mild and bitter he's been taking it for years." Another cartoon, in *The Wall Planet*, showed two German civilians rushing for a bomb shelter as one said to the other "Ja, that man Churchill uses the code M&B—and that means More on Berlin."[28]

In its most emphatic version, the story went as follows: M&B had saved Churchill, Churchill led the nation, therefore M&B had saved the nation. But what was M&B? As noted above, press reports often failed to distinguish between M&B 693 (sulfapyridine) and a related compound also developed by May & Baker, M&B 760 (sulfathiazole). In this they seem to have followed the lead of the doctors and nurses, who often spoke loosely of "M&B." What was certain, in the messages that reached the public, was that M&B was a cure for pneumonia. Other diseases were sometimes mentioned in the press but tended to be eclipsed by the great killer.[29]

The Nature of a Discovery

The British popular press tended to assimilate the story of M&B 693 to a simplified model of discovery that included several elements. Struggling to convey the stunning impact of the new medicine, writers alternated between, or mixed, religious and military metaphors. Lives were saved by the new "miracle drug," or "the intruders were repulsed" (Churchill's phrase) and the foe conquered. Credit could be assigned to a single heroic discoverer. Often in popular press accounts the discovery could be located at a precise moment in time. One day there was no M&B 693, and the next day there was. In these versions of the story, the discovery extended at most from the moment of synthesis to Whitby's first animal experiments.

In one respect at least, the popular press accounts could not be faulted. Against the backdrop of the heavy mortality from pneumonia, M&B 693 did indeed appear to many as a kind of miracle, a wonder drug, a powerful weapon against an enemy of mankind. Only such strong language could adequately convey the impact of a medicine that meant the difference between life and death for hundreds of thousands of people.

In other ways, however, the prevailing popular presentation of the discovery misled. M&B 693 was not discovered by a single person. It was not discovered at a precise moment. It was not a cure for one disease only.

Take just one fragment of the story, the initial synthesis of the compound. Where is credit to be assigned? To Nicholas Grillet, who may have initiated the program to make sulfanilamide derivatives and divided the labor between Ewins and Edmond Blaise? To Ewins, who led his part of the program at May & Baker? To George Newbery, who (probably) asked the lab assistant Alexander to carry out the condensation reaction? To Alexander, who actually carried it out? To Phillips, who came up with a way to deacetylate the product of the condensation reaction? To all of the above? Even if we could answer this in a satisfying way, we have to remember that at this stage, November 2, 1937, T693 was just one more in a long list of compounds entered in the laboratory test book. No one knew that it had any biological activity, much less therapeutic efficacy.

So, was "M&B 693" discovered yet? No. Beyond this lay Whitby's animal studies, Evans's and Gaisford's first series of clinical trials, and years of efforts by many doctors in many countries to probe the potentials of sulfapyridine as a medicine and the nature and extent of its hazards. The questions of who discovered sulfapyridine and when are difficult ones to answer not only because many people were involved over a matter of months or years, but also, and more important, because the nature of the "discovery" was plural, not singular, and changed shape over time. What sulfapyridine was conceived to be in November 1937 was different from what it was conceived to be in December 1937, or March 1938, or July 1938, or November 1939. In fact, its medical identity continued to be in flux right up to the time that Churchill took it, when it was already beginning to be displaced by other sulfa drugs and by penicillin.

To some degree, there was a convergence between popular versions of the discovery and the ways in which it was rewarded by academic and industrial science and medicine. No Nobel Prize followed, although the magnitude of M&B 693's impact on medicine might have justified one. But Ewins was elected a Fellow of the Royal Society and in 1939 was named Director of Research at May & Baker. Whitby, who went on to direct the British Army Blood Transfusion Service during World War II, was knighted, became Regius Professor of Physic at Cambridge University, and as Sir Lionel Whitby served as vice chancellor of the university. In 1939, Whitby was awarded the John Hunter Medal and Prize by the Royal College of Surgeons. May & Baker gained financial rewards and an enhanced reputation. For the most part, however, the other characters in the story here told disappeared from the official account of the discovery and from public view.[30]

One who tried not to disappear was Phillips, who had effected an important step in the synthesis of T693 and whose name appeared with that of Ewins on the original patent. In 1964, the Science Museum in London opened an exhibit on medicinal drugs. The exhibit showcased M&B 693, and curators sought May & Baker's advice on the history of the discovery. The display included a photograph of Ewins but none of Phillips, although Phillips was mentioned in the accompanying text. Phillips, outraged at what he took to be a slight of his own role, went to the press, bringing with him a bottle purportedly containing a sample of the first batch of M&B 693.[31]

It was not the first time that Phillips had gone public in an effort to assert his role, which was rarely mentioned in early press reports on M&B 693. After leaving May & Baker and setting up his own chemical consultancy business, Phillips had given an account to a newspaper in 1944 that made him co-responsible with Ewins for the discovery and that also brought out the element of luck in the form of the presence of the old sample of the compound on the laboratory shelf. Now, in 1964, he was described as angry and bitter as a result of "27 years of frustration and disappointment over his success with M&B 693" and prepared to give "the inside story of how M&B 693 was discovered." The inside story consisted, first, of a debunking of the notion that M&B 693 was the result of 693 experiments, a version that had sometimes appeared in early press reports but that was never put forward by May & Baker or by other participants in the research. Second, Phillips asserted that M&B 693 was the result of "three astonishing accidents": the use of an old chemical from the shelf, Phillips's own "gamble" in using an alkali rather than an acid in one step of the synthesis, and the availability of pneumococcus-infected mice in Whitby's laboratory when the first sample of T693 arrived. Why had credit been withheld? Phillips recalled that "Dr. Ewins was never friendly to me" and speculated that Ewins had looked down on him as a man of working class background who had worked his way up within the company, obtained his degrees by attending evening classes, and held unorthodox ideas in politics. "The result," complained the writer for *The People*, "is this present scandalous insult to a distinguished scientist in the exhibition at the Science Museum."[32]

Phillips was a combative personality. When he died in 1972 he was portrayed as a self-made man who, in his widow's words, "liked to champion the small person against the establishment," was "eccentric and bad tempered," and "always tended to be extreme and was non-conformist in every way." He was a severe critic of the pharmaceutical industry who for many years sought compensation for thalidomide children. No doubt he saw himself as yet another victim of an unjust establishment, and this generalized resentment was part of what drove him to a public attack on the official history of M&B 693.[33]

Also driving Phillips's attack was a particular view of the discovery. Insofar as this view called for more explicit recognition of Phillips's contribution and brought forward the role played by chance, it is consistent with the present study. In making his case, however, Phillips fell into the same error as many of the accounts that drew his ire by equating the discovery with the chemical synthesis of the compound, and indeed even more narrowly with the last step in the original synthesis, the step that he had effected. Only on this view could the reporter for the *Recorder Review* state flatly that "the historic discovery was made on November 2, 1937." And only on this view could credit for the discovery be assigned to one or two individuals.[34]

Whatever the simplifications, selectivity, or outright errors of popular press coverage of M&B 693, there can be little doubt that newspapers, and perhaps other media such as radio, played a role in creating a rapidly increasing demand for the medicine in Britain when it was first introduced. That demand in turn hurried the introduction of M&B 693 into medical practice. The press, the pharmaceutical industry (initially May & Baker), doctors, and the public had convergent interests in embracing M&B 693 and in bringing it into use as quickly as possible. For the press the new medicine was good copy, with drama, intense human interest, local heroes (for local papers covering local doctors and hospitals), and good news for suffering humanity. For May & Baker it held out the prospect of profits and good publicity. For doctors and patients alike it offered hope in the treatment of a disease that still took a heavy toll of mortality despite decades of the best efforts of medical science, and that did so with significantly less trouble and expense than serum therapy. In this context it is not surprising that the main limiting factor on the general availability of M&B 693 was to be found not in the cautions of a few medical researchers and physicians, but rather in the time needed by May & Baker to develop its production capacity.

After sulfanilamide, M&B 693, or sulfapyridine as it came to be known generically, was the first striking success of the second generation of sulfa drugs that appeared in the late 1930s and 1940s. In contrast to the first generation, which included Prontosil and other azo compounds modeled on it, second generation sulfa drugs were (apart from sulfanilamide itself) derivatives of sulfanilamide formed by substitutions in either the amino group or the sulfonamide group of the molecule.[35]

Sulfapyridine's kinship with other members of the second generation extends beyond its chemical identity. Most securely, the overwhelming majority of second generation sulfa drugs were synthesized in laboratories of the chemical or pharmaceutical industry. They emerged as a result of the efforts of industrial laboratories like that of May & Baker to exploit the potential of an already recognized model, sulfanilamide. By focusing their resources on exploration of multiple possibilities within an established framework, industrial laboratories produced thousands of closely related compounds within a few years, variations on a single theme. In this respect, development of the second generation of sulfa drugs, which had a revolutionary impact on the therapeutics of bacterial infections, may be seen as a case of conservative invention in Thomas P. Hughes's sense.[36] Like sulfapyridine, other second-generation sulfa drugs were also beneficiaries of international exchange and diffusion of scientific, medical, and technological knowledge, and probably also serendipity in the research and development process. On these factors it is more difficult to generalize, however, and the extent and nature of their roles must be established for each medicine on a case-by-case basis.

Takeoff

Viewed with a longer perspective, sulfapyridine and other second-generation sulfa drugs that followed it gave powerful additional impetus to an expansion of research and development in the pharmaceutical industry that began with the introduction of Prontosil and sulfanilamide and that would continue unabated for the next three decades and beyond. In this period, which embraced the last prewar years, World War II, and the first two postwar decades, the industry's expanded commitment to research produced a flood of new medicines distinct from its traditional products and of far greater therapeutic range and potency, increased the importance of patents and the prominence of international pharmaceutical companies, and fed dramatic increases in industry output and financial worth.

All of these trends may be glimpsed in the development of May & Baker after introduction of sulfapyridine. M&B 693 was soon tried in veterinary medicine, where it had a dramatic impact comparable to its effect in human medicine. This success was sufficient to propel May & Baker into veterinary products, which for the company was a whole new domain of research and manufacture.[37]

World War II placed great demands on May & Baker, as on all of British industry. Priority was given to war production, and research was slowed except on war-related projects such as antimalarials. In spite of German bombing, however, the company undertook construction that expanded facilities at Dagenham and that created a new plant at Leek. Management began to plan for overseas manufacture and discussed movement into new fields of production. With the appointment of T.B. Maxwell, an American who had come to May & Baker in 1924, as managing director in 1941, the company began to look more decisively toward the reorganization and expansion of its research activities.[38]

Economic troubles in Britain after the war delayed implementation of May & Baker's expansion plans. In the area of medicinal products, however, sulfa drugs continued to be the profitable foundation of the business. M&B 693 had begun to be replaced by sulfathiazole during the war, and the company had made arrangements with Merck for it to manufacture the latter medicine for supply of May & Baker's overseas subsidiaries. The company also obtained licenses from American Cyanamid and from Sharp & Dohme to manufacture second-generation sulfa drugs developed by those companies. In addition to its sulfa drugs manufacture, which remained profitable until sulfas were largely displaced by antibiotics (penicillin and other antibacterial substances derived from microorganisms) in the 1950s, May & Baker worked closely with Rhône-Poulenc in the late 1940s and 1950s to develop and market new medicinal drugs. A fresh stimulus to this activity came in 1948 with the establishment of the National Health Service in Britain.[39]

In 1954, May & Baker began to build a new research institute at Dagenham. When it was completed in 1960, the new facility brought together most of the company's previously scattered research laboratories. It comprised three linked buildings for chemistry (including chemotherapeutics), biology, and administration, respectively, and provided space and equipment for 350 full-time research workers. The institute, which was made possible in substantial part by the medical and commercial success of the sulfa drugs, embodied Maxwell's vision and May & Baker's commitment to research. It also gave formidable expression to May & Baker's participation in a long-term expansion of the British pharmaceutical industry that raised the industry's output by almost 400 percent between 1935 and 1948 and by a further 320 percent between 1950 and 1968, the year of Maxwell's retirement.[40]

The tremendous expansion of pharmaceutical research and production that began in the late 1930s, and that was fueled in part by the success of the sulfa drugs, is exemplified also by the case of Merck, an American company. Between 1936, when it began production of sulfanilamide for clinical trials, and 1953, when it merged with another U.S. company, Sharp & Dohme, Merck carried out a major expansion of its research establishment and production facilities, changes that were supported by, and that helped to drive, surging increases in annual sales. In this transformation, the second generation of sulfa drugs, and sulfapyridine in particular, played a substantial part.

Merck, to be sure, had a research organization in place before the advent of the sulfa drugs. In 1927, the company's president, George W. Merck, had decided to add to Merck's facilities for scientific research, and to that end had hired Randolph T. Major, a Princeton-trained organic chemist, to head a research laboratory. In 1932, the company had begun construction of a new research building that was planned to include a small space for a pharmacological laboratory that would be an adjunct to the more considerable chemical research laboratory. To direct the pharmacological laboratory George Merck and Major hired Hans Molitor, an associate professor at the University of Vienna who had studied with the well-known pharmacologists Ernst P. Pick and Hans Horst Meyer and who already had some fifty publications to his credit. Molitor's laboratory was incorporated as an independent, nonprofit research organization, the Merck Institute for Therapeutic Research, with funding provided by Merck, on January 9, 1933.[41]

In its early years the Merck Institute pursued studies of a variety of therapeutic agents, including local and general anesthetics, alkaloids, hypnotics, antispasmodics, and vagomimetic and sympathomimetic drugs. From the outset, however, investigations on vitamins took a prominent place in the institute's work. Major convinced George Merck that vitamins might be used to enrich white flour or as food supplements to prevent deficiency diseases, and that the company should commit itself to their isolation, structure determination, synthesis, manufacture, and marketing. Synthesis of vitamin C in 1933 added impetus to this program, which Merck pursued with great success through the 1930s and 1940s. Most of the animal studies for this research were designed and carried out by Molitor and the Merck Institute.[42]

Not until 1937 did Merck enter the field of chemotherapy. The novel direction was prompted by the appearance of sulfanilamide, which the company began to manufacture and distribute for clinical testing in 1936 and which it made commercially available in April 1937. No dramatic breakthroughs came out of the early work on sulfanilamide derivatives, but Merck's research path had been broadened in a way comparable to its embrace of the potential of vitamins several years earlier.[43]

With its work on sulfonamides already under way, Merck was quick to embrace sulfapyridine. Even before May & Baker put M&B 693 on the British market in October 1938, arrangements had been made for Merck to make and distribute the compound in the United States. It did not do so commercially until March 10, 1939, but over the eight months preceding its general release, Merck distributed enough of the new medicine, which it called Sulfapyridine Merck, to U.S. physicians to treat some 15,000 patients in clinical trials or emergency cases during the pneumonia season. In many of the emergency cases, sulfapyridine reached hospitals around the country by airplane and special messenger. In April, a month after its general release, several notices appeared in the *Merck Report*, which reached some 69,000 physicians, pharmacists, chemists, and others, praising sulfapyridine and placing it in the context of the sulfonamides as a group. "With full recognition of scientific reserve as the guiding principle in the evaluation of a new remedy," a Merck editorialist wrote, "reflections from authoritative sources indicate that another milestone in chemotherapy has been attained."[44]

In early 1939, Merck's overall sales began to set new records. The company's 1939 report to stockholders attributed much of the increase to "some of the new products in our line," among which sulfapyridine figured prominently. At the same time, research activity at the Merck Institute was undergoing rapid expansion. Experimental work increased by sixty-two percent in 1939 as measured against the previous year, a change that brought the cumulative increase since 1934 to 660 percent. The number of staff rose from twenty-one to twenty-eight. Numbers of experimental animals kept at a given time rose from 3,700 to 4,720, necessitating emergency measures as cages spilled out into hallways and rose in racks toward the ceiling. In May 1939, Merck management authorized a new three-story building to house the institute, and construction began in August. When completed in early 1940, the new building provided a forty-three percent expansion of laboratory space and a 140 percent increase in animal house space. Institute publications also rose sharply, with sixteen appearing in 1939 compared to nine for 1938 and thirteen for the whole period 1935–1938.[45]

In all of this expansion, the sulfa drugs, and especially sulfapyridine, loomed large. While about half of the Merck Institute's research time in 1939 was devoted to vitamins, chemotherapy accounted for much of the remainder. The institute's 1939 report noted that "a considerable number of new synthetic compounds were investigated for pharmacological and toxicological properties." Among the new staff were a biochemist and a histologist to aid in the study of new drugs. Mice for chemotherapeutic research accounted for thirty-five percent of the institute's experimental animals. The publications list for the 1939 report included seven papers on sulfonamides, of which six were on sulfapyridine. Institute researchers made important contributions to the pharmacology and toxicology of sulfapyridine, most notably the finding that solid particles (uroliths) may form in the urine following administration of the drug.[46]

The motivation behind Merck's expansion of research in chemotherapy was given forceful expression in July 1939 by Molitor, director of the Merck Institute and one of the three people (with George Merck and Major) who set research policy at the company. In an article in the *Merck Report* on the experimental evaluation of sulfanilamide derivatives, Molitor noted that the search for new chemotherapeutic agents had been reinvigorated by the discovery of sulfanilamide. "Chemotherapy has entered a new era in the last two years," Molitor pointed out, as enormous efforts were made to synthesize compounds that were related to sulfanilamide but free of its side effects or effective against infections not susceptible to it. The most striking result of this effort was sulfapyridine, which Molitor thought "unquestionably represents one of the greatest advances of all time in the chemical treatment of diseases." Sulfapyridine, too, had its side effects and therapeutic limitations, Molitor observed, and this combination of great success and distinct potential for improvement had given added impetus to chemotherapeutic research. Molitor's observations were couched in general terms but were grounded in his immediate experience in the Merck Institute.[47]

Merck Institute expansion continued unabated in 1940. The institute moved into its new three-story brick building in March, and by early 1941 it had not only filled the new space to capacity but was converting basement areas not originally intended for laboratories in order to begin research on the chemotherapy of malaria and influenza. Use of experimental animals rose by thirty-three percent compared to 1939, and the laboratory went on a seven-day week to meet the demands of animal testing. Outside investigators, mainly academic chemists lacking access to biological testing facilities, sent the institute more than a thousand new compounds to be screened for therapeutic potential. The annual report listed twenty-one publications authored or co-authored by institute researchers. About half of research activity went to vitamins and another third to chemotherapy. The institute examined thirty sulfanilamide-related compounds and conducted study of antibacterial substances derived from microorganisms, including gramicidin, actinomycin, pyocyanin, and penicillin. The shadow of war in Europe is visible in the institute's decision to concentrate its efforts on projects likely to produce results of immediate practical value in the interest of "the national preparedness program." Besides the sulfa drugs work, this meant studies of the effects of vitamins on fatigue, of wound healing, and of the chemotherapy of malaria and influenza.[48]

Once again, research expansion was paralleled and fed by growth in sales. Merck's 1940 report to stockholders announced record revenues, with an important part "played by some of our new products." In particular, demand for synthetic vitamins, sulfapyridine, and sulfathiazole had been increasing rapidly. It was a pattern that would continue for several years. Merck increased its production of sulfa drugs substantially in 1941, in part to meet military needs. In 1942, the company again expanded its production facilities for sulfa drugs, vitamins, and arsenicals and added new ones for the antimalarial Atabrine. Merck's sales of sulfa drugs rose by eight-three percent between 1939 and 1940, by sixty-five percent between 1940 and 1941, by forty-seven percent between 1941 and 1942, and by a further sixty percent between 1942 and 1943. Sales of sulfas peaked in 1943 at $6,177,000. Thereafter, they dropped off as penicillin came into production beginning in 1943. Even so Merck's sales of sulfa drugs remained strong through the rest of the 1940s at levels comparable to those of 1941 and 1942.[49]

After Pearl Harbor and U.S. entry into the war, research at the Merck Institute came to be dominated by war-related projects. Institute personnel and research teams experienced disruption as male staff members left to join the armed forces and were often replaced by less experienced people. On the other hand, a large measure of continuity was assured by the sustained emphasis on vitamins (or nutrition more generally) and chemotherapy, both of which were judged to be of vital importance for the war effort. Some resources previously allotted to other projects were, in fact, shifted into chemotherapy. The latter area, which by 1943 constituted the largest domain of institute activity, included not only sulfonamides but also plant extracts, antibiotics, including penicillin and streptomycin, and antimalarials. Atabrine, the antimalarial introduced by I.G. Farbenindustrie in 1930, became the focus of intense scrutiny at Merck and elsewhere as Allied supplies of quinine were cut off by the Japanese occupation of the Dutch East Indies.[50]

Wartime pressures contributed to increasing elaboration of Merck Institute facilities and research methods. Rapid expansion of research on tropical infectious diseases, for example, led to the setting up of new laboratories and animal facilities, which came into use in the fall of 1943. One focus of research was the influence of climatic conditions on pharmacodynamic and toxic effects of medicines. Among the findings was the demonstration that under tropical conditions use of sulfa drugs was associated with a higher incidence of renal calculi. The increasing variety of infections studied and compounds to be tested led to elaboration and refinement of methods of evaluation. Institute researchers tested compounds in multiple animal species to uncover variations in activity, and research projects increasingly required cooperation among teams of specialists. The discovery that administration of sulfa drugs could induce or aggravate symptoms of vitamin deficiency, coupled with massive use of sulfa drugs in war medicine, led Merck researchers to merge their two major research endeavors in vitamins and chemotherapy to investigate the interaction of drugs and nutrition.[51]

The Merck Institute facilities that were completed in 1940 had been outgrown almost immediately, but although wartime expansion of research aggravated the problem, no new building could be undertaken until after the war. In 1948, Merck began construction of a new institute under a long-range building plan. A chemotherapy building with associated isolation building and animal facilities was finished in 1949, a poultry nutrition building in 1950, and a new laboratory and administration building in December 1952. The carefully designed research complex provided 65,000 square feet of floor space, more than four and a half times the area of the 1940 building. At the opening of the new institute in 1953, total staff amounted to 153 persons, almost three times the number in 1942 and more than fifty times the original staff of three in 1933. At the dedication ceremonies on May 2, 1953, the governor of New Jersey, Alfred E. Driscoll, addressed almost 400 scientists, educators, government officials, and business leaders, including four Nobel laureates (Sir Alexander Fleming, Edward C. Kendall, Otto Loewi, and Selman A. Waksman), and the Vice President of the Rockefeller Foundation, Alan Gregg.[52]

The year 1953 also saw Merck merge with Sharp & Dohme, an American company whose expansion of research and sales since the late 1930s had paralleled Merck's and had been even more squarely based on the sulfa drugs. Until 1929, Sharp & Dohme had been mainly a maker and distributor of ethical drugs, that is, medicines marketed to the medical profession but not directly to the public, but not derived from its own research. With the purchase of the H.K. Mulford Company in that year, it had acquired as products a line of vaccines and serum antitoxins, but even then its research and development facilities had remained small. Only with the appointment of a new president, John S. Zinsser, in 1935, did research move to the forefront of Sharp & Dohme's agenda. Zinsser, who was trained as a chemist and who had worked at Merck as a technical coordinator before moving to Sharp & Dohme, was more attuned to medicinal chemistry than to biologicals and was well prepared to see the opportunity opened by sulfanilamide.[53]

Sometime in the fall of 1936 or spring of 1937, a Sharp & Dohme employee returned from a meeting at which "people from Johns Hopkins" (probably Perrin H. Long and Eleanor A. Bliss) had discussed sulfanilamide, and he "reported glowingly about this new drug." James M. Sprague, an organic chemist, was hired in August 1937 to lead the research on sulfanilamide derivatives. By Sprague's account, the Sharp & Dohme staff prepared a number of compounds, based on sulfanilamide, without striking results. Then in May 1938, they read a report in *Lancet* (no doubt Whitby's article) on M&B 693 and its purported activity against pneumococcal pneumonia. "Well, that directed us to the heterocyclic derivatives of sulfanilamide," Sprague recalled. "For anybody who knew any heterocyclic chemistry at all," he continued, "the door was open."[54]

With the lead provided by sulfapyridine, Sprague and his colleagues turned to intensive preparation of heterocyclic derivatives of sulfanilamide. Their first success was sulfathiazole, which proved as effective as sulfapyridine against pneumonia. In a circumstance indicative of the rapid impact of sulfapyridine, eight other companies also succeeded nearly simultaneously in preparing sulfathiazole. These included May & Baker, which obtained patent rights and assigned them to Merck. Undaunted, Sprague and other Sharp & Dohme researchers pressed on and were rewarded in the early 1940s with a string of successes, notably sulfadiazine, sulfamerazine, sulfamethazine, succinylsulfathiazole, and phthalylsulfathiazole.[55]

Boosted by wartime demand for sulfa drugs, Sharp & Dohme sales increased by 252 percent between 1939 and 1948. Research expenses grew from $184,000 in 1940 to $1,589,000 in 1952. The company built a new research building in 1942, but shortages of materials meant that it was not as large as had been planned. In 1948, Sharp & Dohme began construction of a new, larger research establishment at West Point, Pennsylvania. When completed in December 1951, the new facility was described by James Sprague as "superb, by anybody's comparison. It was even better than Merck's physical facilities at the time." More than 200 research staff occupied the new buildings, up from three in 1930. Sprague's own group of organic chemists grew from about ten in 1937 to twenty-five to thirty in 1953.[56]

The dramatic expansion visible at May & Baker, Merck, and Sharp & Dohme could be traced with variations at numerous other pharmaceutical and chemical companies from the late 1930s to the 1950s. Starting from a foundation of increasing commitment to research in the pharmaceutical industry between the world wars, the boom that began around 1939 propelled the industry, medical practice, and the expectations of the public into a new era in which every year brought many, sometimes scores, of novel and often powerful medicines.[57] At the beginning and center of this boom, acting as exemplar and economic engine, stood the sulfa drugs. Research had made them possible. The ubiquity and cost in death and human suffering of bacterial infections had given them an immediate prominence in medicine. World War II drove forward their development and provided multiple challenges to their production and use.

PART III

Practice and Theory

CHAPTER 9

At War

O n December 3, 1941, New York surgeon John J. Moorhead arrived in Honolulu to give a series of lectures on traumatic surgery. His first lecture, delivered on the evening of December 5, was titled "Treatment of Wounds, Civil and Military." Many of the some 300 people in the audience were Army or Navy doctors. Moorhead's second lecture was scheduled for 9:00 Sunday morning. As he finished his breakfast that day, he heard gunfire in the distance and was told that Pearl Harbor was under attack. When he reached the lecture hall, he found an audience of fifty, with no Navy or Army personnel. Moorhead had barely begun to speak before a local physician rushed in to say that twelve surgeons were needed immediately at the Army's Tripler Hospital. He spent the next eleven hours in the operating room, as a member of one of eight operating teams treating a flood of casualties of the attack. In the midst of this marathon session, Moorhead, who had served with the U.S. Army Medical Corps in World War I, was restored to temporary active duty with the rank of Colonel.[1]

Moorhead's Friday evening lecture, delivered scarcely thirty-six hours before the Japanese attack, could hardly have been timelier. His recommendations for the treatment of wounds, put into practice in the aftermath of the attack, provide a snapshot of the place of sulfa drugs in surgery on the eve of U.S. entry into World War II.

Moorhead told his audience that the adequate cleaning of a wound with soap and water should be followed by debridement (excision of dead or irreparable tissue and removal of foreign bodies) with the goal of obtaining normal color, blood flow, and muscular contraction. After stopping all bleeding, the surgeon should then "place in the wound an adequate amount of a sulfonamide drug, either sulfanilamide or sulfathiazole." Moorhead advised that wounds were not to be immediately sutured but should be covered with a heavy plain gauze dressing. Splints were to be applied if joints were contiguous. Finally, Moorhead enjoined surgeons that as part of aftercare fifteen grains (one gram) of a sulfonamide drug were to be given to the patient "every four hours for three days together with needed sedation."[2]

Most of the numerous casualties received by Moorhead's group of surgeons were victims of bombing or machine gun attack. In contrast to the situation in other medical units where burns predominated, Moorhead's group faced mostly multiple lacerated wounds and compound fractures. The principles Moorhead had outlined in his Friday evening lecture were put to the test in thoracic, abdominal, spinal, and head wounds, in fractures, and in amputations. Surgeons treated the few cases of gas gangrene that developed with a combination of debridement, sulfanilamide in the wound and by mouth, and exposure of the affected areas to X-rays.[3]

Moorhead reported that the results were highly satisfactory. Visiting a large group of evacuated wounded in a San Francisco hospital on January 3, 1942, he found that "they were all doing exceedingly well." Among all the casualties treated at Tripler Hospital in the hours after the Pearl Harbor attack, postoperative mortality was 3.8 percent, with most of the fatalities occurring in patients who had suffered abdominal wounds and were depleted by shock and bleeding. There were no deaths from gas gangrene. Moorhead commented that "the results were better than I had ever seen during nineteen months in France when serving with the French, Belgian, and American medical formations." Writing in the *Journal of the American Medical Association*, he attributed the favorable outcome primarily to treatment of the wounded within six hours, preliminary shock treatment (with transfusion of whole blood, liquid plasma, or saline-dextrose solution), debridement without immediate suturing, and use of sulfonamide drugs in the wound and by mouth.[4]

Moorhead's experience closely paralleled that of another surgeon, Ralph B. Cloward, who treated many Pearl Harbor casualties with penetrating wounds of the head caused by shrapnel. The procedures followed by Cloward in this more narrowly defined surgical domain had much in common with treatment of other kinds of traumatic wounds, including use of sulfonamides at every stage. Preliminary treatment of head wounds included application of a temporary dressing "after the wound has been filled with powder of one of the sulfonamide drugs." Following an operation, the surgeon filled the affected tract of the brain with sulfanilamide powder, and postoperative care included at least a week of chemotherapy. If a postoperative infection occurred, the wound was reopened and packed for drainage with gauze filled with sulfanilamide powder. Although at the time of his report Cloward considered it too early to comment on postoperative complications, he saw a basis for optimism in the consensus of recent surgical literature on principles of treatment for penetrating wounds of the head. These included a recommendation of "generous use of sulfanilamide not only in the scalp and skull wound but in the missile tract in the brain."[5]

Even before publication of Moorhead's and Cloward's reports, local and systemic use of sulfa drugs in treatment of war wounds and burns had been given the official imprimatur of the National Research Council (NRC). Within days after the attack on Pearl Harbor, the NRC had dispatched Perrin H. Long of Johns Hopkins and Isidor S. Ravdin of the University of Pennsylvania (Ravdin was also an Army Medical Corps reserve colonel not on active duty but was later to command the 20th General Hospital in the China-Burma-India theater) to assess the medical response. Long and Ravdin had completed their task by December 22, and on January 18, 1942, they submitted a report to the War Department that painted a glowing picture of the medical service at Pearl Harbor and of the role of the sulfa drugs in particular.[6]

Long's and Ravdin's report had high praise for the use of blood plasma to treat shock and for the role of civilian groups in organizing the supply of plasma and whole blood. In the authors' view, Pearl Harbor also demonstrated beyond question the value of both local and systemic use of sulfa drugs. Wounds that most probably would have been fatal a few years earlier responded readily to treatment with sulfanilamide and sulfathiazole, they noted. In great contrast to World War I, in which patients with perforating abdominal wounds suffered an approximately eighty percent mortality rate, at Pearl Harbor casualties with the same type of wound who survived shock to undergo surgery and sulfonamide therapy nearly all recovered. Navy doctors treating burns (a high percentage of the injuries to sailors) for the first time on a large scale with sulfanilamide or sulfathiazole by mouth reported similar dramatic results in control of infections. Long and Ravdin emphasized the implications for future practice:

> We have been impressed again and again with the incalculable value of sulfonamide therapy in the care of many of the casualties. . . . We believe that it is highly important that physicians—both civilian and military—become familiar with the general and specific considerations which govern the oral and local use of the sulfonamides in the treatment of wounds and burns, and that, in so far as it is possible, routine methods for the use of sulfonamides in casualties be devised and adopted.[7]

The reports by Moorhead, Cloward, and Long and Ravdin indicate that American doctors regarded the medical response to Pearl Harbor as successful both in terms of mortality rates and in terms of control of infections. These reports also show that by the time of the Pearl Harbor attack, use of sulfa drugs for both local and systemic treatment of wounds and burns was becoming routine and that such treatment was credited with an important part in the successful medical response to the attack. This perception reinforced beliefs among doctors as the United States entered World War II that sulfa drugs should be a routine part of treatment of wounds and burns and that these routines should be incorporated into military medicine.

To some, at least, such conclusions did not come as a surprise. Preparations for wartime use of, and research on, the sulfa drugs had begun in May 1940, a full eighteen months before Pearl Harbor, with the establishment of the Advisory Commission to the National Defense Council. The Surgeons General of the Army and Navy had asked the NRC's Division of Medical Sciences to create advisory medical committees as part of war preparation. Long came to Pearl Harbor as the chair of one of these, the NRC's Committee on Chemotherapeutic and Other Agents.[8]

Once the United States was in the war, production of sulfa drugs rose rapidly to high levels that were largely sustained for the duration. Most in demand were sulfanilamide, sulfathiazole, sulfadiazine, and sulfaguanidine. For American military forces, sulfa drugs were mainstays in the treatment not only of wounds and burns but also in treatment of pneumonia, streptococcal infections, meningitis, gonorrhea and urinary tract infections, and bacillary dysentery.

Government-sponsored research, often done by civilians and sometimes organized as cooperative projects, was begun before U.S. entry into the war and ultimately contributed to significant changes in the way sulfa drugs were used. Some of these changes went into effect during the war, but others did not take hold until near the war's end or after it was over. A certain looseness of fit may be observed in the connection of medical research and practice during the war, at least regarding the sulfa drugs. The way the sulfa drugs were used could go in advance of research; that is, practices could be adopted before there was an adequate basis for them in the eyes of researchers. Use could also lag behind research; that is, new practices could be slow to be adopted or practices in place could persist long after research had concluded that there was little or no basis for them.

While the therapeutic revolution initiated by the sulfa drugs had begun well before the war, a number of other important medical innovations occurred during the war and contributed with the sulfa drugs to historically unprecedented low levels of mortality and morbidity among combatants. These included the development of penicillin, use of blood plasma and whole blood, heart and lung surgery, definition and treatment of crush syndrome, rehabilitation medicine, a toxoid vaccine for tetanus, and a combined effort of medicine, entomology, and sanitary engineering to combat typhus and malaria.[9]

The part played by the sulfa drugs in the war must be seen in the context of these innovations. The medical successes of the war were a result of a confluence of prewar developments, including the sulfa drugs, wartime innovations often indebted to government–industry–academic cooperation, and a highly efficient system of organization and delivery of medical services.

Among these changes, the most dramatic and far-reaching in its long-term effects was the development of penicillin, which was accelerated by the war, was completed in time to have an impact on military medicine, and opened the age of antibiotics.[10] Penicillin surely deserves the fame and attention it has received. Yet the very brilliance of the penicillin story has tended to obscure other aspects of the medical history of World War II, not least the major role played by the sulfa drugs.

Contrary to the impression conveyed by some accounts of the penicillin story, penicillin did not supply a treatment for bacterial infections where there was none before, except in a few cases, nor did it suddenly replace the sulfa drugs in therapeutics. Instead, penicillin entered a field of practice for the most part already occupied by the sulfa drugs. Initially because of limited supplies, and because clinical investigations on penicillin were proceeding, penicillin was used in a restricted way, for example, in cases of sulfonamide-resistant infections. Sulfa drugs, supplemented but not supplanted by penicillin, remained part of standard treatment for bacterial infections through the end of the war and beyond.

What follows is an effort to redress the balance, and in so doing to contribute to ongoing studies of wartime medicine that are clarifying the complex connections of practice, production, and research, and of government, industry, and academia, in the medical enterprise. My discussion is confined largely to the United States. The reader should keep in mind that sulfa drugs were heavily used by all combatant states and that patterns of production, use, and research could be different in other national settings.

Preparation for War

Long before Pearl Harbor, American government and industry began planning for production of medicinal drugs in the event of U.S. involvement in the war. In September 1939, shortly after the outbreak of war in Europe, the Army Surgeon General's Office (SGO) asked the American Drug Manufacturer's Association to form a committee to better coordinate government and industry response to the new circumstances. By the end of the month, a Drug Resources Advisory Committee was in existence, chaired by Carson P. Frailey, the American Drug Manufacturer's Association executive vice president and secretary. The committee in turn created subcommittees, and these began investigations on specialized problems.[11]

In the summer of 1940, at the request of the Advisory Commission to the National Defense Council, the committee was reassigned as the Drugs Resources Advisory Committee of the Army and Navy Munitions Board. Its tasks were to study production facilities and raw materials and to cooperate with the National Defense Council Advisory Commission's Drugs and Chemicals Section. Subcommittees considered special commodities such as surgical dressings and instruments, botanicals, biologicals, and vitamins, as well as medicinal chemicals. The subcommittees included members from industry and served to connect drug and related industries to Army and Navy needs.[12]

In 1940, the SGO also established a Requirements Branch within its Procurement Division to assess military needs and to align production facilities and planning with estimated requirements. In February 1941, the Advisory Commission to the National Defense Council was abolished and replaced by the Office of Production Management (OPM). Responsibility for military and other government procurement of drugs and surgical supplies was then vested in the Raw Materials Branch of the OPM's Division of Purchases. As Army and Navy procurement schedules for drugs and related products expanded in the spring and summer of 1941, industry began to have trouble obtaining necessary raw materials and equipment. The result was the establishment of a system of priority ratings in which the Raw Materials Branch played an important part. By October 1941, the increased activity in the area of drugs and surgical supplies led to the creation of a separate Health Supplies Branch under the OPM.[13]

By the time of Pearl Harbor and U.S. entry into the war, preparations for production of medicinal drugs were well advanced. The OPM's Health Supplies Branch had brought in experienced personnel and was assisting industry in obtaining raw materials and needed equipment. It had established working relationships with the OPM's Chemicals Branch, which managed many of the needed raw materials, and with the Army and Navy Munitions Board, the SGO, the Navy Bureau of Medicine and Surgery, and other government agencies.[14]

Preparation for military use of medicinal drugs and related research also stretched back at least eighteen months before Pearl Harbor. Two distinct phases may be discerned in the period of preparation. The first, running from May 1940 to August 1941, was one of increasing civilian–military contact in the field of medicine, organization of personnel, and advice to the military medical services based on the latest current knowledge. In the second, from August to December 1941, the Committee on Medical Research (CMR) was established under the Office of Scientific Research and Development (OSRD), substantial government funds were made available for medical research related to military problems, and CMR-funded research projects were begun.[15]

At the annual meeting of the NRC's Division of Medical Sciences on April 26, 1940, the division's chairman, Lewis H. Weed, spoke of the medical problems of defense and of the division's readiness to assist the government. Liaison officers from the Army and Navy medical services were present. Within a month, German armies invaded Belgium and the Low Countries. In the middle of May, Weed received requests from the Surgeons General of the Army and Navy asking that the Division of Medical Sciences establish committees to advise the medical services on special problems, among which the most urgent were thought to be the use of chemotherapeutic agents in treatment of war injuries and infectious diseases, and the treatment of traumatic shock, especially by transfusion. The first committees organized by the division were, accordingly, those on chemotherapeutic and other agents and on transfusions.[16]

Weed and his colleagues quickly realized that more committees would be needed to cover the military's questions across the whole field of medicine. By the end of 1940, the NRC had established seven main committees (on chemotherapeutic and other agents, transfusions, medicine, surgery, neuropsychiatry, information, and aviation medicine) and numerous subcommittees. The latter were in some cases responsible to more than one main committee where problems overlapped. The committees included contact officers from the Army, Navy, and Public Health Service, respectively. The general assignment of all committees was to give professional advice to the services and to plan and administer research considered necessary to national defense.[17]

An organization had been created, committee members had been recruited, there was a sense of urgency in the leadership, and intentions were good. All of that was not enough, according to John S. Lockwood, who served on the Committee on Chemotherapeutic and Other Agents and its Subcommittee on Surgical Infections. In an article published after the war, Lockwood pointed to three constraints on the action of NRC medical advisory committees before August 1941. One of these was the unfamiliarity of most committee members with the particular medical problems of modern warfare. A second constraint, which reinforced the first, was the lack of provision for "sending teams of experts to the war theaters where our prospective allies were engaged." Finally, the extensive research that committee members thought necessary to fill gaps in existing knowledge could not be undertaken for lack of funds. In another article that appeared after the war, Long, who chaired the Committee on Chemotherapeutic and Other Agents and served on its Subcommittee on Surgical Infections, was more blunt. He referred to the "fumblings which characterized governmental activities in relation to medical preparation for the war in 1940–41" and attributed them to the American people's desire to avoid involvement in the war at almost any cost.[18]

Fumblings or not, medical preparations for possible U.S. involvement in the war took several forms in 1940 and early 1941 apart from the NRC and its committees. In September 1940, the National Defense Council set up a Health and Medical Committee to coordinate "health and medical activities affecting national defense." The new committee promptly established its own subcommittees. The Army Medical Department began planning and preparations to make the department's personnel and facilities commensurate with an ongoing major expansion of the Army. In response to a request from the Army SGO, the American Medical Association (AMA) undertook a census of American physicians, gathering data on age, location, qualifications, and availability for use "in the event of a national emergency."[19]

In the absence of government funding for research on military medicine, the NRC and the AMA moved to gather information already available and to diffuse it to as wide a medical audience as possible. As part of this effort, the first issue of *War Medicine* appeared in January 1941. The new journal was edited by the NRC Division of Medical Sciences through its Committee on Information, whose chairman, Morris Fishbein, also served as chief editor. Fishbein was also editor of the *Journal of the American Medical Association*, and *War Medicine* was published by the AMA. Its subtitle announced that it was "a periodical containing original contributions, news and abstracts of articles of military, naval and similar interest related to preparedness and war service."[20]

Among the articles appearing in the first issue of *War Medicine* was one on "Chemotherapy for infectious diseases and other infections." This was a reprinting, with minor changes, of a circular letter prepared for the Army SGO by the NRC's Committee on Chemotherapeutic and Other Agents and already distributed to Army medical officers in December 1940. Its stated aim was "to summarize the present status of chemotherapy with a view to its application in the treatment of military personnel." In very concise form, the authors recommended treatments, mostly chemotherapy using one of three sulfa drugs (sulfanilamide, sulfapyridine, or sulfathiazole), for seven categories of infections: hemolytic streptococcal infections, scarlet fever, meningococcal meningitis, purulent meningitis, pneumonia, gas bacillus infections, and staphylococcal infections. In each case, the authors made recommendations on dosage and course of treatment, and they concluded with comments on the toxic effects of sulfa drugs and the need for medical officers to monitor treatment carefully. They mentioned local use of sulfa drugs in gas bacillus infections and as "experimental" in chronic staphylococcic suppuration. They presented all of this with the caveat that the rapid development of chemotherapeutic agents would be likely to force modifications of these recommendations from time to time.[21]

Some research on war-related medical problems was done in advance of, or apart from, CMR funding, and some of the results made their way into the pages of *War Medicine*. One focus of attention was venereal disease, especially gonorrhea, which once again—as in World War I—threatened to remove many military personnel from active service. Chemotherapy, especially with sulfa drugs, was prominent among the control measures looked to for assistance.[22] Another problem of great concern was gas gangrene infection, which had claimed many lives in World War I. Supported with funds from the John and Mary R. Markle Foundation, Long and his colleagues at Johns Hopkins studied the effects of various sulfa drugs on gas gangrene infections in mice. They concluded that sulfathiazole and sulfadiazine appeared to have some beneficial effect and recommended local application of either drug (with sulfadiazine preferred) as a prophylactic measure.[23]

With the establishment of the Committee on Medical Research (CMR) under the OSRD in August 1941, the government made available substantial funds for civilian research on military medical problems. The CMR immediately entered into a close relationship with the NRC. Both organizations were headquartered in the same Washington building, and Weed, the chairman of the NRC's Division of Medical Sciences, was made vice chairman of the CMR, under its chairman Alfred Newton Richards. The CMR, which also included representatives from the Army, Navy, and Public Health Service, had the authority to make recommendations for support of medical research to the director of the OSRD, Vannevar Bush. To manage its relationships with civilian investigators, the CMR soon developed an administrative organization with six divisions (for medicine, surgery, chemistry, physiology, aviation medicine, and malaria studies), each with its own chief and deputy chief.[24]

The system that emerged was, in Lockwood's words, "time-consuming and cumbersome." A question from one of the military services would be routed to the appropriate NRC committee. If the committee decided that research was required to give a proper answer to the question, it would suggest individual investigators. The latter would be consulted and asked to submit an application for research funds to the appropriate division chief of the CMR, who might then consult with the NRC committee. The division chief and the NRC would then present a recommendation to the CMR, which could then approve it and ask the director of OSRD to authorize a contract to dispense funds. The CMR required the investigator to submit bimonthly reports, which could be distributed to NRC committees, other researchers, or the military services. If the research reached a definite conclusion, it could become the basis of a formal recommendation from the NRC to the Surgeons General, which would then make the final decision on whether the recommendation would be adopted in military practice. On the positive side, the system permitted maximum freedom to investigators while allowing for consultation with other experts and compliance with legal requirements on the expenditure of public funds.[25]

The transition from the first to the second phase of pre-Pearl Harbor medical preparation is well illustrated by studies of the prevention and treatment of infection in wounds and burns. The problem was considered a top priority by the Surgeon General of the Army, and a Committee on Wounds and Burns was one of the first to be organized by the NRC in the spring of 1940. After its first meeting on June 6, 1940, this committee was quickly reconstituted as the Subcommittee on Surgical Infections, with links to both the Committee on Chemotherapeutic and Other Agents and a new Committee on Surgery.[26]

The Subcommittee on Surgical Infections and the Committee on Chemotherapeutic and Other Agents promptly joined in recommending to the military services that one or another sulfa drug be administered by mouth to a wounded individual as soon as possible after the injury as a means of preventing infection, especially by hemolytic streptococci. The subcommittee did not at first recommend local use of sulfonamides as a prophylactic measure because its members felt that there was no good evidence available to justify the practice. The subcommittee did believe that the problem warranted serious investigation in well-controlled studies. By the end of 1940, it had made plans for a major research project that would examine the use of sulfonamide compounds in treatment of civilian injuries due to accidents, in the hope that firm guidelines would emerge for treatment of war injuries.[27]

The problem was money. No government funds were forthcoming to pay for the needed research units. Such was still the situation in May 1941, nearly a year after planning had begun, when the NRC received an urgent request for advice from the Surgeons General. In response, the Subcommittee on Surgical Infections recommended to the military services that sulfanilamide crystals be placed in all wounds prior to debridement and also later at the time the wound was closed. By the account of one subcommittee member, Lockwood, this advice was based not on new evidence, of which there was none, but "solely upon the current trend of opinion of civilian surgeons, among whom a wave of enthusiasm for this procedure had begun to develop."[28]

Local use of sulfanilamide on wounds was being adopted by British surgeons treating war casualties, also in advance of evidence that the practice was effective. Leonard Colebrook, who was studying surgical infections, wrote to Long from the Royal Army Medical College in July 1941 that "the surgeons have all gone haywire and are shoving the stuff into most of the wounds, and for the most part seem impressed with its value—in fact many of them quite enthusiastic,—but equally quite uncritical." Colebrook asked Long to do what he could to persuade critically minded American surgeons to reexamine the local use of sulfanilamide in compound fractures, noting that "civilian injuries should be just as good for the purpose as war injuries."[29]

Only after the establishment of the CMR in August 1941 could the plans long in place be implemented. In the fall of 1941, the NRC and CMR set up wound study units in eight teaching hospitals in seven cities. Each unit included a responsible investigator and one or more clinical assistants and was equipped with facilities for bacteriological and other clinical laboratory work. The NRC supplied each unit with special forms on which detailed patient records were to be kept. Completed records went to the project's statistical office in New York directed by the chairman of the Subcommittee on Surgical Infections, Frank L. Meleney. At approximately two-month intervals, investigators and clinical assistants met with the subcommittee in Washington. In every study unit, each of the three categories of injury under study—soft part wounds, compound fractures, and burns—was treated with several different chemotherapeutic regimens. One group of patients in each category received sulfadiazine systemically and a mixture of equal parts sulfanilamide and sulfadiazine locally. A second group received sulfadiazine systemically and sulfanilamide locally. A third group received only systemic sulfadiazine. Finally, a fourth group received only the standard surgical treatment given to all groups, with no chemotherapy.[30]

Carefully planned and executed, this ambitious cooperative research project did not begin to yield firm conclusions until the end of 1942. By that time Pearl Harbor had been attacked, the United States had been in the war for a year, and surgeons were treating patients according to guidelines that were in place before the study began.[31]

Production

Pearl Harbor gave a double impetus to U.S. production of sulfa drugs. Whatever preparations had gone before, U.S. entry into the war made the manufacture of war-related products and the availability of their raw materials a matter of fresh urgency. Within days after the attack, the larger American chemical companies involved in the production of raw materials for pharmaceuticals were working on full twenty-four-hour shifts.[32] The perceived success of the sulfa drugs in the medical response to the attack made them objects of special attention. On January 10, 1942, C.F. Shook, an officer in the SGO, wrote to Frailey, chairman of the Drug Resources Advisory Committee, asking the committee to study the "necessity for increased production" of sulfa drugs. Referring to "the wonderful results of the use of Sulfanilamide in the open wounds," Shook reported that the Army Medical Department had decided to increase its supplies of the drug and was of the view that increase of production "is imperative and should be consummated at an early date if possible." In a subsequent memorandum to the OPM, Shook remarked that after Pearl Harbor "it became immediately evident that the requirements of this nation both military, naval, and civilian, for the 'Sulfa' group drugs would exceed production." Another SGO officer, L.L. Gardner, wrote to the Calco Chemical Division of American Cyanamid Company in February 1942 that "the brilliant results from the attack on Pearl Harbor were credited in large measure to the use of the sulfonamide compounds by mouth and in the wounds to control infection."[33]

The Army and Navy were acting on these perceptions. A report on wartime shortages of drugs and medical appliances, submitted to the Surgeon General of the Navy by the New York Academy of Medicine in March 1942, reported that both services were accumulating "vast supplies" of many kinds of drugs and medical equipment, including sulfa drugs. The report cited apparently reliable sources indicating that "within a few weeks the Army ordered 100,000 vials of tetanus antitoxin, 40 million quinine tablets, 35 million sulfadiazine tablets, and 10 million sulfapyridine tablets." It went on to note that "of these sulfa drugs such quantities represent the entire medical requirement of the United States for 2 to 3 months."

The SGO (Army) was also consulting the Drug Resources Advisory Committee on the availability of quantities of sulfadiazine and tannic acid sufficient to make one million one-ounce tubes of an ointment to be used in treatment of burns.[34]

Calls for increased production and supplies of sulfa drugs came in the context of a general reorientation of American production to the war effort. In January 1942, President Franklin D. Roosevelt set the year's production goal at 60,000 airplanes, 45,000 tanks, 20,000 antiaircraft guns, and eight million tons of shipping. Also in January, the OPM was abolished and replaced by the War Production Board (WPB). The Health Supply Branch of the old OPM became part of the WPB's Industry Operations Division.[35]

The most critical period for the WPB and for American industry came in May, June, and July 1942. Rapid expansion of U.S. military and lend-lease requirements for pharmaceutical products put pressure on industry to expand production accordingly, while the WPB struggled to set priorities, establish a workable ratings system for allocation of raw materials, and clarify a sometimes confusing situation to manufacturers. For the sulfa drugs as for many other products, major expansion of production was made possible by continuous monitoring of production, production facilities, and the flow of raw materials. Close cooperation between government agencies and between the WPB and industry ensured that, while allocation controls were necessary for raw materials required to make the sulfa drugs, they were not needed for the sulfa drugs themselves. The sulfa drugs may be subsumed under the statement later made in a government history that "without qualification . . . the Chemicals Bureau [of the WPB] and the chemical industry went to war in 1942."[36]

In late June and early July 1942, the WPB prepared statements on the present status, including uses and production figures, of the most important sulfa drugs. The statement on sulfanilamide described it as of "wide use in the prophylaxis and treatment of infectious diseases caused by bacteria and viruses," adding that "for external application in surgery and wound therapy sulfanilamide is in great demand." The statement concluded that despite an estimated domestic production of more than two million pounds in 1942, production would still lag requirements by more than 200,000 pounds and that production should be stimulated. The statement on sulfathiazole noted that "it may challenge sulfapyridine in the treatment of pneumococcic infections" and that it had the advantages over sulfapyridine of lower toxicity, faster absorption, and apparently greater effect on staphylococcal infections. At the time of the statement (July 3, 1942), the WPB regarded the current and estimated future production of sulfathiazole to be satisfactory. Sulfapyridine presented a different problem. Although U.S. military demand for it was relatively small, and it was possible that in the United States it would be replaced by sulfathiazole in treatment of pneumonia, foreign demand through lend-lease and defense aid was large. The WPB concluded that present production was inadequate and should be increased. The statement on sulfadiazine described it as an "important new chemotherapeutic agent" with possible advantages over sulfathiazole and sulfapyridine. Since the drug was still not thoroughly tested in practice, the statement concluded, demand for it was "fluid." Finally, a statement on sulfaguanidine noted its primary use in acute and mild bacillary dysentery and

other intestinal bacterial infections, and its reported usefulness in operative procedures on the large bowel, in peritonitis, and in ophthalmic infections. The statement
concluded that combined U.S. military, U.S. domestic, and foreign requirements for
sulfaguanidine would far exceed present rates of production and that "production
should be stimulated to meet the estimated demand."[37]

Most in demand in June and July 1942 was sulfanilamide in the crystalline
(powdered) form used in local treatment of wounds. Both the Navy and Army
were determined to obtain adequate supplies for sailors and soldiers, respectively,
and the two services found themselves, temporarily at least, in competition. On
June 8, Shook of the SGO wrote to the Army and Navy Munitions Board
(ANMB) Priorities Committee stating that recent contracts for sulfanilamide
crystals placed by the Navy with Monsanto Chemical Company would effectively
prevent the Upjohn Company from obtaining the bulk crystalline sulfanilamide it
needed to fulfill a prior contract with the Army. Pointing out that "sulfanilamide is
vitally needed to supply the field forces" of the Army, Shook asked the Priorities
Committee to adjust the amounts ordered from Monsanto so that "both services
may secure their just portions." A month later, on July 18, the SGO was urging the
WPB to expand the production of the granular form of sulfanilamide as rapidly as
possible.[38]

The Upjohn Company, together with Hynson, Westcott & Dunning, was under contract from the Army for a very large order of sulfanilamide powder in special sterile envelopes to be included in soldiers' first aid kits. Shortly after Pearl
Harbor, it had become apparent that sulfanilamide powder could become contaminated with microbes against which it was ineffective. Attempts at sterilization of
the powder foundered in the face of its rapid caramelization when heated. An Upjohn bacteriologist, John F. Norton, quickly solved the problem by precise control
of temperature and time in the sterilization process. Upjohn remained a major for-
mulator and packer of sulfonamides produced by other chemical and pharmaceutical companies for the duration of the war.[39]

Other companies were being drawn into the government-directed production
effort. On July 18, 1942, letters went out from Clifford V. Morgan of the Drugs Resources Advisory Committee to Parke Davis & Company, E.R. Squibb & Sons,
and the Calco Chemical Division of American Cyanamid Company. Referring to
the committee's recent study of the production facilities and requirements of the
five most important sulfa drugs, and its review of the data together with the WPB's
Health Supplies Branch, Morgan wrote to Parke Davis that "at that meeting it was
felt that your company would best serve the military as well as civilian needs by
producing amounts of sulfathiazole up to the limit of the capacity of your present
equipment." The annual production target would be 25,000 pounds, and the WPB
would assist the company in meeting the goal. Morgan asked Squibb to aim for annual production of 120,000 pounds of sulfathiazole and 150,000 pounds of
sulfaguanidine and offered the WPB's assistance in carrying out the expansion of
production facilities that this entailed. To Calco Chemical, Morgan expressed the
Drug Resources Advisory Committee's concern that Calco's geographical position
in New Jersey, near the Atlantic coast, could make it vulnerable to enemy attack.
Since Calco was still the sole manufacturer of sulfadiazine, destruction of its plant

could cut off sulfadiazine supplies. Abandoning as economically impracticable the committee's earlier suggestion that new production facilities be built in the Midwest, Morgan instead requested that "your organization arrange to stockpile a minimum of 200,000 pounds of this drug in inland areas not vulnerable to attack." He specified that "at least 50 percent of your output, in excess of that required to fulfill government contracts, should be set aside for this purpose, in order to build up the desired amounts as rapidly as possible."[40]

In September 1942, the WPB underwent a reorganization, one result of which was the dissolution of the Health Supplies Branch and the reassignment of its components. The pharmaceutical, medicinal chemical, biologicals, and botanicals sections were combined with the Toiletries and Cosmetics Branch of the Bureau of Industry and with personnel from a dissolved central Statistics Division to form a new Drugs and Cosmetics Section under the Chemicals Bureau. The Drugs and Cosmetics Section under its Chief, Fred J. Stock, was responsible for "the production, maintenance, and stockpiling of drugs to meet military and essential civilian requirements of [the] U.S." and its allies, and for "assisting the cosmetic industry to convert to products directly needed for war purposes and essential civilian supply." This organization would persist for the remainder of the war.[41]

As expansion of production and demand continued in the fall and winter of 1942, temporary shortages and imbalances in supplies of sulfa drugs occurred that were worrisome to WPB officials. Large orders from the Army for various sulfa drugs led to rumors and panic buying by manufacturers, which provoked WPB controls. When more supplies became available, some companies bought more than they needed. Production then fell in response to soft demand. At a meeting of the Proprietary Drug Industry Advisory Committee on December 10, 1942, Stock, chief of the Drugs and Cosmetics Section, reported temporary shortages of sulfadiazine and sulfathiazole. "There will be some of these drugs in December, more in January, less in February and ample in March," he told the committee. In the background lurked twin specters from World War I: acute and painful drug shortages, and the possibility of a major civilian epidemic comparable to the influenza pandemic of 1918. A memorandum of November 28, 1942, to Robert P. Fischelis, chief of the Medical and Health Supplies Section of the Office of Civilian Supply, referred explicitly to the possibility of an influenza epidemic and to the need for a substantial reserve of sulfa drugs to treat the large number of secondary pneumococcal and streptococcal infections that would accompany it. Fischelis in turn urged manufacturers to set aside part of their production to meet essential civilian demands for normal consumption and possible emergencies.[42]

Whatever problems or uncertainties surfaced in the fall and winter of 1942 came in the midst of an enormous and rapid expansion of production. Taking the aggregate of the nine principal sulfa drugs manufactured in the United States during World War II, total production in 1942 came to more than 4.8 million pounds. This compares to just more than two million pounds in 1941 and to only 760,000 pounds in 1940. Production in 1942 was therefore some 240 percent that of 1941 and some 635 percent that of 1940. The steep upward climb continued, yielding a total 1943 production of more than 8.7 million pounds.[43]

Of the nine sulfa drugs included in these totals, two—sulfanilamide and sulfathiazole—were produced in the largest quantities. Sulfadiazine was manufactured in relatively modest amounts in 1941, but its production increased more than eleven-fold in 1942, and another 3.5-fold in 1943, placing it in the ranks of the two leaders. Sulfaguanidine, more specialized in its uses, nevertheless came into increasing demand and occupied fourth place by 1943. Sulfapyridine continued to be manufactured in the United States, but its production levels dropped after 1941 as it was displaced in use by sulfathiazole and sulfadiazine.[44]

Of the American companies producing finished sulfa drugs during World War II, at least six—Monsanto, Cincinnati Chemical Works, Sherwin-Williams, Calco, Merck, and Winthrop—also produced intermediates needed for manufacture of sulfonamides, while at least four—Abbott, Lilly, Mead-Johnson, and Wyeth—did not. Other U.S. companies were involved in the tableting, packaging, and sale of sulfa drugs. Two of these, Upjohn Company and Hynson, Westcott & Dunning, have been mentioned above. Another example is Sharp & Dohme, which distributed and promoted succinyl sulfathiazole—manufactured by Monsanto—under the trade name Sulfasuxidine. Manufacturers could not take their raw materials for granted. As of September 1943, the WPB listed no less than twenty-six chemicals used in the production of sulfa drugs that were under WPB priority orders.[45]

The record U.S. production level for sulfa drugs achieved in 1943 was not sustained in 1944. Although aggregate production remained high at around four million pounds, this was less than half the 1943 figure. Among the probable contributors to the drop were inventories carried over from 1943, an optimistic turn in the war in mid-1944 that led to a relaxation of control and reconversion plans in the WPB's Chemicals Bureau, and the initial perception that penicillin, which was beginning to enter military medical practice, would replace the sulfa drugs. Production moved up again in late 1944 and the first half of 1945 as the Battle of the Bulge led to sharp increases in military demand, the prospect loomed of a long war with Japan, and manufacturers realized that penicillin would supplement but not replace the sulfa drugs. Sulfaguanidine, to take one example, dropped to production levels in the second and third quarters of 1944 that were lower than those for 1941. Production in the fourth quarter rebounded to surpass 1943 levels and rose even higher in the first quarter of 1945. In January 1945, aggregate production of sulfa drugs was about 300,000 pounds, equivalent to an annual rate of 3.6 million pounds. By June 1945, it had risen to 600,000 pounds, yielding an annual rate, 7.2 million pounds, which was surpassed only in 1943.[46]

Many producers of sulfa drugs were among the thirty American pharmaceutical manufacturers honored with Army and Navy "E" Awards for excellence in production during the war. Given to only five percent of the estimated war production plants in the United States, "E" awards recognized quality and quantity of production, overcoming of obstacles, avoidance of stoppages, maintenance of fair labor standards, and other achievements. One of the awardees, Merck & Company Inc., proudly displayed its award in a 1943 advertisement in its own publication under the heading "Merciful Munitions." "There can be no greater reward for us whose task it is to produce more and still more drugs and chemicals," the ad began, "than to know that somewhere today, on some distant field of battle, these merciful mu-

nitions are easing pain, helping to heal wounds, and saving lives." Next to a picture of a wounded soldier writing home from his hospital bed, the text continued:

> It might be the kid next door . . . or, perhaps, your own boy . . . who may
> write: "I didn't want you to worry, so I didn't tell you sooner, but I ran
> into a piece of shrapnel a few weeks ago. I'm practically as good as new
> now, and will soon be fit as ever. Gee, Dad, those sulfa drugs certainly
> are great stuff. Major Randall, the surgeon who fixed me up, says they
> probably saved my life. I have everything I need here, and am feeling
> fine."[47]

CHAPTER 10

Trial by Fire

As the Merck ad at the end of chapter 9 suggests, the millions of pounds of sulfa drugs pouring from U.S. production lines in each year of World War II were quickly taken up by military and civilian supply networks, and ultimately made their way to doctors and patients at home and in all the military theaters. How were the sulfa drugs used? How effective did practitioners believe them to be, and what problems were associated with their use? Did wartime research on sulfa drugs influence practice, and if so, in what ways? Finally, what effect did the appearance of penicillin on the therapeutic scene have on the place of the sulfa drugs in medical practice?

Answers to such questions may best be sought by tracing the place of the sulfa drugs in the evolving preventive and therapeutic management of a select group of diseases or conditions that figured prominently in the medical practice, and especially the military medical practice, of World War II. Among these were pneumonia, gonorrhea, meningitis, bacillary dysentery, hemolytic streptococcal infections, wounds, and burns. Doctors faced other major problems for which the sulfa drugs were not of significant help, for example, malaria, and others of relatively minor significance in which they were of use, for example, trachoma. The discussion that follows is not a comprehensive survey of therapeutics and preventive medicine in World War II or even of all of the uses of the sulfa drugs during the war. What it does aim to provide is a picture of the evolving pattern of use of the sulfa drugs in the most important diseases or conditions in which they were thought to be effective, and at least a summary assessment of the effect of the wartime introduction of penicillin in each case.[1]

The Coming of Penicillin

To better gauge the impact of penicillin, sulfa drug use must be examined in two periods. The first runs from the prewar time of preparation to May 1943, when clinical investigation of penicillin began in selected military hospitals. The second runs from May 1943 to the end of the war in August 1945, a period in which penicillin was introduced into military use.

The promise of penicillin in treatment of bacterial infections was recognized by Alfred Newton Richards of the Office of Scientific Research and Development (OSRD) Committee on Medical Research in 1941. From that point on, its introduction into medical practice was limited mainly by development of production methods and facilities, and to a lesser extent by the need for clinical investigations.[2]

When the OSRD's Committee on Medical Research was formed in the summer of 1941, there was not enough penicillin available to treat a single case. By the spring of 1942, there was enough to treat one patient, and from June 1942 to February 1943 enough became available to treat 100 patients. Even these slight amounts allowed confirmation of penicillin's great potential in treatment of bacterial infections. Early in 1943, for example, investigators gave verbal report of dramatic successes in treatment of sulfonamide-resistant gonorrhea with penicillin. In May 1943, clinical investigations on the use of penicillin in treatment of gonorrhea began at fifteen Army hospitals. By this time the committee was convinced that the Army and Navy would need penicillin in large quantities, and Richards met with members of the War Production Board's Drugs and Cosmetics Section to plan the first production program.[3]

On July 16, 1943, the War Production Board issued an allocation order controlling distribution of the limited supplies of penicillin and restricting deliveries to the Army, Navy, OSRD, and Public Health Service. Penicillin for treatment of U.S. civilians could be released only through OSRD. On the same day, the Surgeon General of the Army released a Circular Letter informing medical officers on the present status of penicillin. The letter told officers that penicillin was apparently nontoxic and that it was highly effective in low concentrations against acute infections due to staphylococcus, hemolytic streptococcus, pneumococcus, meningococcus, and gonococcus. At the same time, it warned them that "one of the most important factors limiting the clinical application of penicillin is its productibility." Most of the available supplies, the letter stated, were to go to a select group of hospitals in which investigations on wound infections and sepsis or on gonorrhea were being conducted. Officers requesting use of penicillin were instructed to make arrangements with one of the designated hospitals and to confine use to cases "with grave life-endangering infections that have resisted other appropriate forms of therapy, especially the sulfonamides, and to the type of cases in which it has been found effective."[4]

The War Production Board's Penicillin Producers Industry Advisory Committee met for the first time in September 1943. By October, eighteen U.S. companies were producing penicillin, but although some companies had large plants under construction, none was yet operating beyond the pilot plant stage. Supplies were not available in significant amounts for overseas military use, and although clinical investigations on penicillin were proceeding in some twenty civilian hospitals, supplies for civilian use were very limited. Penicillin did not play a notable role in the medical response to the epidemic of respiratory tract infections that occurred in the United States from late November 1943 to February 1944.[5]

The gap that still existed between perceived present and future needs for penicillin and actual supply is visible in a conference held in March 1944, under the auspices of the War Production Board, that included representatives from the government and the penicillin producers. The purpose of the meeting was to consider the terms of a contract under which the penicillin producers would agree to share among themselves technical information and patent rights. The motive behind it was to speed production. The War Production Board's Fred J. Stock, who chaired the meeting, stated that "production is not adequate to meet military and essential civilian demands; and while that condition prevails, everything possible must be done to get maximum production." The Army's Major J.A. Purinton told the conference that "the Surgeon General would like to have a product that can be taken into the front lines, but as yet the Army has not been able to explore the use of penicillin under combat conditions," presumably due to inadequate supplies.[6]

The year 1944 witnessed a dramatic surge in penicillin production that all but eliminated such problems. By June, when the invasion of northern Europe began, monthly production in the United States was more than nine times what it had been in January. By December 1944, it was more than twenty-three times the January figure. At 1,600 billion Oxford Units, total penicillin production for 1944 was seventy-seven times what it had been in 1943. The climb continued into 1945, with monthly production in June more than twice what it had been at the end of 1944.[7]

By the time of the Normandy landings, enough penicillin was available to treat all Allied casualties who needed it. The U.S. civilian population was served by a system set up by an advisory panel composed of members from the War Production Board (including the chairman), the Public Health Service, OSRD, and the American Medical Association. The panel initially named 1,000 hospitals as "depot hospitals" that were to receive, store, and further distribute available supplies of penicillin according to assigned monthly quotas. A Civilian Penicillin Distribution Unit, which administered the system, operated from May 1, 1944, to March 15, 1945. The number of designated depot hospitals increased with the supply of penicillin, reaching 2,700 by December 1944.[8]

It is in this context of a limited supply of penicillin from May 1943 through early 1944, followed by rapid expansion of its availability from the spring of 1944 through the rest of the war, that the impact of penicillin on sulfa drug use must be seen. Since the strengths and failings of the sulfa drugs, and of penicillin, varied with the conditions they were used to treat, the evolving relationships of the two kinds of therapies must also be viewed on a case-by-case basis.

Pneumonia

Pneumonia had been a major killer in World War I. Together with influenza and measles, with which it was often associated as a secondary (and lethal) infection, pneumonia accounted for seventy-three percent of all deaths from disease in a war in which just over half of all deaths among American troops were due to disease. As a new war began in Europe in the fall of 1939, American doctors aware of the earlier experience with pneumonia saw renewed cause for concern. Speaking to the Johns Hopkins Alumni Association in December 1939, Perrin H. Long, who had served with an ambulance unit in World War I, recalled the virtually uncontrolled ravages of influenza and pneumonia in 1918. At the same time, he held out the hope that pneumonia, at least, would be controlled in the new war by sulfanilamide and its derivatives, which by this time included sulfapyridine.[9]

Well before the appearance of sulfapyridine, Army doctors at Walter Reed General Hospital in Washington, DC had been using sulfanilamide in treatment of bacterial pneumonia. From 1936 to February 1939 they treated one group of lobar pneumonia patients with antipneumococcal serum. A second group received sulfanilamide, and a third the standard nonspecific therapy. They found lower mortality rates and fewer complications in the groups treated with serum or sulfanilamide.[10]

By February 1939, Walter Reed doctors were in touch with Merck & Company Inc. to obtain supplies of sulfapyridine for use "on a controlled experimental basis" during the pneumonia season. Over the next year they treated seventy-three cases of pneumonia with only two deaths and concluded that "sulfapyridine therapy in pneumonia has been the most effective and satisfactory type of treatment that has been generally accepted to date." They were impressed with sulfapyridine's military potential. Probably thinking of the sulfa drug's relative ease of use compared to serum therapy, which required typing skills and equipment, they wrote that sulfapyridine "is a very effective and practical therapeutic agent for the treatment of pneumonia in the Theater of Operations in time of war, and could be instituted as far forward as the Battalion Aid Station [near the front lines] if advisable."[11]

Use of sulfapyridine in pneumonia therapy spread rapidly, but even as Walter Reed physicians reported on its successes in February 1940, they also noted the appearance of another new sulfa drug, sulfathiazole. At that time, they had treated few patients with sulfathiazole but reported it to be as effective as sulfapyridine in pneumonia while producing much less nausea, vomiting, and toxicity. In the United States, sulfathiazole rapidly overtook sulfapyridine in civilian and military practice. By December 1940, when the Surgeon General of the Army released the circular letter produced by the National Research Council (NRC) titled "Chemotherapy in Infectious Diseases and Other Infections," sulfathiazole had become the recommended drug of choice by medical officers in all cases of primary pneumococcal pneumonia and in most cases of secondary pneumonia in which bacteria were thought to be involved. A report in *Military Surgeon* based on 209 pneumonia cases treated prior to November 1941 featured sulfathiazole and emphasized its advantages (with sulfapyridine and sulfadiazine) for treatment of pneumonia in "tent hospitals, in small infirmaries in outlying posts or in field medical installations, even in those that are necessarily without X-ray equipment or laboratory apparatus."[12]

Now it was sulfathiazole's turn to be overtaken. In 1940, another new sulfa drug, sulfadiazine, was introduced by American Cyanamid. Early clinical tests showed sulfadiazine to be as effective as sulfapyridine or sulfathiazole in treatment of pneumonia and other bacterial infections but much less likely to cause nausea, vomiting, mental disturbances, or other undesirable reactions. By the time of Pearl Harbor, sulfadiazine had begun to be introduced into military practice. When the Surgeon General of the Army released a revised version of the Circular Letter on "Chemotherapy of Infectious Diseases and Other Infections" in February 1942, sulfadiazine had replaced sulfathiazole as the drug of choice in most pneumonias. Sulfathiazole continued to be used, but sulfapyridine was increasingly relegated to a distant third place in pneumonia therapy after 1941. Sulfadiazine remained the standard treatment for most pneumonias through the end of the war.[13]

Penicillin had entered the scene of pneumonia therapy by July 1943, when the Surgeon General's circular letter listed pneumococcal infections among those most amenable to treatment by the new medicine. Pneumonia was among the conditions treated with penicillin in hospitals selected for its clinical investigation in 1943 and 1944. For example, among the patients treated for a total of twenty-nine different diseases at the U.S. Naval Hospital in Portsmouth, Virginia, between August 1, 1943, and June 30, 1944, thirteen received penicillin for pneumococcal pneumonia or pneumococcal empyema. The cure rate in these cases was 100 percent. Such successes earned penicillin a permanent place in pneumonia therapy and contributed to the Office of the Surgeon General decision in May 1944 to drop antipneumococcal serum from the Army supply tables.[14]

Without more detailed study than is possible here, it is not possible to weigh exactly the relative roles of sulfa drugs and penicillin in the treatment of pneumonia in the last two years of the war. What is clear is that penicillin did not replace sulfadiazine as the standard therapy in most instances. At least until the spring of 1944, penicillin was not available in substantial quantities, even for military use. Thereafter, the effectiveness of sulfadiazine and its ready availability continued to make it an attractive choice except in cases of sulfonamide-resistant pneumonia.[15]

An official history of U.S. Army medicine in World War II acknowledged the difficulty of obtaining reliable figures for the incidence of bacterial pneumonia during the war, since accurate bacteriological diagnosis was not accomplished in many cases. Nevertheless, it was clear to all that pneumonia in World War II was a disaster that did not happen. The incidence, severity, and mortality of pneumonia were much less than they were expected to be, and much less than they had been in World War I. To give only one illustrative figure, the death rate for lobar pneumonia among American troops in World War I was estimated to be 259 per 100,000 per year. Army figures for 1942–1945 gave the comparable death rate as less than 2 per 100,000 per year.[16]

What accounts for the enormous contrast? Part of the answer was the absence of an influenza pandemic comparable in severity and scope to that of 1918, which had created many cases of pneumonia among its weakened victims. Another part was the entire absence of measles epidemics, which could also give rise to pneumonia, among American troops. One author of the Army's medical history, Yale Kneeland, Jr., speculated that "an inexplicable fluctuation in the nature of the disease" making it less severe, might also have played a role. All of that considered, there was no doubt in the minds of analysts after the war that the use of chemotherapeutic agents, especially the sulfa drugs, had played a significant role in minimizing both the severity and the mortality of the disease.[17]

Gonorrhea

Venereal diseases cast another long shadow from World War I over preparations by American physicians for possible entry into another great conflict. Here the problem was not the lethality of the diseases, which was slight, but the cost they exacted in disability and lost manpower. Gonorrhea, in particular, had been third among causes of noneffectiveness in American troops in World War I, with a rate of 2.59 per 1,000. An editorial in *War Medicine* in January 1942 noted that in World War I "an appalling total of more than seven million man days was lost on account of venereal disease." Prevention and control of gonorrhea had been a major problem for American military medicine in the earlier war, and there was little reason to believe that things would be different in the one that now threatened to involve the United States.[18]

One of the first subcommittees to be formed by the NRC Division of Medical Sciences in June 1940 was that responsible for venereal diseases, under the Committee on Chemotherapeutic and Other Agents. The subcommittee met frequently, and its recommendations were incorporated into the Surgeon General of the Army's Circular Letter number 18, released on March 10, 1941.[19]

As the first statement of official policy in the period of preparation before U.S. entry into the war, Circular Letter number 18 attempted to bring order into a field of therapeutics then characterized by a diversity of practices. Sulfa drugs were not effective against syphilis. Although gonorrhea had been treated with sulfanilamide as early as 1937, and later with sulfapyridine with more success, Army guidelines left use of these medicines to the discretion of individual medical officers. Circular Letter number 18 called for laboratory confirmation of the diagnosis of gonorrhea and for a clearly defined regimen of treatment with sulfathiazole, supplemented with sulfapyridine if necessary. It also defined criteria for cure and for a follow-up test three to four months after the initial infection.[20]

Despite the rapid expansion of the Army in 1941 and 1942, effective implementation of Circular Letter number 18 was favored by the presence of most troops in training camps in the continental United States, by the existence of well-staffed hospitals in the camps, and by the hospitalization of all cases of gonorrhea. Deviations from the guidelines occurred, but the overall result was a greater standardization of therapeutic practices in the Army.[21]

Experience with Circular Letter number 18 in the field led the NRC Subcommittee on Venereal Diseases to recommend revisions, and these were incorporated in Circular Letter number 74, released by the Surgeon General on July 25, 1942. Circular Letter number 74 made sulfadiazine an alternative to sulfathiazole as a drug of choice in treatment of gonorrhea and reduced the role of sulfapyridine. It revised recommended dosages and reduced the time to follow-up examination. Most notably, and ominously, it recommended that "carefully selected patients with sulfonamide-resistant infections be given ten hours of sustained fever therapy," in which doctors artificially induced fever in patients in the hope that it would destroy residual gonococci not affected by chemotherapy, a sign that even the best available sulfa drugs could not effect cures in all cases.[22]

Standard Army practice early in the war was to hospitalize all patients with gonorrhea. This policy was reconsidered during 1942 in response to the filling of hospital beds and the loss of training time. Attempts to treat soldiers with sulfa drugs while on duty status proved successful and became the basis for a circular letter issued on February 1, 1943, authorizing such treatment wherever feasible. The new policy was widely implemented in the United States and overseas.[23]

Meanwhile, resistance of gonorrheal infections to treatment with sulfa drugs was increasing, with average rates of cure falling below seventy-five percent and the appearance of more and more chronic cases. At the Surgeon General's request, the NRC's Subcommittee on Venereal Diseases presided over a conference in April 1943 to examine the use of combined chemotherapy and fever therapy in cases of sulfonamide-resistant gonorrhea. The result was a circular letter issued in May 1943 that defined the procedures to be followed in fever therapy and increased the numbers of hospitals in which it could be done.[24]

Verbal reports in early 1943 of the effectiveness of penicillin in cases of sulfonamide-resistant gonorrhea, and confirmation of these reports in clinical investigations in fifteen Army hospitals beginning in May 1943, opened the possibility of an efficient alternative to fever therapy. In September 1943, prompted by these studies, the Surgeon General authorized the treatment of sulfonamide-resistant gonorrhea with penicillin. Short supplies of penicillin placed constraints on use of the new medicine, however. Not only did sulfa drugs continue as standard therapy for gonorrhea, but dosages were increased, and beginning in August 1943 the Surgeon General authorized administration of sulfathiazole as a prophylactic measure. Even when penicillin was used, dosages were held to a minimum to conserve supplies.[25]

Penicillin use in gonorrhea therapy expanded in parallel with the explosion of penicillin production in 1944. Both numbers of cases treated and dosages per case increased. A major turning point was signaled in September 1944 when a War Department Technical Bulletin (Technical Bulletins having replaced Circular Letters) directed that penicillin henceforth be the drug of choice in treatment of gonorrhea. Sulfa drugs were now to be used only when patients failed to respond to penicillin. Replacement of sulfa drugs by penicillin in military practice did not occur suddenly or uniformly, but the motivation was clear. According to one Navy doctor reporting in November 1944, as many as fifty percent of gonococcal infections in the Navy were thought to be at least partially resistant to sulfonamides.[26]

For World War II as a whole, the venereal diseases were by far the leading cause of disability or ineffectiveness among military personnel due to infectious or parasitic diseases. Of the venereal diseases, gonorrhea accounted for about

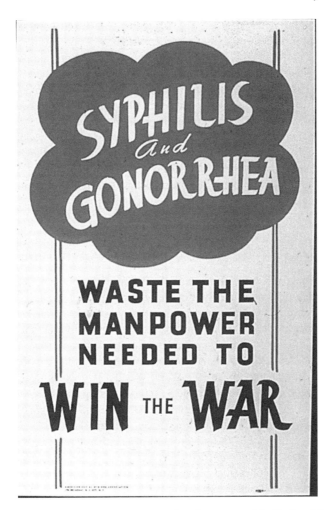

Figure 10.1. U.S. World War II poster (reprinted courtesy of the National Archives).

eighty percent of the problem. In the Army alone there were over 880,000 cases of gonorrhea, an incidence rate of more than thirty-four cases per year per 1,000 persons. This compared to less than half that number and incidence rate for the next largest category, malaria.[27]

In this context, the therapeutic use of the sulfa drugs, and later penicillin, had a major impact. Long before the war, the systemic use of sulfanilamide, then sulfapyridine and sulfathiazole, and the abandonment of older, local methods of treatment of gonorrhea had sharply reduced both the complications of the disease and the numbers of days lost from active duty because of it. The trends continued in the early years of the war and were given an additional boost by the introduction of penicillin. In 1937, when sulfanilamide was first tried, twenty-eight percent of gonorrhea cases in the U.S. Army involved complications. With the introduction of the sulfa drugs, the percentage of cases with complications dropped to 24.5 percent in 1938, 23 percent in 1939, 8 percent in 1940, 6.6 percent in 1941, and 2 percent in 1942. With combined sulfa drug and penicillin therapy the rate of complications dropped still further, to 1.5 percent in 1943 and 1 percent in 1944. In 1939, soldiers with a venereal disease (about eighty percent of the cases were gonorrhea) lost an average forty-two days to the disease. Treatment with sulfa drugs, and later penicillin, brought time lost down to twenty-two days in 1941, ten days in 1943, and seven days in 1944. Little wonder that Hugh J. Morgan, a Brigadier General and Chief Consultant in Medicine to the U.S. Army, speaking in November 1944, stated that "from the military standpoint no more important development in therapeutics has occurred than in the field of the venereal diseases."[28]

Meningitis

The experience of World War I pointed to yet another potential threat to American service personnel: meningitis (inflammation of the meninges, the membranes surrounding the brain and spinal cord), especially that caused by the meningococcus bacterium. In contrast to the case of gonorrhea, the threat from meningitis came not from high incidence and days lost to service, but from the suddenness and unpredictability of its appearance and its high mortality. Within months of U.S. Army mobilization in World War I, a serious outbreak of meningitis had occurred among soldiers. In the 33 months during and after U.S. participation in the war, there were approximately 5,900 cases of meningitis in the Army, with a case mortality rate of thirty-one percent, despite the use of meningococcal serum. Although meningitis ranked only seventy-sixth as a reason for admission to hospitals in World War I, it ranked sixth as a cause of death. Uncertainty about the mode of transmission of meningitis and the apparent ineffectiveness of prevention and control measures occasionally led to panic that could disrupt training or other military operations.[29]

A major break in the treatment of meningitis and in the outlook for its victims came in 1937 with the recognition of sulfanilamide as an effective chemotherapeutic agent in the disease. By 1940, the case fatality rate for meningitis in the United States had dropped dramatically, to one-third or one-fourth of what it had been. Most medical observers attributed at least a large part of the change to use of the sulfa drugs.[30]

When the war broke out in Europe in 1939, sulfanilamide was an established part of treatment of meningitis in the U.S. Army. The first circular letter on "Chemotherapy in Infectious Diseases and Other Infections," put out by the Surgeon General in December 1940 on the basis of NRC recommendations, named sulfanilamide as the drug of choice in most meningitis cases, with sulfapyridine to be used in cases of purulent meningitis.[31]

Despite the availability of chemotherapy, anxiety about possible meningitis outbreaks rose as the United States began mobilization in the fall of 1940. Early in 1941 the Preventive Medicine Office of the Army's Office of the Surgeon General organized a Commission on Meningococcal Meningitis, headed by

Long, that included civilian as well as military members. In April 1941, the Surgeon General received a report based on the recommendations of the commission that specified how military and civilian groups would act cooperatively to study and control the disease.[32]

For more than two years after the beginning of mobilization in September 1940, incidence of meningitis remained low, and the feared epidemic failed to materialize. Therapeutics continued to evolve. Starting from an insight first gained in World War I, doctors now recognized two stages to the disease. In the first stage, called meningococcemia, the blood became infected. In the second stage, the infection could become localized, most dangerously in the meninges, giving rise to the classic symptoms of meningitis. Early recognition of the first phase and prompt treatment became a primary goal of therapy. By February 1942, sulfadiazine began to replace sulfanilamide, sulfapyridine, or sulfathiazole as the drug of choice in treatment of meningitis. Although some doctors still used meningococcal serum in some cases, there was increasing inclination to use chemotherapy alone. In July 1942, Long presented a report for the Commission on Meningococcal Meningitis in which he gave an "extraordinarily low" case fatality rate of 4.1 percent for the U.S. Army over the previous year, a success that he credited to early diagnosis and treatment.[33]

In December 1942, the incidence rate for meningitis at Army bases in the United States moved sharply upward. By March 1943, it had peaked at 2.9 cases per 1,000 persons per year, the most severe epidemic of meningitis among U.S. troops since World War I. By early fall of 1943, the incidence rate had fallen back to close to preepidemic levels, only to rise again in the winter of 1943–1944 to a second, lower peak of 1.1 in February 1944. Highest rates of infection were recorded among recently inducted soldiers.[34]

Well before the outbreak of the first meningitis epidemic, some Army doctors had tried giving subtherapeutic doses of sulfa drugs to healthy soldiers as a preventive measure. At Fort Eustis, Virginia, between January and June 1942, for example, fifty-six soldiers determined to be meningococcus carriers were isolated and treated with sulfathiazole over several days, with the result that all showed negative cultures for meningococcus. During the first outbreak, from December 1942 to February 1943, medical officers administered low dosages of sulfadiazine to an entire Army cantonment, including military and civilian personnel, at Camp Adair, Oregon. They found an immediate reduction in incidence, without disruption of training or other operations. On May 21, 1943, all 18,000 men at an Army base in Greensboro, North Carolina, were "diazined," that is, given about five grams of sulfadiazine within nineteen hours. Doctors pronounced the trial a success in the first eight weeks after the event.[35]

Experiences such as these, and the threat of a new epidemic in the coming winter, led the Surgeon General to issue Circular Letter number 170 on September 30, 1943. This circular letter made prophylactic treatment of new recruits with sulfadiazine part of official Army policy.[36]

Sulfadiazine prophylaxis did not prevent a second meningitis epidemic among U.S. troops in the winter of 1943–1944, and the overall impact of the program was difficult to assess after the war. Nevertheless, doctors were convinced that it helped to control specific outbreaks and to prevent disruption of Army operations in which large numbers of people were moved from place to place and required to act under very diverse circumstances. Given the panic that meningitis could cause, it is likely that the psychological effect of organized preventive measures combined with effective therapy had an important role apart from reduction of the rates of incidence and mortality. As two Army doctors at Fort Eustis, Virginia, put it, "questions of morale may dictate many of the policies to be adopted, regardless of their medical value. This post has had the familiar experience of finding the hysteria caused by the meningitis almost as difficult to handle as the disease itself."[37]

Late in 1943, small amounts of penicillin became available at some Army hospitals for treatment of meningococcal infections. In February 1944, the Surgeon General issued a technical bulletin recommending use of penicillin in addition to sulfadiazine in fulminating (very sudden and intense) infections and in place of sulfadiazine in cases that failed to respond to the sulfa drug or in which the patient had a strong reaction to it. Thereafter, although supplies of penicillin increased, its place in the treatment of meningitis remained limited. Not only was sulfadiazine thought to be highly effective, and relatively free of toxic effects compared to other sulfa drugs, but some studies suggested that penicillin was less able than sulfadiazine to maintain effective concentrations in the spinal fluid. Sulfadiazine remained the drug of choice in meningococcal infections through the end of the war, with penicillin in a supplementary role.[38]

Even with increasingly efficient diagnosis, effective chemotherapy, and eventually chemoprophylaxis, meningococcal infections still accounted for 559 deaths in the U.S. Army during World War II. Where meningococcal infections had been second only to pneumonia as a cause of death from disease among U.S. troops in World War I, they were now, in World War II, second only to tuberculosis in that role. This much said, without the sulfa drugs, later joined by penicillin, the outcome almost certainly would have been far worse. A total of 559 deaths among almost 14,000 cases represents a case mortality rate of four percent. Had the World War I mortality rate of thirty-one percent held again, nearly eight times as many American soldiers would have died of meningococcal infections. Although massive doses of sulfa drugs were often given to patients with the most severe infections, only three deaths were judged by doctors to be drug induced, a rate of 0.04 percent. So effective was sulfadiazine that in January 1944 the American Medical Association's Council on Pharmacy and Chemistry removed antimeningococcal serum and meningococcal antitoxin from its list of New and Nonofficial Remedies. To these effects must be added a less measurable one: the boost to morale given by medicines that brought a degree of control to what had been a frightening and unpredictable illness.[39]

Bacillary Dysentery

Less frightening and more predictable, but also potentially disruptive of military operations, bacillary dysentery and related diarrheal conditions posed another challenge to military medicine. Diarrheas and dysenteries were among the most characteristic maladies of armies in wartime. Crowding and poor sanitation, especially in field operations, facilitated the fecal contamination of food and water that was the most common route of transmission for the causative bacteria. Until World War I, diarrheas and dysenteries were a significant cause of deaths as well as illness. As William Osler put it at the end of the nineteenth century, "[Dysentery] has been more fatal to armies than powder and shot." In the U.S. Army in World War I, the case fatality rate from these conditions was low, at 0.043 percent, but more than 48,000 cases were seen by doctors.[40]

By the beginning of World War II, doctors were aware of the importance of good sanitation as a preventive measure but had little to turn to in the way of therapy. Efforts were under way to develop serums or vaccines, but so far these had been unsuccessful. In an article published in 1940, Eli Kennerly Marshall, Jr., opened the possibility of help from a new direction, the sulfa drugs. While investigating sulfanilamide derivatives in a search for a compound as effective as sulfapyridine against pneumococcus infections, but less toxic, the Johns Hopkins pharmacologist had come across several compounds that were water soluble but poorly absorbed from the gastrointestinal tract. He reasoned that these properties together with antibacterial action might indicate a medicine that could be used to treat bacterial infections that were mainly or entirely localized in the intestine. Such a drug, Marshall thought, would represent "a new principle in the use of the new bacterial chemotherapeutic agents; the fundamental principle involved is the achievement of a high concentration of the drug in the intestine and a low concentration in the blood and tissues," a combination that would presumably maximize therapeutic action while minimizing toxicity. From among these compounds, Marshall selected a sulfanilylguanidine (the name was later shortened to sulfaguanidine) for closer investigation.[41]

In his original study, Marshall stopped short of trying sulfaguanidine on human patients. By January 1941, he was able to report favorable results from its use in treatment of seventeen children suffering from acute bacillary dysentery. By this time also he had arranged for samples of the medicine to be sent to medical officers with the British Middle East Forces. Tried first against severe cases of bacillary dysentery, sulfaguanidine proved to be a specific cure in these and also in milder cases. Doctors often delayed treatment in the early cases for three or four days to allow for laboratory confirmation of the infective organism. Later experience showed that if sulfaguanidine was given within hours of the appearance of symptoms, it could quickly stop the diarrhea and prevent damage to the lining of the colon. Many patients could be cured without a hospital stay, an especially important result for an army at war. In a letter to Marshall dated February 5, 1941, G.A.H. Buttle wrote that "this seems to be a really important discovery" and asked Marshall to convey to the manufacturer (Lederle Laboratories) that the British forces had an urgent need for large quantities of the medicine. On March 10, Buttle wrote to Marshall again, this time enclosing a report on the favorable results obtained from treating nine patients with sulfaguanidine and adding that "we have now only a few ounces of the drug left, but I hope there is some more on the way." American shipments of sulfaguanidine to British Middle East Forces were under way by April 1941.[42]

By the summer of 1941, sulfaguanidine had been added to the U.S. Army Drug Supply Catalog and had begun to enter military practice as a prophylactic and therapeutic agent. A year later, in July 1942, the War Production Board regarded its range of uses as still under investigation but noted its place in treatment of bacillary dysentery.[43]

In 1942–1945, more than half a million cases of diarrhea and dysentery were recorded by the U.S. Army. Although field conditions often precluded the laboratory work needed for confirmation of a diagnosis of bacillary dysentery, doctors analyzing the available data after the war concluded that a sizable proportion of all diarrheal conditions should be placed in that category. Incidence was highest among troops stationed overseas, where seventy-five percent of reported cases occurred among a population that represented forty percent of the average strength of the Army. The highest rates of incidence occurred in the summer of 1943 as large numbers of fresh troops entered areas where diarrheal diseases were endemic and sanitation poor. Hardest hit were Army personnel in the North Africa and Mediterranean, Middle East, and China-Burma-India theaters. Although the overall incidence of diarrheas and dysenteries was comparable to that of World War I, the case fatality rate of 0.02 (116 deaths among all reported cases) was considerably lower than the earlier war's figure of 0.043.[44]

Treatment with sulfa drugs to eliminate infection remained a standard part of Army management of bacillary dysentery through the end of World War II. Sulfaguanidine was widely used, as war correspondent Ernie Pyle discovered when he fell sick early in the Sicily campaign in 1943. It was joined by sulfathiazole and especially sulfadiazine, which had become the drug of choice by early 1945. Attempts at mass screening of carriers and their treatment with sulfa drugs foundered on practical obstacles. Results of mass prophylaxis using sulfa drugs were encouraging, but trials were not well controlled and the practice was not generally adopted. What was constant was that a soldier diagnosed with or presumed to be suffering from bacillary dysentery would be very likely to receive a sulfa drug as part of his treatment.[45]

Some sense of the disruptive potential of bacillary dysentery and the impact of sulfa drugs may be gained from reports published during and after the war. "Montgomery says the Eighth Army won, but Rommel claimed the victory for dysentery," wrote Sir Sheldon Dudley of the battle of El Alamein, a major turning point in the war in North Africa. General Erwin Rommel's claim was supported by British medical officers, who were appalled by the poor sanitary practices of the otherwise well-disciplined *Afrikakorps* and who estimated that forty to fifty percent of Rommel's troops were weakened by dysentery.[46]

Far from North Africa but also in 1942, Australian and Japanese forces were fighting in New Guinea, on the Kokoda trail, in the Owen Stanley Ranges. Good sanitary measures were impossible on the narrow and fiercely contested jungle trail, and both sides suffered from severe dysentery. Alarmed by the increasing casualties from the disease, Australian medical officers arranged for all available reserves of sulfaguanidine in Australia to be rushed by air to Port Moresby. From there, the medicine was moved to the forward area and was used to treat all soldiers with diarrhea or symptoms of dysentery. Within ten days, the epidemic on the Australian side was completely controlled. Lacking sulfaguanidine, the Japanese forces continued to be decimated by dysentery. Many Australian medical officers believed that sulfaguanidine gave the advantage to the Australian forces and saved Port Moresby.[47]

A less dramatic but quietly effective role for sulfa drugs is indicated in published wartime reports from U.S. forces in diverse locations. Army doctors used sulfaguanidine and sulfathiazole to successfully treat seventy-nine percent of bacillary dysentery cases at Camp Claiborne, Louisiana, between September 1941 and October 1942. Sulfaguanidine controlled an outbreak of the disease in an army garrison in Puerto Rico in 1942 or early 1943. At an overseas Army station hospital (the published article does not give the name or location), doctors used sulfaguanidine or sulfadiazine to treat 1,120 cases of diarrhea or dysentery between May and November 1943. The response "appeared to be almost miraculous," with almost all patients showing marked improvement within twenty-four hours. A general report on the status of the sulfonamides from November 1944 noted that "during the past year, in the field, the sulfonamides have continued to prove of great value in the treatment of dysentery."[48]

Penicillin brought no additional relief. A War Department Technical Bulletin published in January 1945 stated simply that "penicillin has been demonstrated to be ineffective on dysentery organisms *in vitro*, and clinical trials to date indicate that the drug is useless for treatment."[49]

Hemolytic Streptococcal Infections

Also characteristic of troops in wartime and potentially disruptive of military operations were diseases caused by the hemolytic streptococcus, such as scarlet fever and streptococcal sore throat (tonsillitis and pharyngitis), and their complications or sequelae, including pneumonia, ear infections, endocarditis, arthritis, and rheumatic fever (which could lead to permanent damage to heart valves). Although hemolytic streptococcal diseases and their complications were not well differentiated in World War I, their incidence, and in some cases their case mortality rates, were apparently high.[50]

By the time the United States entered World War II, the sulfa drugs had been used effectively for several years against streptococcal infections, and mortality rates remained low through the first year of the war. Nevertheless, in the Navy alone there were more than 47,000 streptococcal infections in 1942, and more than 2,700,000 man-days were thought to be lost from this cause. Incidence remained high in 1943 as large numbers of new recruits arrived at training centers. Crowding, frequent movement of populations, the presence of highly communicable strains of hemolytic streptococcus, and the occurrence of respiratory viral infections converged to favor streptococcal illness. At some naval training centers, incidence rates were two to six times those in the civilian population. Scarlet fever reached the highest levels ever recorded in the U.S. Navy.[51]

Methods to control streptococcal infections included isolation of carriers during the period in which they were thought capable of transmitting the infection, air sanitation including oiling of barracks floors and processing of blankets with mineral oil to minimize airborne dust, siting of training away from geographical areas of high incidence, and avoidance of overcrowding. Medical analysts pointed out that the effectiveness of isolation was vitiated early in the war by failure to recognize that sailors or soldiers with streptococcal sore throat were as likely as those with scarlet fever to spread the infection. Resiting of training camps and avoidance of overcrowding were impractical under conditions of a wartime emergency. Air sanitation, though useful, was insufficient by itself.[52]

By the fall of 1943, the Navy faced a failure of control measures, rapidly rising rates of infection, a strain on medical facilities, and the possibility of a streptococcal pandemic. The war demanded not only the continuation but also the expansion of recruit training. This objective could be achieved only if hemolytic streptococcal infections were controlled.[53]

In these circumstances, the Navy held a conference in September 1943 at which a decision was taken to undertake a program of chemoprophylaxis using sulfa drugs. Some precedent was available in the work of civilian clinicians who, beginning in 1939, had reported that streptococcal throat infections and recurrences of rheumatic fever could be prevented in rheumatic fever patients who took small daily doses of a sulfa drug. Mass chemoprophylaxis to prevent meningitis epidemics had been tried in the Army in 1942 and 1943.[54]

The Navy program was nevertheless unprecedented in its sheer scale and duration if nothing else. Beginning on December 1, 1943, recruits at five naval training centers began to receive doses of one gram of sulfadiazine daily. Other recruits at the same centers were observed as controls. The effects were swift and dramatic. At one center where 20,000 men were studied, the incidence of scarlet fever and tonsillitis in the 10,000 receiving daily doses of sulfadiazine dropped to about fifteen percent of that in the control group within one week. The number of cases of rheumatic fever fell sharply in the treated group after two weeks, while it rose in the control group. Similar results were observed at other centers. In February 1944, the Navy decided to extend the program to three additional training centers and to discontinue use of controls at the five original centers. Between December 1943 and June 1944, about one million men participated in the program, 600,000 as recipients of chemoprophylaxis and 400,000 as controls.[55]

The program was judged to be a striking success. Not only did incidence rates for scarlet fever, tonsillitis, and rheumatic fever drop dramatically, but rates of hospitalization for all types of respiratory disease also declined sharply, and the spread of infection from one naval activity to another was apparently suppressed. Alvin F. Coburn, the author of one analysis of the program published during the war, estimated its dollar savings to the Navy at between $50 million and $100 million (1944 U.S. dollars), and its savings in the time of medical personnel at one million man-days. Coburn also concluded that "without chemoprophylaxis to prevent *implantation* of respiratory pathogens, the training programs of the U.S. Navy would have been impossible of maintenance. With mass chemoprophylaxis, training programs have been completed."[56]

When the initial Navy program was completed in June 1944, medical officers did not consider sulfonamide-resistant strains of streptococcus to be a sig-

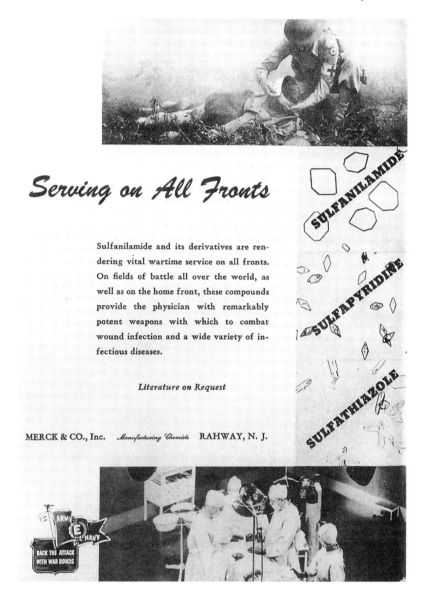

Figure 10.2. Merck advertisement that appeared in *Annals of Surgery* and other American medical journals in 1943 (reprinted courtesy of the Merck Archives).

nificant problem. By September 1944, evidence was available that resistance was becoming a serious obstacle to the Navy's prophylaxis program, and when Coburn published his detailed analysis of the initial program in January 1945, he acknowledged the presence at naval training centers of strains resistant to prophylactic doses of sulfadiazine. Such strains were able to spread quickly among recruits receiving chemoprophylaxis because competing bacteria had been suppressed. In the last months of the war, the spread of resistant strains of streptococcus forced the Navy to abandon mass chemoprophylaxis as a control method.[57]

Although the Army took an early interest in chemoprophylaxis of streptococcal infections, and the Army Air Forces especially carried out intensive studies of its effectiveness in early 1944, it was never adopted on the scale of the Navy program. War Department Technical Bulletin number 112 was issued in November 1944 authorizing use of chemoprophylaxis under certain circumstances, but by this time the effectiveness of the method was being undermined by the spread of resistant strains.[58]

As penicillin became more widely available in 1944, it came into use in treatment of streptococcal infections, especially those resistant to sulfonamides. In March 1945, an NRC conference considered its possible prophylactic use as a replacement for the now compromised sulfa drugs, but studies under field conditions outlined at the conference were not undertaken, and prophylactic use of penicillin was not adopted.[59]

Wounds and Burns

For obvious reasons, the treatment of wounds and burns was among the highest priorities of the Army and Navy medical services. An important part of the problem was the prevention and control of bacterial infections, which were especially likely and could be especially dangerous under combat conditions. The medical response to Pearl Harbor dramatized the problem and at the same time held out the hope that a major part of the solution had been found in the prophylactic and therapeutic use of the sulfa drugs. The search for a solution had begun much earlier, however, and, as noted above, included a major civilian study begun in the fall of 1941 and sponsored by the Committee on Medical Research of the OSRD.[60]

Experience in the Spanish Civil War had suggested that oral doses of sulfanilamide could help to prevent infections in wounded soldiers. In November 1939, the British Army, by this time at war, made oral prophylactic doses of sulfanilamide part of standard practice in the management of wounds. The French Army also made early use of sulfanilamide or its derivatives in both local and systemic treatment and prophylaxis of war wounds.[61]

In 1940, the British Army continued and expanded its use of sulfa drugs in management of wounds. In March, Colonel Leonard Colebrook gave a talk to British Army doctors in France in which he emphasized the role of sulfanilamide and sulfapyridine and the special dangers posed by hemolytic streptococcus infections of wounds. A British War Office memorandum issued in August directed that sulfanilamide should be given orally or locally to all wounded who might have a septic infection or gas gangrene. When war wounds were discussed at the Medical Society of London in December, the value of the sulfa drugs was affirmed by those present, including Colebrook, and one speaker described the positive difference they had made in the treatment of the wounded evacuated from Dunkirk.[62]

As early as 1939, a few American surgeons had begun to experiment with local application of sulfanilamide in tissues where infections existed or might occur, and some reported favorable results. Also in 1939, E.R. Squibb & Sons began to supply a few physicians with sulfapyridine, sulfathiazole, or sulfanilamide in oil suspensions or in powdered form for local application, and by December 1940 the Office of the Surgeon General of the Army was expressing a keen interest in the outcome. An Army medical officer wrote to Squibb that "for some time it has been our ambition to secure a satisfactory medium whereby sulfanilamide or its derivatives could be used locally."[63]

In June 1940, the NRC had recommended to the Surgeons General of the Army and Navy that wounded soldiers or sailors receive prophylactic oral doses of a sulfa drug. By the last months of 1940, Army doctors had heard reports of successful local use of sulfanilamide by dentists treating tooth infections and by surgeons treating wounds and compound fractures. An Army Surgeon General's Office Circular Letter issued in December 1940 mentioned the local use of sulfanilamide in gas bacillus infections, and in January 1941 Army doctors were in correspondence with Abbott Laboratories about supplies of sulfanilamide and sulfathiazole in powdered form for trials of local prophylaxis and treatment of wound infections at Walter Reed Hospital. By July 1941, more than four months before Pearl Harbor, the Surgeon General's Office was making plans to supply each soldier with tablets of sulfanilamide that he was to take on his own in the event that he was wounded and medical aid was not immediately available. In September 1941, the Surgeon General's Office was making arrangements for Army surgeons to be supplied with powdered sulfanilamide and sulfathiazole in five-gram sterile envelopes with shaker tops.[64]

By the time the United States entered the war in December 1941, systemic and local use of sulfa drugs in prophylaxis and treatment of wound infections was well established in surgical practice. It was supported by a small number of animal experimental studies, reports of British and French military experience since the beginning of the war, and the testimony of American surgeons based on their own clinical observations. In lieu of well-controlled clinical studies, the NRC's Subcommittee on Surgical Infections preferred to reserve judgment, especially regarding the value of local use of sulfa drugs in wounds. In the face of surgeons' enthusiasm and urgent requests for advice from the Army and Navy, however, even the Subcommittee on Surgical Infections felt compelled to recommend local use of crystalline (powdered) sulfanilamide in wounds in May 1941. When John Moorhead and his colleagues entered the operating rooms to treat wounded soldiers and sailors at Pearl Harbor, they could feel confident that they had behind them a consensus of surgical practice and the sanction of the highest medical authorities in the land.[65]

In these circumstances, it is not surprising that in spite of all the fanfare surrounding the medical success at Pearl Harbor, the effect of this experience as far as the management of wounds was concerned was to confirm and reinforce existing surgical practice, not to take it in a new direction. In 1942, the use of sulfa drugs in prevention and treatment of wound infections was consolidated and extended in American military surgery and medicine.

Circular Letters issued by the Surgeon General of the Army in February 1942 affirmed that sulfa drugs given locally and by mouth had proved of value in wound infections and recommended their use specifically in gas bacillus (gas gangrene) infections, local staphylococcal infections such as boils or carbuncles, and peritonitis secondary to appendicitis or bowel perforation. By March 1942, plans were being made to include packets of powdered sulfanilamide in soldiers' first aid kits for self-administered local use.[66]

An authoritative statement on the prevention of infections in wounds and burns, prepared by the NRC's Committee on Chemotherapeutic and Other Agents and Committee on Surgery, appeared in *War Medicine* in May 1942. Noting that infections of wounds and burns were a major problem of military surgery, the document asserted that recent experiences had "demonstrated beyond doubt the value of the application of crystalline sulfanilamide to wounds which are awaiting debridement" and that oral sulfanilamide should be started immediately after wounding. It also recommended extensive and routine use of crystalline (powdered) sulfanilamide in the postoperative treatment of wounds.[67]

That this document reflected current Army and Navy practices at the same time that it sanctioned and reinforced them is indicated in wartime publications by medical officers of both services. Although these reports were usually careful to emphasize that chemotherapy was no substitute for proper surgical procedures, they agreed that local and systemic use of sulfa drugs was routinely employed and had proved useful. The experience of one Navy hospital ship, the *Solace*, may serve as example. A passenger liner converted to a floating hospital of 450 beds with seventeen medical officers, two dental officers, twenty-one nurses, and 160 hospital corpsmen, the *Solace* was at Pearl Harbor at the time of the Japanese attack and treated many naval casualties there. It went on to receive thousands of wounded sailors and marines in the battles of the Coral Sea and the Solomon Islands campaigns of the spring and summer of 1942. First aid prior to arrival at the ship usually included a sprinkling of one of the sulfa drugs in powdered form into the wound. Treatment on the ship included local use of sulfathiazole powder or suspension, while sulfa drugs (usually sulfathiazole) were given by mouth only when there was evidence of spreading infection. Treatment of patients who survived gas bacillus infection included "generous use of sulfathiazole locally and by mouth," and sulfathiazole was given orally for a week to all those with compound fractures. The burn treatment of choice on the *Solace* included local application of sulfathiazole either as an ointment or a dusting powder.[68]

As the advantages of sulfadiazine over other sulfa drugs for systemic use became known in 1942, it began to replace sulfanilamide in military medical practice and in the small packages issued to soldiers going into combat. Sulfanilamide in crystalline (powdered) form remained the drug of choice for local application.[69]

The idea of self-dosing by soldiers caught the imagination of civilians and prompted thoughts of emulation. In August 1942, a doctor wrote to the Surgeon General of the Army on behalf of the Boy Scouts of America, stating that the youth organization was considering the inclusion of sulfanilamide powder in its first aid kits. The Surgeon General's Office responded firmly that "the use of sulfanilamide in first aid kits for the immature was not regarded as advisable."[70]

In fact, it was only in combat conditions, in which a wounded man might not have access to immediate medical attention, that self-administration of sulfa drugs was considered appropriate by the medical services. At other times, sulfa drugs were to be taken only under the supervision of a physician. Behind this caution lay the recognition that sulfa drugs were capable of producing what were commonly called toxic effects or toxic reactions. These included (but were not limited to) nausea, vomiting, dizziness, fever, rash, acute agranulocytosis (with decrease of granular white blood corpuscles), hemolytic anemia, and anuria (inability to urinate). Medical officers were expected to monitor patients taking sulfa drugs as thoroughly as wartime conditions and facilities permitted. Laboratory procedures included measurement of the concentration of the sulfa drug in the blood, body fluids, and urine; blood counts and hemoglobin determinations; urine examinations; and bacteriological studies. The medical officer then had to decide on appropriate action, which might include adjustment of dosage or regimen or suspension of sulfa drug treatment altogether.[71]

Concerns about possible inappropriate use of sulfa drugs by soldiers and uncertainty about the efficacy of self-administered doses in preventing infection led the Canadian Army to decide against inclusion of sulfa drugs in soldiers' first aid kits, at least until the fall of 1942. In October 1942, E.W. Archibald, a Canadian Army medical officer, wrote to James C. Magee, Surgeon General of the U.S. Army, asking for clarification of current American practices. The inquiry was prompted in part by pressure from the Canadian public to consider the adoption of measures that might enhance the safety of Canadian troops. In his reply, Magee outlined current U.S. Army practice, pointing out that sulfadiazine tablets for oral administration were issued to soldiers only when they were on the way to combat zones and that medical officers attached to units were expected to monitor the use of tablets by soldiers. In reply to Archibald's questions about the basis for the practice, Magee remarked that "the many factors which influence wound infection in battle casualties including type of terrain, climate, the condition of the men, and the type of missile which inflicts the wound, make it difficult to evaluate the influence of the sulfonamides." He admitted that there was no "definite clinical proof " that a single four-gram dose of sulfadiazine had a significant effect in preventing wound infection but maintained that there was "presumptive evidence" that systemic infection could be prevented by sustained oral administration of sulfonamides, beginning with the tablets taken by the soldier on his own.[72]

The Canadian Army's hesitations reflect an undercurrent of uncertainty amidst the general consensus on the value of the sulfa drugs in prevention and treatment of wound infections. For a small minority of physicians, uncertainty as to efficacy of the sulfa drugs combined with their known toxicity and the presumed existence of alternative therapeutic measures to produce outright antagonism. One whose opposition to the sulfa drugs was especially strong was James F. Kelly, a professor of radiology at the Creighton University School of Medicine in Omaha, Nebraska. Kelly was a pioneer in the use of X-rays to treat gas gangrene and other wound infections. In 1940, he had tried to persuade the NRC to include X-ray treatment in the large-scale cooperative civilian study of wound therapy then in the planning stage. Although the proposal apparently had some support within the NRC, the study begun in the fall of 1941 focused exclusively on the sulfa drugs.[73]

Angered by what he regarded as a brushoff by the NRC, and especially by the Committee on Chemotherapeutic and Other Agents chaired by Long, Kelly appealed to a higher authority in the person of Secretary of War Henry L. Stimson. In a letter to Stimson of October 6, 1942, Kelly attacked the sulfa drugs as, at best unproven, at worst harmful. In the treatment of wound infections, they were "going along for a ride on soap and water and adequate debridement," he said, and were also, contrary to the claims made by their advocates, useless against gas gangrene. In Kelly's view, the wide popularity of the sulfa drugs was due largely to media attention cultivated by promoters in the medical community, a state of affairs that he compared to the "mercurochrome racket of twenty some years ago." He threatened (with apparent inconsistency) to go to the media himself to make known what he regarded as a proven alternative to sulfa drugs, namely, X-ray treatment of wounds. If this were not enough, he concluded that "the sulfonamides (which come out of Germany) may cost us this war unless they are controlled."[74]

Kelly's proposals for X-ray therapy had some support in Army medical circles, and in 1940 two Army reserve doctors had proposed the placement of portable X-ray units with mobile surgical hospitals. Others opposed the practice, however, citing the dangers of possible overdosage of radiation and the apparent success of sulfa drugs in combating wound infection. In its reply to Kelly's letter, the Surgeon General's Office (which was asked to respond on behalf of Stimson) regretted that Kelly did not wish to resubmit his case to the NRC but offered no alternative course of action.[75]

The almost desperate tone of Kelly's letter to Stimson reflected his position on the margin of current medical practice. By the time that he wrote it, however, the large civilian study of the role of the sulfa drugs in the prevention of infections in wounds, compound fractures, and burns was beginning to arrive at conclusions that would vindicate some of his criticisms.

Launched just weeks after Pearl Harbor, this study, sponsored by the OSRD's Committee on Medical Research and supervised by the NRC's Subcommittee on Surgical Infections, began with high optimism that the value of local and systemic use of the sulfa drugs would be confirmed. One subcommittee member, John S. Lockwood, recalled that "there was little doubt in the minds of some of us associated in this study but that prophylactic sulfonamides would both reduce the mortality from infection in war wounds, and also permit uncomplicated healing of most penetrating wounds subjected to debridement and closure within a reasonable time after injury."[76]

Great care was taken by the study's planners to assure the credibility of its findings. The participation of nine units at nine different hospitals (two of these considered only burns) allowed for large enough numbers of cases to permit statistical analysis. Investigators used uniform methods of collecting data so that the study could differentiate factors that might favor or minimize wound infections. All cases received the best standards of surgical care. Research units carried out bacteriological analyses of tissues and materials from wounds. Cases treated with sulfa drugs were compared to parallel series of cases that did not receive drugs. Over the twenty-two months between January 1, 1942, and October 31, 1943, the study compiled 2,191 complete records of cases, of which 926 were soft-part wounds, 674 were compound fractures, and 591 were burns. To assist in analysis of the results, the NRC enlisted John Fertig, a biostatistician at Columbia University.[77]

After six months of the study, it was evident to investigators that the drug-treated cases were no freer of local infection than were the controls. Since local use of sulfadiazine and sulfanilamide together produced profuse exudation in the wound and since sulfadiazine placed in a wound could cake and act as a foreign body for several weeks, investigators decided to discontinue local use of sulfadiazine and to proceed with local sulfanilamide alone. After another six months, it was clear that local sulfanilamide by itself had no advantage over the controls, and the researchers discontinued all local use of sulfa drugs for the remainder of the study.[78]

In his presentation of the study's findings, its director, Frank L. Meleney, reported that the main factors in the development of infections in soft-part wounds and compound fractures were the amount of tissue damage, contamination by dirt and foreign bodies, time between the injury and surgical care, the nature of the bacteria in the wound, and the thoroughness with which dead tissue and contaminants were removed from the wound. In burns, the first four of these factors also applied, but they were secondary to the extent of the deep burn.[79]

The study had found no evidence that sulfa drugs in any form or combination had a significant effect on the development of wound infections. "The use of sulfonamides as employed in these cases either systemically alone or locally alone, or combined, has not materially reduced the incidence or the severity of local infections in the wounds," Meleney wrote, "nor have they delayed the development of infection nor have they eliminated the pathogenic organisms from the wounds." Mortality from infections was extremely low in all three categories, however, a result that Meleney attributed to the effectiveness of the sulfa drugs in preventing the spread of local infections into the bloodstream. This beneficial effect could be obtained, Meleney reported, even if sulfa drugs were given systemically only after the appearance of an infection. Therefore, no benefit derived from either local or systemic prophylactic use of the drugs, and "omitting the routine early use of these drugs would avoid a great waste of material and many toxic reactions."[80]

The study concluded that the main burden for the prevention of wound infections must be placed squarely on accepted principles of surgical practice. This meant above all the removal of dead tissue and contaminants at the earliest opportunity and the rapid restoration of the normal physiology of the affected part.[81]

This was emphatically not the result that participants in the study had anticipated or desired. It seemed to offer little recourse to military practice when combat conditions produced contaminated wounds that could not be promptly treated by surgeons. Having reached this negative conclusion, however, the architects of the NRC study drew back from it. Meleney pointed to important differences between civilian accidental wounds such as those found in the study and war wounds. Civilian patients varied widely in age and general condition, whereas wounded soldiers were typically young and in good condition. Civilian wounded were usually treated quickly, while the time between injury and treatment could vary widely in war conditions. Finally, transportation of a wounded civilian to the hospital was usually quick and atraumatic, while transport of a wounded man from the battlefield could add to his injury. The civilian study was not able to examine uses in which wounds were treated immediately with local sulfa drugs and surgery was delayed, as could happen on the battlefield. Meleney also pointed out that if sulfa drugs were not given routinely as a prophylactic measure, infections might be overlooked "in a rush of military hospital work," and septicemia could develop before the medicines could be used effectively. In his introduction to Meleney's report, Allen O. Whipple spoke for the NRC when he wrote that because of such differences between civilian and military conditions, "no comparisons are made for the use or disuse of bacteriostatic drugs as prophylactic agents in the prevention of local wound infection in war wounds."[82]

Penicillin began to become available for clinical research on wound infections in January 1943. The limited quantities at first led the Committee on Chemotherapeutic and Other Agents to restrict its use to treatment of established infections in compound fractures of the long bones. For this purpose, two units were set up at Army hospitals, first a small one at Bushnell General Hospital in Utah and, when this proved successful, a large one at Halloran General Hospital. Both units were directed by Champ Lyons, a member of the Subcommittee on Surgical Infections. Their work established the principles involved in the use of penicillin to treat infected compound fractures. Also in 1943, several of the units already in place to study the use of sulfa drugs in prevention and treatment of wound infections expanded their scope to include penicillin and sulfathiazole crystals. Although the studies confirmed the power of penicillin in treatment of general infections, neither penicillin nor crystalline sulfathiazole was significantly more successful than the sulfa drugs already tested (sulfanilamide, sulfadiazine) in the prevention of wound infections.[83]

The full report on the wound infection study, including statistical analysis, did not appear until 1945 and so was not available to practitioners until the end of the war. Meleney published a preliminary report on 1,500 cases studied through April 1943, however, and this was published in the *Annals of Surgery* in the same year. In this early statement, Meleney emphasized the value of the sulfa drugs in preventing systemic infections but also reported evidence that the sulfa drugs did not reduce the incidence of local infections.[84]

From this point on, the clinical research status of local use of sulfa drugs in wounds could at best be described as problematic. The point was underlined in a talk given by Lockwood in November 1943. Noting the many variables involved in the incidence and healing of wounds, Lockwood argued that clinical research on the sulfa drugs was subject to a confusion "compounded because of the rapid succession of new drugs which have been introduced, the diversity of physical forms, vehicles, doses, and time schedules in which they have been employed, and, fundamentally, to a failure to recognize the limitations of local sulfonamide therapy." Citing Meleney's preliminary report, he emphasized that confusion in clinical research on local chemotherapy would end only when research objectives were defined in specific terms and when investigators used proper controls. Since military practice had so far produced mixed opinions on the value of local chemotherapy, and since controlled studies had not yet been conducted with war casualties, Lockwood saw no need to discontinue current practices. "The most that can honestly be said for prophylactic sulfonamide in wounded soldiers," he wrote, "is that the practice is entirely rational, and that no evidence has been brought forward to contraindicate its use. Therefore, in the opinion of the writer there is every reason to continue the practice."[85]

Lockwood's views were echoed in two discussions of the current status of the sulfa drugs published in 1944, one by Lyons and the other by W.W. Hall, a captain in the U.S. Navy Medical Corps. While both authors emphasized the medical consensus behind the systemic use of sulfa drugs in treatment of wounds, Lyons wrote that "good clinical evidence for or against the continued local use of sulfonamide preparations in wounds is not available," and Hall remarked that "considerable confusion exists with respect to the value of the sulfonamides when applied locally in wounds."[86]

Lyons and Hall in 1944, like Lockwood in 1943, made it clear that whatever doubts had been thrown up by civilian research, Army and Navy practice in all theaters of war included routine local use of sulfa drugs. Lyons thought that he perceived "a distinct trend away from local sulfonamide therapy" but conceded that individual preference and opinion guided practice and that many excellent military surgeons continued local chemotherapy. Citing Lockwood, Hall even gave his approval to current practice, concluding that "as there appear no contraindications to the first-aid local use of sulfanilamide, it seems logical that it be continued." Only in treatment of burns, both authors agreed, was local use of sulfa drugs "definitely contraindicated."[87]

Published reports reflecting U.S. military practice from 1943 through the end of the war in 1945 confirm the ubiquitous use of sulfa drugs in both local and systemic treatment of wound infections. The same reports make clear that penicillin was introduced, especially in 1944–1945, as a supplement to the sulfa drugs and not, in most cases, as a replacement for them in the treatment of wound infections. Army and Navy doctors occasionally voiced doubts about the value of local use of sulfa drugs in wounds. Even when they did so, however, they often continued with local use in their own practices.[88]

Several examples may be taken from the Pacific campaigns of late 1944 and 1945. Jerome F. Grunnagle, an Army medical officer, described the treatment of ninety-three men with open head wounds received during fighting in the Philippines from October 1944 to May 1945. Grunnagle questioned the value of local application of sulfanilamide as part of first aid treatment, but sulfanilamide dressings were applied in at least some of the cases. He strongly favored early systemic treatment with a sulfa drug or penicillin and thought that such treatment would allow adequate debridement to be done with a longer delay after wounding than would otherwise be possible. He routinely used continued systemic treatment with a sulfa drug or penicillin and thought that this helped to prevent the spread of local infections. He mentioned dusting of sulfonamide crystals into wounds when the nose or accessory nasal passages were involved.[89]

Navy medical officer H.A. Barnes gave an account of his treatment of men wounded in fighting on a coral island in the Palau Islands group. Injuries included thoracic, abdominal, and head wounds. Barnes emphasized the problems and limitations of the sulfa drugs and pointed out that their toxicity could be especially dangerous in a tropical climate in which it was more difficult to maintain body water. Having stated these reservations, he reported routine systemic use of both sulfa drugs and penicillin and noted that "the synergism of drug action combining sulfonamides with penicillin often produced gratifying results." He used penicillin locally in the pleural cavity in certain types of thoracic surgery and thought that topical application of sulfa drugs was useful in first aid between the initial injury and the beginning of definitive surgical therapy.[90]

Handling of battle casualties aboard an attack transport ship during "a recent amphibious operation" (probably a Pacific island, since volcanic soil is mentioned) was the subject of a published report by Navy medical officer E.S. Groseclose. Medical personnel on the ship treated 284 men, most having sustained multiple gunshot or shrapnel wounds. First aid treatment included application of sulfanilamide powder to wounds, and surgeons also applied sulfanilamide powder to wounds as part of surgical treatment on board the ship. In all cases of serious wounds, the men were given a sulfa drug or penicillin systemically to prevent infection.[91]

The assault on Iwo Jima that began on February 19, 1945, produced many casualties. Navy medical officers M. Baldwin and C.W. Reynolds described the experience on one ship with medical facilities that received 239 of the wounded. Corpsmen and a doctor went ashore and gave immediate treatment to wounded men on the beach. Envelopes of sulfanilamide crystals were among the "irreducible minimum of supplies" taken ashore, and all extremity (arm and leg) wounds were sprinkled with sulfanilamide as part of first aid treatment. The violence of the battle, the large number of casualties from mortar and small arms fire, and the minimal cover on the beach made rapid evacuation of wounded a priority. The ship itself was within range of enemy fire. On the morning of the third day, the ship was so extensively damaged that it was thought for a time that it would sink, but it stayed afloat and continued to receive casualties. Doctors made extensive use of sulfa drugs. In treatment of fractures and open head wounds, they applied sulfanilamide powder locally, and after operations all patients received sulfathiazole by mouth or intravenously. For perforated chest wounds and some extremity wounds with extensive tissue damage, they gave intramuscular dosages of penicillin. They treated burns as wounds, with compression dressings and sulfathiazole emulsion. Even in their published report, the officers raised no questions about the efficacy of either local or systemic treatment with sulfa drugs.[92]

As far as the chemotherapy of wounds is concerned, it might be said that practice began the war ahead of research and ended the war behind it. In the spring of 1941, the NRC endorsed the local use of sulfa drugs in wounds not on the basis of research but under the influence of the convergent pressures of a wave of enthusiasm from civilian surgeons and urgent requests from military medical services that wanted to have the best possible tools in place before U.S. entry into the war. The

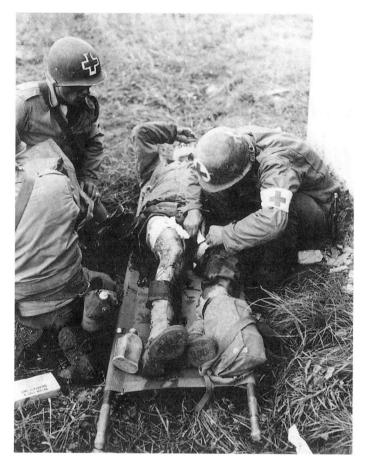

Figure 10.3. U.S. Army medics treat a soldier's leg wound with sulfanilamide powder, near Metz, France (reprinted courtesy of the National Museum of Health and Medicine, Armed Forces Institute of Pathology).

perceived success of the sulfa drugs at Pearl Harbor speeded their adoption in the military management of wounds, which was consolidated in 1942. By the time the NRC-supervised civilian study of the use of sulfa drugs to prevent wound infections began to publish preliminary conclusions that questioned the value of chemoprophylaxis in mid-1943, U.S. Army and Navy practices were already in place. Thereafter, from about mid-1943 to the end of the war, the findings of a large, well-conducted civilian study that had found little value in chemoprophylaxis of wounds coexisted uneasily with military practice that made extensive and routine use of it.

Only in September 1945, a month after the end of the war, did the Office of the Surgeon General of the Army issue a statement that, while based on experience in combat conditions, reached conclusions on the value of prophylactic chemotherapy of wounds that were similar to those of civilian researchers. The statement affirmed sulfa drugs and penicillin administered systemically to be of value in prevention and control of general infections. At the same time, it declared flatly that "no presently available chemotherapeutic agent can sterilize a contaminated or infected war wound" and reported that the routine local use of chemotherapeutic agents had been abandoned.[93]

Why was there a persistent divergence between the findings of civilian researchers and the practices of military doctors from mid-1943 to the end of the war? Part of the answer has already been given: civilian researchers lacked confidence that their conclusions were valid for wounds received and treated under combat conditions. The lack of confidence may in turn have been exacerbated by inadequate communication between civilian and military physicians. After the war, Lockwood maintained that there were unnecessary barriers between civilian investigators and military practitioners. "It must be remarked," he wrote, "that the war was almost over before the civilian investigators were permitted to become even partially familiar with the details of some of the medical problems in the combat zones." Lockwood also made the significant claim that research progress reports were never widely distributed to medical officers in the field.[94]

Probably also at work was the tendency of therapeutic practices, once in place and declared successful, to persist even in the face of evidence that they are flawed or ineffective. Such tendencies may be observed in peacetime and could be expected to be even more conspicuous under the sometimes extreme pressures of wartime practice on or near the battlefield.

Two more specific circumstances probably also favored prophylactic use of sulfa drugs, including local application in wounds. One of these was the close fit between the sulfa drugs and the military system for delivery of medical services developed during World War II. Among the hallmarks of this highly effective system were its mobility, its adaptability to varied conditions in the field, and its rapid provision of medical attention to wounded men at or just behind the front lines. To work within this system, medical supplies and equipment had to be made portable and as easy to use as possible. The sulfa drugs were light, occupied little space, were easy to administer, and could be issued to soldiers as tablets or packets of powder that could be used in the field even in the absence of an aid man or corpsman. They were frequently incorporated into the most essential supplies.[95]

One example, recorded by war correspondent Pyle during mountain fighting in the Italy campaign of December 1943 to April 1944, is telling. A battalion was fighting on a rocky ridge at an elevation of almost 4,000 feet. Every ounce of its supplies had to be carried up the mountain by mules and, for the steep last two-thirds of the distance, on the backs of men. Only the most essential items could be taken. By Pyle's account "on an average night the supplies would run something like this—85 cans of water, 100 cases of K ration, 10 cases of D ration, 10 miles of telephone wire, 25 cases of grenades and rifle and machine gun ammunition, about 100 rounds of heavy mortar shells, 1 radio, 2 telephones, and 4 cases of first-aid packets and sulfa drugs."[96]

Also at work in the persistence of prophylactic use of sulfa drugs was the less tangible but emphatically real matter of morale. Taking a tablet or sprinkling powder on a wound was something a wounded soldier or someone near him could

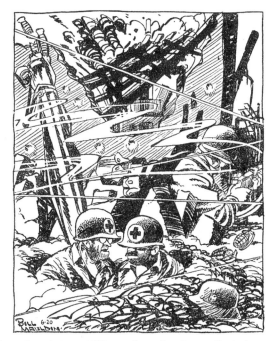

"Quit beefin' or I'll send ya back to th' infantry."

Figure 10.4. Cartoonist Bill Mauldin, who spent several years in the U.S. Army during World War II, was keenly aware of the presence of medical aid on the front lines. From Bill Mauldin, *Up Front*, New York: Henry Holt & Co., 1945 (reprinted courtesy of United Media).

do immediately. Sulfanilamide acquired an early and high reputation among American troops. In the North Africa campaign of 1942–1943, Pyle reported that "doctors and men both talked about it constantly, almost with awe," and credited it with preventing infections even when wounded men were otherwise untreated for twenty-four hours. Apparently, use was easier to master than pronunciation, as soldiers called the medicine with the five syllable name everything from "snuf-falide" to "sulphermillanoid." By whatever name, once the attachment was formed, it would be difficult to dislodge from practice.[97]

The men who took comfort in the presence of the sulfa drugs on or near the battlefield were not wrong. As far as bacterial infections were concerned, the sulfa drugs, imperfect as they were, carried the main burden of treatment and played an important role in prevention throughout World War II. They were there at Pearl Harbor to help prevent or to treat general infections and kept that role through the last battles in the Pacific. They minimized mortality from the great killers, pneumonia and meningitis, and in the case of the latter reduced the panic that often accompanied it. They brought down the incidence of complications in gonorrhea and prevented the loss of many days from active duty because of that disease. They helped to control one of the plagues of armies, bacillary dysentery, and by doing so in at least one battle may have enabled an Allied victory. Applied in mass prophylaxis in the middle of the war, they made possible the successful completion of large-scale U.S. Navy training programs that were threatened with disruption by streptococcal infections.

When penicillin appeared on the scene in 1943, it quickly proved its effectiveness in all of the conditions considered here, with the exception of bacillary dysentery. At the same time, limitations of supply, at least until the spring of 1944, and the perceived success of established practices with the sulfa drugs limited penicillin's role until the end of the war. Its impact was probably greatest in treatment of gonorrhea, where the sulfa drugs had encountered high percentages of resistant cases by 1943. In the other categories of infection here considered, penicillin was used alongside of, and sometimes together with, the sulfa drugs, supplementing but not replacing them. After the war penicillin, streptomycin, and other antibiotics would open a new era of bacterial chemotherapy that would place the sulfa drugs in a distinctly secondary role. While the war continued, it was the sulfa drugs that the Allied soldier, sailor, marine, or airman was most likely to encounter and that might well save his life.

CHAPTER 11

A Mechanism Revealed

As evidence mounted during World War II that sulfa drugs could not prevent or eliminate localized wound infections, doctors often explained the failure by referring to a theory of the mode of action of sulfa drugs first advanced in 1940 by British medical bacteriologist Paul Fildes and biochemist Donald D. Woods. According to this view, sulfanilamide and, by extension, other sulfa drugs exerted a deleterious effect on bacteria by interfering with an enzyme that helped synthesize a nutrient the bacteria needed for growth and reproduction. Sulfanilamide closely resembled a compound (a "substrate") acted upon by the enzyme to produce the needed nutrient, so sulfanilamide was able to compete with the substrate and displace it. In this way, Woods and Fildes claimed, sulfanilamide prevented the formation of the nutrient and thereby blocked the growth and reproduction of the bacteria. Unable to increase in numbers, the invading bacteria were then destroyed by the defenses of the human or animal host.[1]

With the Woods-Fildes theory in mind, doctors surmised that sulfa drugs in wounds failed to act against bacteria because wounds contained unusually high concentrations of the substrate that sulfanilamide competed with in bacterial metabolism, effectively neutralizing the local action of the drugs. Bacteria continued to grow and reproduce—so went the theory—and the local infection persisted, even though sulfa drugs could prevent the spread of the infection to the rest of the body.

Explanation of the resistance of wound infections to chemotherapy was but one of the applications of the Woods-Fildes theory in the 1940s. After its publication in 1940, the theory rapidly gained widespread acceptance among medical researchers and physicians as an explanation of the effectiveness of the sulfa drugs against bacterial infections. This achievement alone would have assured the fame

251

of the theory, but its significance for medical and biological research proved to be far wider. Above all, the theory's ability to explain the action of an enormously successful class of medicines provoked the formulation of the concept of an antimetabolite. According to this concept in its most general form, a compound chemically similar to a compound needed by a cell or organism could interfere with the cell or organism's use of the needed compound, and thereby prevent normal functioning or growth. So stated, the idea had potential applications far beyond the realm of the sulfa drugs or even bacterial chemotherapy.

Formulated in conjunction with the Woods-Fildes theory, and with the explanation of the mode of action of the sulfa drugs as its leading exemplar, the antimetabolite concept had multiple effects on medical research in the 1940s. It brought together and clarified what had been scattered and sometimes puzzling research findings from the 1930s. It added a new explanatory tool to chemotherapeutic and pharmacological theory. It opened the way to rationalize and improve the use of existing medicines, including the sulfa drugs. Finally, it provided a basis for new research programs aiming at rational drug design.

Background

The first sulfa drugs, Prontosil and sulfanilamide, entered medical practice without benefit of understanding of their mode of action. Gerhard Domagk, who had earlier sought a compound that would act against bacterial infection by stimulating the host's immune system, conceded in his first publication on Prontosil that its action was more specific, in that it affected only certain types of bacteria. The idea of specific action made slow headway among German physicians, many of whom continued to adhere to the idea of an indirect action through the immune system.[2]

The Pasteur Institute team's 1935 demonstration of the efficacy of sulfanilamide separated Prontosil's therapeutic activity from its nature as an azo dye in the eyes of most physicians and researchers, but left open the question of the mode of action of sulfanilamide.[3]

Interest in the mode of action of the sulfa drugs rose rapidly with the arc of their therapeutic success. Between 1936 and 1940, numerous theories were put forward by investigators in Europe and North America. As Daniel Bovet has pointed out, many of these theories were later forgotten because they did not contribute to the line of investigation that ultimately proved successful. While increasing numbers of investigators embraced the idea that the drugs had a direct action of some kind on microbes, the precise nature of this action remained open to debate, and others were unwilling to rule out some kind of stimulus to the host's immune system. Competing views included suggestions that the medicines acted through the host's nervous system, that they neutralized microbial toxins, that they inhibited the formation of bacterial capsules, or that they contributed to the formation of compounds highly toxic to the microbes. Still other researchers looked for the basis of the sulfa drugs' effect in their interference with enzymes necessary to bacterial survival, growth, or reproduction.[4]

While those ideas were being advanced and considered, John Hopkins pharmacologist Eli Kennerly Marshall, Jr., was approaching the problem of the therapeutic action of sulfanilamide and other sulfa drugs from a different angle. Convinced that understanding of the action of a medicine depended on knowledge of its fate in the human or animal host, Marshall first developed a colorimetric method for measuring the concentration of sulfanilamide in body tissues. Applying the method in experimental studies of animals and humans, Marshall was able to make quantitative determinations of absorption, blood concentration, and excretion of sulfanilamide against time and as a function of dose, animal species, and mode of administration. These studies provided a rational basis for determining therapeutic dosages, and Marshall's further development of methods to gauge the quantitative effectiveness of sulfa drugs in experimental bacterial infections was applied to more than 100 sulfonamides by 1941.[5]

The methods Marshall developed for the sulfonamides became part of standard practice in chemotherapy and pharmacology, but their application left open the question of the mode of action of sulfanilamide and other sulfa drugs on bacteria. Some degree of convergence occurred between 1936 and 1938 as leading French, British, and American investigators concluded that sulfanilamide was bacteriostatic, not bacteriocidal. That is, in contrast to previous antibacterial agents, which were thought to kill bacteria outright, sulfanilamide was thought by those researchers to inhibit bacterial growth, making the microbes vulnerable to the host's defenses, especially phagocytosis.[6]

While the consensus supporting a bacteriostatic action of sulfanilamide and related compounds and rejecting their stimulation of the host's defenses held between 1938 and 1940, in other respects considerable uncertainty remained regarding mode of action. In a survey of the field published in 1939, Perrin H. Long and Eleanor A. Bliss judged the theories so far advanced to be "composed mainly of unconfirmed findings" that were largely the result of "the multiplicity of avenues of approach which have been followed and the profusion of observations which have been made." Examples of uncertainty were not hard to find. Long and Bliss pointed to continuing doubts as to whether sulfanilamide was responsible for all or only part of Prontosil's therapeutic effect. No definitive conclusions could be drawn as to whether sulfanilamide caused morphological changes in bacteria, such as interference with capsule formation. Nor could researchers say with assurance whether or not sulfanilamide neutralized the toxic products of bacteria.[7]

On the key question of how sulfanilamide and its derivatives inhibited bacterial growth, Long and Bliss's view was that "we enter the realm of pure fancy." One theory, derived from the work of R.L. Mayer, held that within the host organism sulfanilamide gave rise to an oxidation product that in turn acted on invading bacteria. Another theory, advanced by Arthur Locke, E.R. Main, and R.R. Mellon, asserted that a sulfanilamide-derived substance interfered with catalase, an enzyme present in the growth medium of bacteria. The catalase was therefore unable to prevent the buildup of the hydrogen peroxide normally produced by the bacteria, which in turn inhibited bacterial growth.[8]

Long and Bliss gave little credence to these ideas, concluding instead that "probably the most plausible theory is that the drug interferes in some way with the metabolism of susceptible bacteria." They cited as principal spokesmen for this line of thinking the Paris-based medical researcher Constantine Levaditi and the American surgeon and bacteriologist John S. Lockwood. Levaditi had suggested that sulfanilamide and other sulfa drugs were transformed in the body into an unknown substance that he called the active principle X. He thought that this substance, probably a sulfur–protein complex, somehow altered the nutrients that the bacteria would ordinarily take up from the body in such a way that the bacteria were unable to use them. The germs stopped multiplying, were unable to produce capsules, and became vulnerable to the body's defenses, phagocytosis in particular.[9]

Lockwood had found that peptone, a product of the partial breakdown of protein, had an antisulfanilamide effect when streptococci were observed in blood serum. He had concluded that the invasiveness of streptococci depended on their ability to split proteins by enzymatic activity and that noninvasive strains were those that had somehow lost this ability. According to this view, sulfanilamide and other sulfa drugs acted by interfering with a specialized metabolic activity of invasive bacteria, preventing the microbes from utilizing protein as a nutrient.[10]

Lockwood had begun investigation of the mode of action of sulfanilamide with clinical studies, on the view that "a study of the drug's effect on various types of hemolytic streptococcus diseases as they occur in man might lead to a hypothesis which could then be subjected to experimental tests." With colleagues Alvin F. Coburn and Herbert E. Stokinger, he collected observations in 1936 and 1937 on the first 250 patients treated with sulfanilamide at Presbyterian Hospital-Columbia University Medical Center and Willard Parker Hospital in New York City. The investigators noted that relapses of treated infections were more frequent in patients with localized infections containing necrotic tissue, such as mastoiditis or abscesses, and less frequent in cases in which there was not a local concentration of bacterial or human tissue debris. The variations in effectiveness of the drug seemed to have more to do with the character of the lesion than with the nature of the infecting organism. Lockwood and his colleagues did not claim to know whether the debris itself had a protective action on the bacteria or whether it merely prevented a sufficient concentration of sulfanilamide in the local site. They were willing to speculate that "sulfanilamide may alter the total metabolism of the microorganism or may interfere especially with some specific function, such as its capacity to digest protein. In either case the presence of necrotic tissues appears to be of importance."[11]

In tandem with these clinical studies, Lockwood pursued experimental investigations on the effect of sulfanilamide on hemolytic streptococci in serum and blood *in vitro*. These were carried out in the Laboratory of Surgical Bacteriology at the University of Pennsylvania School of Medicine and were motivated in part by Lockwood's belief that failure to understand the mode of action of sulfanilamide had blocked both rational therapy with the drug in different kinds of lesions and the development of new antibacterial compounds. In the course of his experiments Lockwood noted that the bacteriostatic effect of sulfanilamide was counteracted by the presence of peptone in the serum or blood. Believing that he had also shown that sulfanilamide interrupted the ability of invasive bacteria to use protein, he concluded that "the effect of sulfanilamide in the serum may then be to interfere with the protein-splitting mechanism of the young invasive strepto-coccus, leading to progressive reduction in population unless peptone-like sub-stances are present." Whether the sulfanilamide acted on the substrate or on the production or activity of the enzymes themselves Lockwood did not pretend to know. He did believe the evidence sufficient to indicate that "the essential action of sulfanilamide will be found to lie in this general realm."[12]

Long and Bliss regarded Levaditi's and Lockwood's theories as more plausi-ble than were competing ideas but still tentative because they were based on the doubtful and slimly supported premise that virulent streptococci possessed a spe-cial protein-splitting enzymatic activity lacking in the nonvirulent streptococci. They concluded that no adequate theory of the mode of action of the sulfa drugs was yet available but that "the speculations of Levaditi, Lockwood, and Mellon and his associates, while not in themselves providing the final answer to the ques-tion, should prove a stimulus to other workers."[13]

This last prediction was being fulfilled even as Long and Bliss's book ap-peared in print. Between 1938 and 1940, several investigators in Britain and the United States moved toward the view that sulfanilamide and related compounds acted by interference with enzyme action in bacteria. For this work, Lockwood's ideas provided a direct or indirect stimulus.[14]

In a lecture to the Royal College of Physicians in November 1938, Lionel Whitby lamented the lack of theoretical understanding of the mode of action of the sulfonamides and the consequent "tedious empirical trial and error" of re-search. Reviewing current ideas, he noted that the lag phenomenon, that is, the frequently observed delay between the administration of the sulfonamides *in vivo* or *in vitro* and the beginning of their bacteriostatic effect, suggested that the drugs acted by interference with food assimilation by bacteria. To explain this interfer-ence Whitby resorted to the language of Paul Ehrlich, visualizing a kind of "re-ceptor" in the bacterium with which the drug combined to block the organism's use of essential nutrients. Whitby did not refer in this lecture to Lockwood's the-ory but did cite the latter's work in support of the assertion that certain common constituents of laboratory media could prevent the action of sulfanilamide.[15]

In a subsequent paper co-authored with his colleague James McIntosh, the di-rector of the Bland-Sutton Institute of Pathology at Middlesex Hospital, Whitby distanced himself from Ehrlich's model, pointing to the lack of evidence that sul-fonamides were fixed in any way by the bacteria on which they acted. Instead, he and McIntosh moved toward the view that "the mode of action of the sulphonamide drugs is most probably bound up with the inactivation of bacterial enzymes, but for the complete solution of the problem we must depend on the activities of the bacte-rial chemist. In this conclusion we are in agreement with Lockwood (1938) and Locke, Main, and Mellon (1938)."[16]

Lockwood's theory and experimental findings were taken as starting point for the investigations of T.C. Stamp, a University of London bacteriologist. Stamp set out to determine whether there were substances other than peptone that could counter the bacteriostatic effect of sulfonamide, on the view that such a substance need not be a nutrient but might be instead an "enzyme factor." His approach was to prepare different fractions of bacteria and to test each fraction for its antibacteriostatic effect in various media, hoping to finally isolate the effective compound. Stamp succeeded in identifying an active fraction, which he characterized as free of protein and consisting of "a mixture of substances of low molecular weight, including free amino acids." Acknowledging the need for further chemical analysis, he nevertheless concluded that the active substance might be either a necessary nutritive factor, such as an amino acid, or a coenzyme.[17]

Citing Lockwood, Alexander Fleming—not yet drawn back to penicillin work—compared Lockwood's findings on the effect of peptone on the bacteriostatic action of sulfanilamide to his own experimental results on the similar effects of thick suspensions of different kinds of bacteria on the action of sulfanilamide and M&B 693 (sulfapyridine). Fleming took note of Stamp's "very interesting" paper in which the latter had "carried the subject further in regard to the hemolytic streptococcus by isolating the active fraction."[18]

In parallel with but separately from Stamp and Fleming, University of Sheffield bacteriologist H.N. Green was also pursuing the elusive antisulfanilamide factor. Beginning with studies of the sensitivity of *Brucella abortus* to sulfanilamide, Green became convinced that the bacteria themselves contained such a factor. His efforts to extract it met with small success until he read Stamp's paper and adopted his methods. That done, he obtained an active preparation that proved to be a powerful growth stimulant not only in *Brucella abortus* but in other kinds of bacteria. Green thought it likely that the active substance stimulated the reproductive process in the bacterial cell, and named it "P factor," the P standing for pullulation or proliferation.[19]

On the basis of further studies with the active preparation, he concluded that there was a direct quantitative relationship between the effects of P factor and those of sulfanilamide, that P factor specifically antagonized the action of sulfanilamide and so was not simply a general growth stimulant, and that P factor did not appear to combine with sulfanilamide, both substances remaining intact in each other's presence.

Green also found that mild heat accelerated, and cold retarded, the bacteriostatic action of sulfanilamide, a result that he viewed as "strong evidence" that the reaction the drug inhibited was enzymic in nature. He finally concluded that P factor might be a coenzyme, as Stamp had suggested, and that in any case the enzyme reaction involved appeared to be "a fundamental one in bacterial metabolism."[20]

The Woods-Fildes Theory

Within a month of Green's submission of his paper for publication on January 18, 1940, Fildes and Woods announced that they had identified the antisulfanilamide factor. It was *p*-aminobenzoic acid, a compound very close in structure and composition to sulfanilamide. Speaking to a meeting of the Biochemical Society in Sheffield on February 17, Woods and Fildes presented for the first time their hypothesis that sulfanilamide worked by competing with and displacing *p*-aminobenzoic acid, the usual substrate in an enzyme reaction essential to bacterial cell growth and reproduction.[21]

In reaching this conclusion, Fildes and Woods were indebted to earlier work on the mode of action of the sulfonamides, and in several important respects their own investigations paralleled those of contemporaries such as Stamp and Green. At the same time, they were able to move beyond the results obtained by others by virtue of earlier research or training not directly related to the sulfonamides, or even to the general problem of drug action.

By far the more senior member of the team, Fildes had spent a long career developing and implementing an innovative research program in bacterial physiology and nutrition. His Unit in Bacterial Chemistry at London's Middlesex Hospital, set up in 1934, played a leading role in the identification of "essential metabolites," substances required by the bacterial cell for normal function. Fildes concentrated on pathogenic bacteria but conceived of them in a broad evolutionary and biological framework. In his view, bacteria had originally been able to synthesize all of their essential metabolites out of simple compounds in their environments. Adapting to richer organic environments and to biological hosts, some bacteria had lost the ability to synthesize their own requirements. The result was the evolution of parasitism and infectious disease.[22]

Woods had taken his Ph.D. at Cambridge in 1937 as a student of Marjory Stephenson, leader of the other important school of bacterial chemistry in Britain. As student and collaborator of Stephenson, Woods had been closely involved in work on amino acid metabolism in bacteria and had become expert in the use of the Warburg manometer in biochemical research. When offered a fellowship to work with Fildes in 1939, Woods readily accepted, in part because he saw it as an opportunity to expand his experience of bacterial chemistry in the direction of nutritional studies.[23]

Not until 1939 did Fildes become involved with the question of the mode of action of sulfanilamide. His first contact with the problem came through Middlesex Hospital colleagues Whitby and McIntosh, who were conducting animal trials and clinical tests of sulfa drugs supplied by May & Baker and who, as noted above, had come to the conclusion that their mode of action probably involved inactivation of bacterial enzymes.

Woods later suggested that this hypothesis had been inspired by informal teatime discussions between Whitby, McIntosh, and Fildes and his colleagues. While these may have played some role, it seems more likely, given the prior speculations along these lines by investigators directly involved in the mode of action question and Whitby and McIntosh's mention of those investigators in their 1939 paper, that Whitby and McIntosh's views were prompted by those of Lockwood and others.[24]

Fildes's prior work in the 1930s had included studies of other ways in which bacterial growth could be inhibited by interference with essential metabolites. One way involved a decrease in the intensity of chemical reduction in the medium or within the bacterial cell, for example, by a dye such as methylene blue. The dye oxidized a substance that had to be reduced in order for metabolism to proceed. Another way involved the molecular combination of the antibacterial agent with

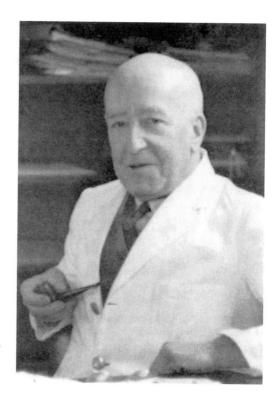

Figure 11.1. Sir Paul Gordon Fildes (1882–1971) (*Biographical Memoirs of Fellows of the Royal Society*).

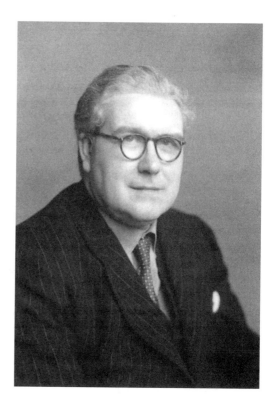

Figure 11.2. Donald Devereux Woods (© The Godfrey Argent Studio, reprinted with permission).

some essential metabolite in the cell, thus rendering it inactive. Such was the case when mercury combined with sulfhydryl groups ($-SH$), which were known to be required for cell growth.[25]

Moved by Whitby and McIntosh's suggestions on the mode of action of sulfanilamide, Fildes in early 1939 undertook investigations to determine whether any known essential metabolite could be shown to inhibit the action of sulfanilamide. These were unsuccessful. Then Stamp's publication in early July 1939 made it known that an extract of hemolytic streptococcus reversed the action of sulfanilamide. Stamp's paper indicated that a substance or substances that reversed the action of sulfanilamide could be isolated from microorganisms, and provided a key laboratory technique (use of a weakly alkaline extract) to do so.[26]

Stamp and Fildes both assumed that the extract contained an essential metabolite for streptococci. This could not be a growth factor for streptococci since all of these growth factors were already known. Stamp had not determined the chemical nature of the substance, probably because (according to Woods) he attempted chemical analysis at too early a stage of purification.[27]

On the basis of his prior experience and biological views, Fildes believed that an essential metabolite was not likely to be specific to one organism, but common to many. For this reason, he decided to use yeast to try to extract the essential metabolite. Available cheaply and in large quantities from baker's shops or breweries, yeast had the added advantage of harmlessness compared to pathogenic bacteria. About mid-July 1939, Fildes, using Stamp's method, prepared an extract of yeast and found it to have strong antisulfanilamide activity. At the end of July 1939, Fildes turned the task of identifying the essential metabolite over to Woods, who conducted his first experiment with yeast extract on August 8, 1939.[28]

Woods had joined Fildes's unit on April 1, 1939, and had spent the first four months working "without much success" on the nutrition of the gonococcus. When he began working on the problem of extracting the antisulfanilamide factor from yeast in August, war seemed imminent, and the prospect of discovering something that might help develop better sulfa drugs gave urgency to the work.[29]

Woods began with the hypothesis that the antisulfanilamide factor in yeast might be a substance essential to the growth of the organism, and therefore employed methods routinely used to characterize such substances. Two lines of investigation went on simultaneously. One was biological: different extracts of yeast were tested for antisulfanilamide activity using as test organism a virulent strain of *Streptococcus hemolyticus*. The second line of investigation Woods described as "a straightforward attempt to concentrate, purify and isolate the factor itself and establish its chemical nature," using what were by then traditional methods for the isolation of substances from natural sources.[30]

Woods concluded from both lines of investigation that the antisulfanilamide substance had certain chemical characteristics in common with sulfanilamide. The biological tests also ruled out nonspecific growth stimulation of the bacteria by the yeast extract and combination of the antisulfanilamide substance with sulfanilamide, and showed a strict quantitative relationship between concentration of sulfanilamide and the amount of extract needed to overcome its action, results that paralleled closely the independent and almost simultaneous findings of Green.[31]

To Woods, the result of the chemical and biological work together "was reminiscent of the competitive inhibition of enzyme reactions by substances chemically related to the substrate or product," a kind of phenomenon first described by biochemists at Cambridge in 1928 and familiar to Woods through his own Cambridge training and experience. This suggested that the antisulfanilamide factor was a substrate or product of an enzyme reaction in the bacterial cell and that sulfanilamide inhibited this reaction by virtue of its similarity in chemical structure to the substrate. If so, the question was: what substances are structurally similar to sulfanilamide and have chemical characteristics similar to the extract substance?[32]

One obvious candidate was p-aminobenzoic acid, a compound to be had at small cost from British Drug Houses Ltd. Woods later recalled that "the test was put up at 1 P.M. on 14 December 1939 and I must admit that 12:30 P.M. on 15 December, when I took the tubes out of the incubator, was (and still is) the most exciting moment in my scientific life." Test tube cultures to which both sulfanilamide and p-aminobenzoic acid were added clearly showed that the inhibitory effect of the former had been overcome by the latter. Further work showed the antisulfanilamide activity of p-aminobenzoic acid to be greater than that of some sixteen chemically related compounds. Although p-aminobenzoic acid could not be isolated in pure form from the yeast extract, the multiple chemical similarities of the two substances provided strong circumstantial evidence of their identity. Woods concluded that p-aminobenzoic acid was essential for the growth of the cells, that "the enzyme reaction involved in the further utilization of p-aminobenzoic acid is subject to competitive inhibition by sulphanilamide, and that this inhibition is due to a structural relationship between sulphanilamide and p-aminobenzoic acid (which is the substrate of the enzyme reaction in question."[33]

At the end of the 1940 article in which he presented these results, Woods stated that his investigation was based "on a general working hypothesis that antibacterial substances act by interfering with some substance essential to the bacterial cell ('essential metabolite,' Fildes, 1940)." At the same time, he noted that "the experiments are also in accord with the suggestion, based on indirect evidence, that the interference is connected with inactivation of bacterial enzymes (Lockwood, 1938; McIntosh and Whitby, 1939)." While a consistent case can be made for both assertions, it should be clear from the preceding discussion that advocates of one or another enzyme-interference hypothesis played a leading role in prompting and framing the investigations that finally led to an explanation for the mode of action of sulfanilamide.

Although Fildes had previously considered ways in which antibacterial agents could work by interfering with essential metabolites, these did not include interference with enzymes or enzyme reactions. Not until early 1939 did Fildes become interested in the mode of action of sulfanilamide. When he did so, the stimulus came from Middlesex Hospital colleagues McIntosh and Whitby, who were conducting their own studies on the sulfonamides and who were at least partially persuaded by the enzyme-interference ideas proposed by Lockwood and others.

A comparison with Stamp is instructive. Independently of Fildes, but moved by a serious interest in the enzyme-interference theory of Lockwood, Stamp set out to determine whether substances other than peptone were antibacteriostatic. Concluding that sulfanilamide acted by interfering with a necessary nutritive factor or an enzyme in the bacterial cell, Stamp had succeeded in preparing an extract with antisulfanilamide effect and in partially characterizing it in chemical terms. Only after Stamp published his results in early July 1939 was Fildes able, using Stamp's methods, to prepare his own extract with marked antisulfanilamide activity from yeast.[34]

Green, too, independently of Fildes, came to the conclusion that his bacterium, *Brucella abortus*, contained an antisulfanilamide factor. With the assistance of Stamp's extraction methods, Green went far in characterizing his P factor, describing its interaction with sulfanilamide in ways that paralleled Woods's description of his yeast extract. Green concluded that his P factor might be a coenzyme and that, in any case, he had strong evidence that the reaction inhibited by sulfanilamide was an enzymatic one.

What, then, did Fildes contribute that was distinctive? One thing was surely his willingness to use yeast to extract the antisulfanilamide factor. As Robert E. Kohler has emphasized, this was a decision grounded in Fildes's broadly biological vision and prior experience with essential metabolites.[35] Another was his assignment of Woods to the problem. With Woods came his experience with Cambridge biochemistry, and especially the crucial idea of competitive inhibition that took Woods beyond Stamp, Green, or anyone else seeking to understand the mode of action of sulfanilamide.

Fildes clearly acknowledged prior and current views on enzyme interference as a probable explanation for the antibacterial activity of sulfanilamide, and placed his findings with Woods among them. The first paragraph of his May 1940 article in *Lancet* mentioned by name Lockwood, McIntosh and Whitby, Stamp, and Green.[36]

At the same time, in the assertively titled "A Rational Approach to Research in Chemotherapy," Fildes boldly went beyond the others, including Woods, both in generalizing the findings and in proposing a new basis for chemotherapeutic research. Building on his earlier work, Fildes now subsumed the results with sulfanilamide under a broader framework of possibilities for antibacterial action:

> Antibacterial substances function by "interfering" with an essential metabolite and thus inhibit growth. The interference may be (1) by oxidising a substance which requires to be reduced, (2) by molecular combination forming an inactive product, or (3) by competition for an enzyme associated with the essential metabolite. It is claimed that sulphanilamide acts as in (3), the essential metabolite being *p*-aminobenzoic acid.

The last category, in particular, pointed beyond itself. Fildes emphasized that "Class (3) inhibitions require an inhibitor so closely related in formula to the essential metabolite that it can fit the same enzyme, and sufficiently unrelated to be devoid of essential metabolic activity." Couched in such abstract terms, the third category invited the conclusion that "chemotherapeutic research might reasonably be directed to modification of the structure of known essential metabolites to form products which can block the enzyme without exhibiting the specific action of the metabolite." Fildes had converted a particular, if spectacular, result with a known antibacterial agent into a proposal for a research program that might identify many others yet unknown.[37]

Reception of the Woods-Fildes Theory

By the time the Woods-Fildes theory made its appearance in 1940, frustration had been building for several years over the lack of rational guidelines in the search for new, more effective sulfa drugs. The very success of those that did exist threw their deficiencies and limitations into sharp relief and thus increased the desire for some compass for research. Hans Molitor, director of the Merck Institute of Therapeutic Research, expressed the mood well. In an article published in July 1939, Molitor stated flatly that "chemotherapy has entered a new era within the last two years" and that "sulfapyridine unquestionably represents one of the greatest advances of all time in the treatment of diseases." Yet both sulfapyridine and sulfanilamide had undesirable side effects, Molitor added, and even considered together they left important infectious diseases untouched by chemotherapy. How to proceed? "If the search for new chemotherapeutic agents is to be elevated from the present empirical procedure of laboriously testing thousands of drugs and finding by mere luck one which is valuable," Molitor asserted, "it would seem desirable first to investigate the mode of action of sulfanilamide and sulfapyridine and attempt to correlate their different antibacterial properties with their chemical structure." He concluded that "we may hope that the time is not too distant when the research chemist will base his work on the knowledge of reactions between the infectious microorganisms and the cells of the host, and on the basis of this knowledge deliberately synthesize chemicals which are likely to interfere with these processes." Molitor's views were shared by many involved in research in chemotherapy.[38]

In this situation, acceptance of the Woods-Fildes theory was driven as much by the pent-up desire for a rational direction to chemotherapeutic research as it was by preparation of the ground by prior ideas of enzyme interference or the experimental evidence offered by its authors. One investigator who quickly adopted the theory on all three grounds was Lockwood. As of June 1940, Lockwood still maintained that no satisfactory explanation of the mode of action of the sulfonamides in biochemical terms was yet available. By October he had read the Woods and Fildes papers and was persuaded, although at first he wished to preserve continuity with his earlier ideas by seeing *p*-aminobenzoic acid as one of a class of sulfonamide inhibitors somehow bound up in tissues and in need of release by enzymatic degradation of protein. By 1941, he was emphasizing the unadorned Wood-Fildes theory and had embraced Fildes's general statement as the basis of a rational research program in chemotherapy.[39]

Lockwood was not alone. Other investigators quickly embraced the Woods-Fildes theory, and by the mid-1940s it was by far the most widely held view of the mode of action of the sulfonamides.[40]

Acceptance of the Woods-Fildes theory boosted optimism in chemotherapeutic research not only in the search for new and better sulfonamides but also in
the pursuit of antibacterial agents of other kinds. In 1950, Woods estimated that in
the previous ten years more than 100 analogs of bacterial growth factors, including B vitamins, amino acids, and nucleic acid derivatives, had been synthesized
and found to have various kinds of inhibitory action on bacterial growth.[41]

Some of the earliest efforts to apply the theory came in Fildes's own renamed Department for Research in Bacterial Chemistry at London's Middlesex
Hospital. During 1940 the department's work shifted to a nearly exclusive focus
on the theory and its extension. In addition to the Woods and Fildes papers described above, Fildes also published his findings on the mode of action of mercury as an antiseptic, and H. McIlwain, a researcher in Fildes's department,
showed that pyridine-3-sulfonic acid acted as a bacterial inhibitor by antagoniz-
ing nicotinic acid. In 1941, Fildes published his demonstration that indoleacrylic
acid antagonized the growth-stimulating properties of tryptophan in the typhoid
bacillus.[42]

In September 1940, Fildes and Woods departed for war work, leaving the exciting application of their theory to others. McIlwain became director of the department, which moved to the University of Sheffield for the duration of the war.
McIlwain's wartime research continued the study of synthetic analogs of bacterial
metabolites and explored the biochemical foundation of their specificity of action.
Contrary to early expectations, no new chemotherapeutic agents comparable to the
sulfonamides emerged from this research.[43]

Although the Woods-Fildes theory was widely accepted in the 1940s, it was
also subject to criticisms and revisions. A small minority of investigators rejected
the theory. Richard J. Henry, for example, did so on the grounds that *p*-
aminobenzoic acid could not be demonstrated by rigorous methods to be an essential metabolite for bacteria inhibited by the sulfonamides. Henry pointed out
that antagonism of sulfonamides by *p*-aminobenzoic acid did not mean that the
latter was necessarily an essential metabolite of the bacteria. Henry proposed instead that sulfonamides acted by "interfering with a specific fraction of the total
oxidative metabolism of [dividing] cells."[44]

More common was acceptance of the Woods-Fildes theory in its general form
joined to criticism and modification of it in detail. In 1943 and 1944 American investigators P.H. Bell and Richard O. Roblin, Jr., combined the Woods-Fildes theory with observations linking the chemotherapeutic activity of sulfonamides with
their ionization and molecular structure. The resulting theory proved able to predict for the first time approximate *in vitro* antibacterial activities of new sulfonamides prior to their synthesis. Given the early high hopes that a good theory
would provide a rational basis for synthesis of new sulfonamides, there was irony
in the conclusion reached by Bell and Roblin that the most active sulfa drugs had
already been made. Northey called this finding "a *post mortem* of the sulfa
drugs."[45]

In the course of its statement and acceptance, the Woods-Fildes theory underwent two steps of generalization. The first was taken by Fildes in his 1940

Lancet paper when he stated three different ways in which interference with essential metabolites could occur, one of which was competitive inhibition of enzyme action, and proposed a general research program in bacterial chemotherapy based on these three kinds of interference. Fildes thus went beyond explanation of the particular case of the mode of action of sulfanilamide in two ways: by positing two other kinds of interference with essential metabolites, and by defining a research program that applied to bacteria in general, not only those acted on by sulfa drugs.

The second step was taken by researchers other than Woods and Fildes sometime between 1940 and 1942. It involved definition of the concept of antimetabolite as a substance that interfered with the action of an essential metabolite in a living cell. This could mean bacteria, but it could also mean other kinds of infectious microorganisms or neoplastic (cancerous) cells that appeared within an organism. The beginnings of a transition to the broader concept may be seen as early as 1941 in a paper presented by Lockwood to a conference on chemotherapy. Lockwood found grounds for optimism in the probable validity of the Woods-Fildes theory, and ventured in conclusion that

> it is perhaps pardonable to suggest that we may be provided with a new method of approach to the treatment of cancer, a disease in which unrestrained proliferation of tissue cells is similar in some respects to the proliferation of bacteria in invasive infections. If the difference between malignant cells and normal cells should be found to be due to the local activity of some chemical growth factor, a compound of similar chemical configuration might be administered to cancer patients which would block the activity of the proliferative factor without exhibiting its physiological effects.

Similar ideas were soon taken up by other investigators, and the search for antimetabolites become a major theme of cancer research in the 1940s.[46]

The Woods-Fildes theory therefore provoked, though it did not itself state in full generality, an important addition to chemotherapeutic and pharmacological theory. In the 1940s, the concept of antimetabolite was applied not only to the attempt to design new drugs but also as a tool to elucidate cell metabolism, that is, to advance fundamental knowledge in biochemistry.[47] The concept also allowed researchers to begin to bring together and make sense of scattered and sometimes puzzling findings from the 1930s on the antagonism of structural analogs of vitamins, hormones, and amino acids for their respective metabolites. Pharmacologists had been at a loss to explain the antagonism in physiological action between acetylcholine and structurally related compounds including atropine. In 1937 A.J. Clark proposed as explanation that antagonistic compounds competed for a specific reaction site in the target cell. In 1938, D.W. Woolley and his collaborators found that two derivatives of nicotinic acid, which they were investigating as possible substitutes for this vitamin, instead had toxic effects on animals with nicotinic acid deficiency. Also in 1938, H.M. Dyer was surprised to find that ethionine, an ethyl analog of the amino acid methionine, had toxic rather than beneficial effects when given to rats in place of methionine. In 1940, Richard Kuhn published results of studies on algae showing that male or female behaviors could be elicited depending on the ratio of two chemically closely related hormones, which therefore acted as antagonists to one another. By the mid-1940s, all of these results and similar ones could be subsumed under the new concept of antimetabolite.[48]

Rational Drug Design Based on the Woods-Fildes Theory and the Antimetabolite Concept

Although no antibacterial agents of stature comparable to that of the sulfa drugs emerged from application of the Woods-Fildes theory or the more general antimetabolite concept, research programs based on these ideas yielded useful chemotherapies and established the long-term value of this approach to rational drug design. Notable examples are the efforts that led to *p*-aminosalicylic acid (PAS) as a component of tuberculosis chemotherapy, to 6- mercaptopurine as a drug treatment for leukemia, and to trimethoprim-sulfamethoxazole as an effective combination therapy for bacterial infections.

In the early 1940s, Jörgen Lehmann, a Swedish medical researcher, noticed a paper in *Science* by Frederick Bernheim showing that salicylic acid and benzoic acid each increased the oxygen consumption of the tubercle bacillus *in vitro*. Bernheim concluded that similar compounds might play a role in the metabolism of the bacillus. Reasoning along the lines of the Woods-Fildes theory, Lehmann arranged for a chemist at the Ferrosan Research Laboratories in Malmö to synthesize more than fifty derivatives of benzoic acid in the hope of finding one or more that would antagonize salicylic acid or benzoic acid and that would therefore have a bacteriostatic effect on the tubercle bacillus. Test-tube experiments indicated that the most active of these derivatives was PAS. By March, 1944 Lehmann was conducting parallel animal experiments and clinical tests on twenty patients using the new compound. Patients under treatment showed an improvement in general condition and no deleterious effects. Only later was it found that PAS is an antagonist of the metabolite *p*-aminobenzoic acid.[49]

Numerous clinical studies of PAS in treatment of pulmonary tuberculosis followed over the next several years, including a controlled and statistically analyzed trial conducted in Sweden that ended in 1949. All reported favorable results, and the controlled study concluded that patients treated with PAS improved more rapidly than those in the control group. PAS's beneficial effects were limited, however, and streptomycin, a new antibiotic first announced in 1944 and widely available by 1946, soon became the chemotherapy of choice in tuberculosis. By 1949, limitations of streptomycin and problems of resistance were leading researchers to try combination chemotherapies. Large-scale trials such as those conducted by the U.S. Veterans Administration soon demonstrated that PAS and streptomycin together were distinctly more effective and less prone to develop resistance than either given alone. In the 1950s, PAS became a routine part of combination chemotherapy in tuberculosis.[50]

In 1942, George H. Hitchings and his colleagues at the Wellcome Research Laboratories in Tuckahoe, New York, made the antimetabolite concept the basis of an extensive study of compounds closely related to or derivatives of naturally occurring purine and pyrimidine bases of the nucleic acids. By the time they began this investigation, other research had demonstrated a variety of purine and pyrimidine requirements in various microorganisms. This implied the existence of biochemical pathways for the incorporation of preformed constituents of nucleic acids and also differences in these pathways between different species. Starting with this knowledge, Hitchings and his collaborators decided to undertake systematic study of purine and pyrimidine analogs with two aims. First, they would try to elucidate the roles of purine and pyrimidine bases in nucleic acid synthesis and thus in growth, and of the part played by folic acid in the synthesis of these bases. Second, they would seek to identify among the analogs new chemotherapeutic agents, on the theory that parasitic tissues dependent for survival on rapid growth should be especially sensitive to compounds antagonistic to substances needed for growth. As Hitchings and his colleagues later pointed out, this logic "applies equally well to bacterial, viral, rickettsial, and neoplastic diseases [cancers], so that, in a sense, one might say we have been searching for the philosopher's stone, the universal panacea, of the ancients."[51]

Hitchings and his collaborators set out to study "the relationship between chemical structure and biological activity in order to determine the biochemical significance of each chemical feature." Taking as starting point the natural purine and pyrimidine bases, they synthesized variants of each in an effort to establish the biochemical significance of each atom on the molecule. The questions were, first, what changes in chemical structure or composition produce what changes in biological activity? And, as a particular case of the first question, what changes in the chemical structure or composition of the natural purine and pyrimidine bases produce antimetabolites or antagonists? Soon they were able to make a number of generalizations on structure–activity relationships.[52]

While this research was under way, other investigators were pursuing studies of folic acid, a vitamin already implicated in nucleic acid metabolism. Successful determination of the chemical structure of folic acid in 1946, joined with the antimetabolite concept, led to an intensive search for folic acid antagonists. In 1947, Sidney Farber and his colleagues at the Children's Medical Center in Boston began trials of folic acid antagonists on children with acute leukemia. Compounds were supplied by Y. SubbaRow of the Research Division of Lederle Laboratories, and by the Calco Chemical Division, both part of American Cyanamid Company. One of these, called aminopterin, the product of a slight modification of the folic acid molecule, produced temporary remissions in some patients. It was the first leukemia drug of significant promise.[53]

Even the partial success with aminopterin and other folic acid antagonists boosted optimism that effective cancer chemotherapies based on the antimetabolite concept might be found. By 1949, the Division of Chemotherapy of the Sloan-Kettering Institute for Cancer Research in New York was testing hundreds of analogs of folic acid and of pteridines, pyrimidines, and purines against a variety of experimental cancers in mice and rats. Lederle and Calco supplied some of those compounds, while others came from the Hitchings group at Wellcome Research Laboratories. By 1954, the Sloan-Kettering Institute had tested more than

1,000 purines and pyrimidines, most supplied by Hitchings and his colleagues, against experimental cancers.[54]

A few of these compounds showed promise. Among them was 6-mercaptopurine, an analog and antagonist of adenine and hypoxanthine. Hitchings and his colleague Gertrude B. Elion submitted 6-mercaptopurine and a related compound, thioguanine, for animal testing in January 1951. Both animal tests and the initial clinical studies carried out by Sloan-Kettering staff showed 6-mercaptopurine to be a useful leukemia drug that produced remissions in a significant number of patients with acute leukemia and chronic granulocytic leukemia. Since 6-mercaptopurine differed from the folic acid antagonists in its mode of action, it came with the added benefit of lack of cross-resistance with that group of drugs. Some patients who no longer responded to other drugs were able to benefit from 6-mercaptopurine. By 1954, wider clinical studies were confirming the early findings, and thereafter, 6-mercaptopurine entered the standard arsenal of chemotherapies in leukemia.[55]

In the 1950s and 1960s, the Hitchings group's antimetabolite program yielded other results of medical importance, including discovery of the antibacterial agent trimethoprim. In 1948, they published their finding that diaminopyrimidine derivatives acted as folic acid antagonists. In the early 1950s, they studied the action of these compounds in a variety of organisms and concluded that they displayed enough selectivity of action from species to species that among them might be found useful chemotherapeutic agents. Knowledge of the mechanism of action of folate antagonists and of the biochemistry of the folate pathway advanced rapidly in the 1950s, and at the same time the Hitchings group put forward three diaminopyrimidine compounds for brief clinical testing. While these compounds produced unacceptable nausea and malaise in patients, all demonstrated antibacterial action and the promise of the research program.[56]

Further study of the diaminopyrimides yielded trimethoprim, a compound with higher antibacterial activity and fewer side effects than the compounds previously examined. In 1965 Hitchings and James J. Burchall found that trimethoprim and other diaminopyrimidines acted by inhibiting an enzyme, dihydrofolate reductase, involved in the conversion of dihydrofolic acid (folic acid) to tetrahydrofolic acid (folinic acid). Because trimethoprim acted as an inhibitor of folate utilization, while sulfonamides were known to act as inhibitors of folate biosynthesis, Hitchings and his colleagues reasoned that combination therapy using trimethoprim and a sulfonamide might produce a more powerful antibacterial effect, a concept later termed "sequential blockade." Laboratory studies confirmed the prediction, with the combinations showing effectiveness against a broader spectrum of bacterial species and less vulnerability to the development of resistant strains than either drug alone.[57]

In 1968, the combination drug trimethoprim sulfamethoxazole was made available to physicians, and numerous clinical studies over the next dozen or so years confirmed its value in bacterial chemotherapy. Writing in 1982, Adrian J. Salter of the British division of Wellcome Research Laboratories called the trimethoprim-sulfamethoxazole combination with some justice "the first major non-empirical development in the field of anti-bacterial chemotherapy."[58]

According to the mechanism of action theory held by its originators, trimethoprim worked as well as it did because of its selective affinity for the bacterial enzyme as against the corresponding mammalian enzyme. In the eyes of Hitchings and his colleagues the effectiveness of the medicine also confirmed the concept. As Bushby and Hitchings put it, "the development of trimethoprim supports the theory expressed a number of years ago (Hitchings. et al., 1952) that specific cell receptors vary sufficiently, from species to species, to provide a basis for the selective toxicity required of a chemotherapeutic agent." Indeed, by the 1970s specific inhibitors of dihydrofolate reductases were the basis not only of antibacterials but also of several antiprotozoal, anticancer, and diuretic drugs in clinical use.[59]

Conclusion

Formulation of the Woods-Fildes theory of the mode of action of sulfanilamide brought about a sharp break and redirection of research in chemotherapy. Most narrowly, it created the basis for a broad consensus among researchers on the mode of action of the most successful new medicines of the time. More important, it provoked two steps of generalization that opened up a broad horizon of future research. The first was taken when Fildes proposed a rational program for research in bacterial chemotherapy. The second was taken when other researchers formulated the antimetabolite concept, which applied to other microbes and to cells of larger organisms as well as to bacteria and which was seen by researchers as a method for doing fundamental biochemistry as well as for identifying new chemotherapeutic agents. Once defined in clear and general terms, the antimetabolite concept also allowed researchers to make sense of findings from the 1930s that had previously seemed puzzling or anomalous and to make more rational use of existing medicines, including the sulfa drugs. Neither Fildes's program for bacterial chemotherapy nor the research based on the broader antimetabolite concept met the high expectations with which it began. No class of medicines emerged that was comparable in stature to the sulfa drugs, and penicillin soon provided a spectacular opening for bacterial therapeutics in an entirely new direction. By the early 1950s, however, the antimetabolite program could claim at least two modest practical successes, in PAS for tuberculosis therapy and 6-mercaptopurine for the treatment of leukemia. More successes would follow, as investigators followed the antimetabolite concept into new territory. In seeking to explain how the sulfa drugs worked, researchers had opened the way to decades of future investigation.

CHAPTER 12

The Sulfa Drugs and Twentieth-Century Medicine

The sulfa drugs stand at the center of a major transformation of medicine in the twentieth century. They initiated a revolution in the therapeutics and management of bacterial infections. They gave a powerful impetus to the expansion of the pharmaceutical industry, and to its research and development component in particular. They contributed heavily to the opening of an era of miracle drugs, with its attendant optimism, increased rate of appearance of new medicines, regulatory dilemmas, and unanticipated therapeutic problems. Finally, the sulfa drugs, apart from their place in the treatment of bacterial infections, also had numerous and often unanticipated ramifying effects on the development of different medicinal drugs or compounds with other practical uses.

A Therapeutic Revolution

The magnitude of the break with the past was plainly visible to contemporaries. Referring to Prontosil, Lionel Whitby wrote of "the most remarkable recent advance in modern therapeutics—namely, the discovery of the antistreptococcal activity of an azo dye containing a sulphonamide group." Eli Kennerly Marshall, Jr., regarded the introduction of sulfanilamide into medicine as ranking with "two really great therapeutic discoveries of all medicine—the discovery of anesthesia and that of antiseptic (or aseptic) surgery." Surveying fifty years of medicinal chemistry in the *Merck Report* for 1941, C.R. Addinall dated the "renaissance of chemotherapy" from Gerhard Domagk's findings on Prontosil and the subsequent development of the sulfa drugs. Writing in the 1980s of the first clinical use of sulfapyridine in 1938, Ronald D. Mann recalled "the frequent comment of the physicians of a generation ago that there was always someone on the ward dying of lobar pneumonia." Lewis Thomas, too, describing his internship at Boston City Hospital in the late 1930s, remembered "the astonishment when the first cases of pneumococcal and streptococcal septicemia were treated" with sulfa drugs. "The phenomenon was almost beyond belief," he recalled. "Here were moribund patients, who would surely have died without treatment, improving in their appearance within a matter of hours of being given the medicine and feeling entirely well within the next day or so."[1]

The views of contemporaries were echoed by later commentators. Writing on the occasion of the fifty-year anniversary of the Association of the British Pharmaceutical Industry in 1980, Nicholas Wells reflected that "in many ways, looking back over the last 50 years, the discovery of the sulphonamides was the outstanding therapeutic advance which revolutionized attitudes to pharmaceutical progress." In his extensive historical survey, *Modern Drug Use*, Mann concurred, crediting Prontosil with "ushering in the modern chemotherapeutic era" and calling the introduction of the sulfa drugs "from some points of view, the most notable therapeutic advance" of the half century after 1935.[2]

The therapeutic impact of the sulfa drugs may be viewed in terms of effects on mortality from bacterial infections, or in terms of the practices of doctors, nurses, and hospitals. As Harry F. Dowling has emphasized, assessment of the effects of a specific chemical or biological agent on overall mortality figures is beset with numerous difficulties. While it is clear that decline of infectious diseases played a major role in the increase of life expectancy in the United States between 1900 and 1971, the role of chemotherapy in this decline must be weighed against other factors, including industrialization, increasing national wealth, rising levels of education, and improved public health measures. Nevertheless, some idea of the impact of specific agents can be gained from careful examination of geographically localized sites and from controlled studies carried out at the time the agents are introduced.[3]

The sulfa drugs had a clear impact on the maternal mortality from childbirth and its complications, a major health problem in the 1930s. Studies done in the United States in the 1920s and 1930s showed maternal mortality rates ranging from 4.9 to 6.7 per 1,000 live births. These rates translated into more than 20,000 deaths a year among American mothers at the time the first sulfa drugs were introduced. By 1941, the U.S. rate had dropped to 3.2 per 1,000 live births, and by 1950 it had fallen to one-fifth of 1935 levels. Most of this drop can be credited to control of streptococcal septicemia by sulfa drugs at first, then antibiotics.[4]

A Merck document on drug research released in 1959 reached similar conclusions, referring to public health reports to support the claim that between 1937 and 1952 some 1.5 million lives were saved in the United States "as a result of the accelerated decline of mortality due largely to sulfonamides and antibiotics." The same document estimated that had the rate of decline in mortality in the fifteen years preceding 1937 continued in the fifteen years after 1937, some 76,000 more mothers would have died of puerperal fever, and approximately 29,000 additional deaths would have occurred due to other streptococcal infections in the United States.[5]

Sulfa drugs and, later, antibiotics also produced dramatic drops in case mortality rates for one of the major killers, pneumonia. From a rate of 30.5 percent in a typical U.S. city hospital for patients receiving no specific treatment, the mortality dropped to 12.3 percent for patients receiving sulfa drugs, then to 5.1 percent for those receiving penicillin or a tetracycline. Empyema (fluid in the pleural cavity), a condition often associated with pneumonia, and serious complications such as endocarditis and meningitis became rare. Use of typed serums, which could reduce mortality rates for pneumonia to less than fifteen percent, was gradually abandoned over a several-year transition period. Timing of the replacement of serotherapy with chemotherapy varied by place, institution, and individual practitioner.[6]

Early in the twentieth century, outbreaks of meningococcal meningitis in the United States killed between seventy percent and ninety percent of those who contracted the illness, making it one of the most feared of bacterial infections. Antimeningococcal serum, introduced in the 1910s by Simon Flexner, reduced the mortality rate to about thirty percent in treated patients and became the standard therapy until the introduction of the sulfa drugs. Following the first report in the U.S. medical literature on the use of sulfanilamide in meningococcal meningitis in 1937, the sulfa drug rapidly displaced serum therapy. Sulfanilamide was displaced in turn by sulfadiazine, which by the mid-1940s had reduced overall mortality from the disease to around ten percent. Sulfadiazine would remain the standard therapy for meningococcal meningitis until 1965.[7]

Some of the literature cited above merges the effects of the sulfa drugs and the antibiotics. That the impact of the sulfa drugs alone was substantial and well in advance of the appearance of penicillin is shown by the experience of the U.S. military services during World War II. Impact of the sulfa drugs alone was also highlighted in an analysis of the vital statistics of England and Wales for 1939–1942. A report prepared by Percy Stokes, a medical statistician in the government's General Register Office, concluded that the notable decline in death rates in the civilian population in these years, which by 1942 resulted in an annual saving of lives "well into five figures," was primarily due to use of sulfa drugs.[8]

Introduction of the sulfa drugs brought correspondingly dramatic changes in the practices of doctors and nurses. Previously, faced with bacterial infections, American physicians tended to favor a therapeutic conservatism that supported the natural healing powers of the body with rest, good nutrition, and hygiene. With the notable exception of the typed serums used in a minority of cases, they employed drugs as little as possible. With few therapeutic options available, medical training emphasized diagnosis and prognosis. "The medicine we were trained to practice was, essentially, Osler's medicine," Thomas recalled. "Our task for the future was to be diagnosis and explanation."[9]

The change to an active therapeutics of bacterial infections, or for some physicians from serum therapy to chemotherapy, did not occur immediately in 1936 and early 1937. American physicians might hesitate to embrace the sulfa drugs for a number of reasons. Much effort and many resources had been invested in serum therapies, and with all their difficulties, they could be very effective. Some ambivalence toward the role of science in medicine persisted in spite of

changes in medical education and rising professional standards in the early decades of the twentieth century. Physicians differed on whether the source of medical authority lay in science or in a doctor's experience and position in the
community. Some doctors feared deskilling by what at first appeared to be one-
size-fits-all medicines that were initially available over the counter, especially in
the midst of a depression that encouraged self-dosing and the avoidance of doctor's bills.[10]

The uneasiness that persisted even after doctors accepted the sulfa drugs is
partially captured in a poem that appeared in the *Journal of the American Medical
Association* under the title "Sulphanilamide and the Doctor":

> The Doctor now sits in his big office chair,
> With his feet on the top of the table;
> His brow is all furrowed with deep lines of care,
> (Just picture him there, if you're able)—
> His office is filled, but with big empty chairs,
> And his office force all now are idle . . .
> No gall-bladders to drain, no disease of the brain
> From absorption of toxins malicious;
> No more chills in the night, many parents to 'fright,
> And no more infection so vicious.
> We revolve in our mind the reason to find
> For the loss of all means for a living,
> And the reason we see can nothing else be
> But Sulfanilamide we are giving—
> So with nothing to do, and the prospect so blue
> We can only sit down and discuss
> NOT what have we done with this product,
> BUT—WHAT HAS IT DONE WITH US?[11]

If they stopped to answer the question posed in the last line, American doctors
would have found much that was positive. By the summer of 1937, physicians and
patients in large numbers had embraced sulfanilamide, to be followed by sulfapyridine in the pneumonia season of 1938–1939. Expensive and difficult serum
treatment programs for pneumonia could be reevaluated and, over a period of
some eight years, abandoned, even if after hesitation on the part of doctors who
had used the treatments extensively, in favor of chemotherapy. Beginning with
sulfanilamide, sulfa drugs supplied a solution to a major threat to medical authority in the 1930s, the high rates of maternal mortality due to puerperal septicemia.
Even before the Elixir Sulfanilamide disaster in the autumn of 1937, physicians
were emphasizing the need for medical supervision for patients taking the powerful new medicines. With the passage of the U.S. Food, Drug, and Cosmetic Act in
1938, sulfa drugs were among the first members of the category of prescription
drugs that provided a new role for physicians and a new basis for medical authority and prestige.[12]

The sulfa drugs initiated dramatic changes in the disease patterns and patient
populations of American hospitals, changes reinforced by the introduction of

penicillin and other antibiotics. In the mid-1930s, infectious diseases typically accounted for the greatest number of hospital cases, required the most time from doctors and nurses, and were responsible for most fatalities. By the early 1950s, this pattern had been replaced by one in which noninfectious diseases and conditions predominated.[13]

Nursing practice also changed in significant ways with the introduction of sulfa drugs. Nurses were often the first to notice toxic side effects in patients, effects that might require modifications in dosage or administration or even suspension of sulfa drug therapy. Sulfa drugs also brought sharp reductions in patients' recovery time, and thus in the proportion of nursing time devoted to care of patients with bacterial infections.[14]

The introduction of the sulfa drugs brought the beginnings of wide-ranging changes in the practices of medical specialties, including, notably, surgery, orthopedics, otolaryngology, obstetrics, and pediatrics, as infectious diseases or the threat of infection receded in importance.[15]

With the revolution in the therapeutics of bacterial infections came also a transformation of the pharmaceutical industry that was given a major impetus by the exemplary success of the sulfa drugs. A key component of this change was an expanded commitment to research and development. In the United States, the two decades after the end of the First World War had witnessed an increasing engagement with research on the part of pharmaceutical companies, with rising research budgets, the establishment of in-house research staffs and facilities, and contacts with academic scientists. In 1938, and coincident with the success of the first sulfa drugs, that process began a dramatic acceleration that was reinforced by the demands of World War II. Exemplified in this volume by the cases of Merck and Sharp & Dohme (for the U.S.) and by May & Baker (for Britain), the industry's accelerated commitment to research resulted by the 1950s in industrial research establishments that far exceeded in size and cost the scale of their mid-1930s predecessors.[16]

The introduction of the sulfa drugs also provoked a qualitative shift in pharmaceutical research and development regarding bacterial infections, away from serums, antitoxins, and vaccines and toward medicinal chemistry. Penicillin and other antibiotics further reinforced the movement away from the older biologicals. In the 1940s and 1950s, enthusiasm for sulfa drugs and antibiotics had a negative impact on funding and positions for vaccine research.[17]

Viewed in a wider framework, the accelerated expansion of research and development in the pharmaceutical industry had its most striking result in the kinds and numbers of new drugs that entered medicine and commerce. Beginning with the first sulfa drugs in the late 1930s, a steady stream of new medicines, and even new classes of medicines, made their appearance. They included in addition to the sulfa drugs and antibiotics, antihistamines, psychotropic drugs, diuretics, and cancer drugs. In the United States, the numbers of new single drugs introduced each year averaged fifty in the 1950s. Although the annual average dropped to around twenty in the 1960s, the flow continued. As in the case of the sulfa drugs, so in these cases, invention and discovery depended on wider networks of innovation that included academic, governmental, and private nonprofit institutions as well as an industry committed to research. Only with such an industry in place, however, could these medicines be developed, produced, and placed in the hands of doctors and patients. The prominence of industry in drug innovation after 1938 is reflected in the increasing importance of patents.[18]

Driven by the new drugs emerging from research laboratories and in turn supplying the financial resources for further expansion of research, pharmaceutical production also underwent tremendous expansion. As is indicated by the cases of May & Baker, Merck, and Sharp & Dohme, this accelerated growth began well before U.S. or even British entry into World War II. As this volume also documents, World War II gave an enormous boost to U.S. pharmaceutical production, including most conspicuously first the sulfa drugs, and then penicillin. Expansion did not end with the war. By 1957, total drug sales of U.S. ethical drug manufacturers were seven times what they had been in 1939.[19]

With the expanded volume of production came also qualitative change, as the pharmaceutical industry entered a new age of large-scale high-precision manufacturing techniques required by the new research-derived medicines. The industry soon learned, moreover, that reliance on research-based innovation came with a price, namely, obsolescence of older medicines. Again sulfa drugs showed the way. As sulfapyridine and other sulfa drugs displaced serum treatment of pneumonia, serum production became unprofitable, and companies lost capital investments in production facilities.[20]

As important as the transformation of therapeutics and the expansion of the pharmaceutical industry brought about by the sulfa drugs was the accompanying sense of a sharp break with the past and the opening up of a new horizon of possibilities. In 1937, at least one American press report referred to Prontosil and sulfanilamide as "a modern miracle," and similar language greeted the appearance of M&B 693 (sulfapyridine) in the British press starting in 1938. In his preface to Iago Galdston's *Behind the Sulfa Drugs: A Short History of Chemotherapy* (1943), a book written for a nonspecialist audience, Perrin H. Long wrote that "the last six years have a witnessed a modern miracle in the treatment of infectious diseases . . . never before has there been a group of drugs which have benefited so many people." Galdston echoed Long's language, remarking that "chemotherapy is, to employ an all too common phrase, the miracle of miracles in modern medicine," although he hastened to add that chemotherapy "is miraculous only in the sense that birth is miraculous," in that it is the product of a long gestation.[21]

In 1938, no less a personage than Sir Edward Mellanby, Secretary of Britain's Medical Research Council, ventured to predict that within fifty years the rapid progress of medicine would transform the functions of hospitals by eliminating many diseases currently considered important. In his foreword to another book for a lay audience, F. Sherwood Taylor's *The Conquest of Bacteria: From Salvarsan to Sulphapyridine* (1942), historian of medicine Henry Sigerist noted that the sulfa drugs "have revolutionized medicine" and added that "there is no doubt that more drugs can be found that will destroy more bacteria, and we are justified in hoping that chemotherapy may also cure diseases that are caused by a filterable virus." It was in this climate of renewed optimism that Howard Florey and Ernst Chain undertook their study of antibacterial substances produced by molds and bacteria, recovering and extending Alexander Fleming's early work on penicillin.[22]

The appearance in the 1940s first of penicillin and then of streptomycin and other antibiotics reinforced the sense of a new age dawning. In a book published at the end of the decade and titled simply *The Miracle Drugs*, American medical writer Boris Sokoloff summarized what he called the "phenomenal advances" of the previous ten years and concluded that "we are still only at the beginning of the new era of chemotherapy . . . one cannot doubt that sooner or later our armament of anti-microbial substances will become so rich and powerful that only a few, if any, disease producing germs may remain beyond the reach of the weapons in the arsenal of science."[23]

Expressions of intense optimism came also, significantly, from those most closely involved in the research. Writing in 1950 Richard O. Roblin, Jr., director of the Chemotherapy Division of American Cyanamid, rejoiced that "the past ten years have seen a spectacular revival of interest in chemotherapy after more than a generation of scientific poverty and disappointment." Crediting Prontosil and sulfanilamide with initiating the revival, Roblin went on to trace numerous ramifications of these beginnings in work related to the sulfa drugs. He called for a broad and flexible definition of chemotherapy, reaching beyond infectious to non-infectious diseases, and predicted that the greatest progress of the coming decade would come in the latter field, in the treatment of diseases such as hypertension, asthma, rheumatic fever, cancer, and diabetes.[24]

The flow of new, powerful, research-based medicines into the marketplace and medical practice that began with the sulfa drugs created pressure to improve methods of evaluation of new drugs and, in the United States, to strengthen drug control legislation. Sulfanilamide played an incidental role in passage of the 1938 U.S. Food, Drug, and Cosmetic Act through the Elixir Sulfanilamide disaster. As the first new drug considered under the 1938 law, sulfapyridine became a paradigmatic case for the implementation of therapeutic reformers' ideas in the handling of new drugs through the immediate postwar period by the U.S. Food and Drug Administration (FDA). By the 1950s, as sulfa drugs and antibiotics were joined by other new classes of medicines and myriad medicinal drug combinations, therapeutic reformers began to look to statistics and especially the randomized clinical trial as a rigorous method of evaluation that would supplement or replace reliance on clinical judgment and experience. Concerns about costs and hazards of new medicines, and about perceived inadequacies of the FDA's oversight, led to Congressional hearings and, against the background of the thalidomide disaster, to passage of the 1962 Kefauver-Harris amendments to the 1938 Act. By the late 1960s, the randomized clinical trial had became an integral part of the FDA's revamped drug approval process.[25]

The sulfa drugs were also behind the inclusion in the 1938 Food, Drug, and Cosmetic Act of new requirements for manufacturing standards and controls for nonbiological drugs. Such controls already existed for biologicals such as antitoxins and vaccines as part of the 1902 Biologics Control Act. FDA concern with the explosive and sometimes indiscriminate use of sulfanilamide, a powerful new nonbiological drug, in 1937 led to efforts by the agency to monitor the production processes, dosage forms, quality controls, and possible harmful effects of sulfanilamide even before the Elixir Sulfanilamide disaster in the fall of that year. Although sulfanilamide was not the toxic component of Elixir Sulfanilamide, the episode dramatized the lack of adequate manufacturing standards and further reinforced the FDA's motivation to write such standards into the 1938 law. Once the law was in effect, the nature of the controls needed was further clarified by responses to a second disaster that occurred in 1940, this time as a result of faulty procedures in the manufacture of sulfathiazole. The 1962 Kelfauver-Harris amendments simply extended the manufacturing control provisions of the 1938 law to apply to all drugs, not only new ones.[26]

Diseases of Medical Progress

As noted above, the magnitude of the early successes, first of the sulfa drugs and then of the antibiotics, led to much talk of an era of miracle drugs or wonder drugs and inspired some to imagine a future largely free of disease. The widening of the therapeutic revolution in the 1950s to include new classes of powerful medicinal drugs reinforced the sense of a break with the past and of an opening to a future of unbounded possibilities.

By the late 1950s, however, physicians had accumulated enough experience with the new medicines to induce a sense of sobriety and to seriously call into question, if not eliminate, the more utopian tendencies of the age of miracle drugs. As early as 1937, the American Medical Association had warned of the need for vigilance in regard to the "undesirable side reactions" of sulfanilamide and its derivatives. In 1939 Thomas Parran, then Surgeon General of the U.S. Public Health Service, had warned that "the wide publicity accorded to the remarkable therapeutic efficacy of sulfanilamide has resulted in the creation of a public health problem of considerable gravity," with many individuals suffering toxic reactions made worse by consumption of the medicine outside of medical supervision. Subsequent years of practice with sulfa drugs and other new medicines gave substance to the early warnings.[27]

Some of this experience and doctors' reflections upon it may be found in Robert H. Moser's *Diseases of Medical Progress: A Contemporary Analysis of Illness Produced By Drugs and Other Therapeutic Procedures* (1959; second edition, 1964). No muckraker or casual critic of medicine or the pharmaceutical industry, Moser was a U.S. Army physician and avowed therapeutic rationalist. He acknowledged "the remarkable therapeutic armamentarium now at our command" but also pointed out that "there has been an increasing awareness by physicians throughout the Western world of the wonders and hazards of modern therapeutic agents" and concluded that "we have reached a point in medical history when we must reappraise the status of drugs and patients." The reappraisal brought to physicians in Moser's edited volume comprised, by the second edition, sixteen chapters by thirteen authors, with many references to published literature, on a wide range of diseases, conditions, and drugs. Much of it concerned adverse reactions of patients to medicines introduced over the previous two decades and employed in an appropriate way, that is, "diseases-which-would-not-have-occurred-if-sound-therapeutic-procedure-had-not-been-employed."[28]

The increasing awareness of adverse reactions to the new medicines embodied in Moser's book was but one of the accumulating problems besetting the new age of miracle drugs. Resistance of some infectious organisms to chemotherapy or antibiotics was widely recognized and studied by physicians by the mid-1950s. New opportunities for infection could be opened up by innovative medical or surgical interventions. While older kinds of infections were brought under control by therapy, new kinds might be discovered. Investigators or pharmaceutical companies seeking new anti-infective agents seemed to run up against a law of diminishing returns, with each innovation requiring greater investments of time and resources. The very success of anti-infective agents could lead to complacency, the relaxation of government or private efforts at control, and the resurgence of infections, as occurred in the case of venereal diseases. On a broader scale, successful control of the major infectious diseases contributed to an aging population and increasing prominence of chronic diseases.[29]

Consider only the problem of resistance. That bacteria could become resistant to drugs was recognized by Paul Ehrlich, but the absence of effective antibacterial agents rendered the issue moot for decades. Resistance first emerged as a practical problem during World War II, with mass use of sulfa drugs in treatment or prophylaxis of infections by the U.S. military. By 1943, increasing resistance of the gonococcus to sulfa drugs had substantially reduced their therapeutic effectiveness and led to their replacement with penicillin as sufficient quantities of the antibiotic became available in the latter part of the war. The U.S. Navy's successful use of sulfadiazine in the mass prophylaxis of hemolytic streptococcal infection and their sequelae foundered in the last months of the war with the emergence of sulfonamide-resistant strains of streptococcus. These events prompted investigations into the sources of resistance that began during the war and continued thereafter.[30]

By 1955, resistance of pathogenic bacteria to sulfonamides and antibiotics was generally recognized by the medical community and had already been the subject of numerous investigations. A review of the literature published by Maxwell Finland, a professor of medicine at Harvard and a clinician at Boston City Hospital, listed 564 publications, and this did not include coverage of some important aspects of the resistance problem.[31]

On the whole, bacterial resistance to sulfonamides did not increase in the first two postwar decades, even as they continued to be used, for example, in prophylaxis of streptococcal infections to prevent recurrences of rheumatic fever. A major exception surfaced in 1963 with an outbreak of meningococcal meningitis at the San Diego Naval Training Center. Since World War II, sulfadiazine had been used routinely in treatment and prophylaxis of meningococcal meningitis, with substantial success. Sulfonamide-resistant meningococci were now implicated in the San Diego outbreak. In an investigation published in 1965,

Theodore G. Eickhoff and Finland concluded that due to the existence of sulfonamide-resistant strains of meningococcus in both military and civilian populations, "a sulfonamide drug alone can no longer be considered adequate therapy for clinical cases of meningococcal meningitis" and also that "except when the isolates are demonstrated to be sensitive, sulfonamide drugs can no longer be relied upon for effective chemoprophylaxis." Over the next several years, the incidence of sulfonamide-resistant strains of meningococci continued to increase. One consequence was a revival of interest in development of meningococcal vaccines, work on which had been discontinued with the arrival of the sulfa drugs in the 1930s.[32]

After years of work and reflection on the problem, Finland concluded that increasing bacterial resistance to sulfonamides and antibiotics was mainly due to overuse or misuse of the drugs and that the trend could be corrected. Nevertheless, he went on to caution that "each new discovery of an antibiotic, of a device, or of a procedure, carries risks that must be evaluated and weighed for possible untoward effects, among which the occurrence of serious, drug-resistant infections must always be borne in mind."[33]

By the time that Finland wrote these words in 1972, the unalloyed enthusiasm of the early age of miracle drugs had been tempered by experience and reflection to a sober if still resilient optimism. Already in 1955, British bacteriologist Ronald Hare had warned a general audience that "the virtual elimination of infectious diseases as a cause of death and disablement" that then seemed on the horizon, although desirable in itself, "will bring a host of serious problems in its train."[34]

A few years later, a similar cautionary line of thinking was taken much further by René Dubos, a French-born and -trained microbiologist long on the staff of the Rockefeller Institute for Medical Research. In *The Dreams of Reason: Science and Utopias* (1961), Dubos argued that one of the most characteristic aspects of the modern world, and "its most lasting illusion," was initiated by Francis Bacon's "utopia of happiness based on application of scientific knowledge." As one manifestation of such thinking, Dubos pointed out, medical utopias looking to the elimination of all disease had been put forward in the past but had been given new life in the twentieth century by advances in nutrition and the control of infectious diseases. These undoubted successes had been extrapolated into predictions of the eventual control or elimination of all disease through the progress of experimental medicine.[35]

While Dubos believed that the achievements of scientific medicine were real and substantial, and that they would continue to be so, he regarded the extrapolation from these achievements to the conclusion that all diseases could and would one day be eliminated to be utopian and an illusion. It was utopian in his view because, like all utopias, it assumed a stable and unchanging reality. In fact, he argued, both natural and social conditions change, and therefore no adaptation to them could be permanent. The same proposition applied also to diseases. As old ones are controlled, new ones appear. Medical science overcomes challenges only to be faced with new ones. Dubos went so far as to say that his personal view was that "the burden of disease is not likely to decrease in the future." Rather, it would simply change in its particulars.[36]

Dubos's critique of medical utopias may be compared with Thomas P. Hughes's characterization of the utopias sometimes associated with other kinds of technological change. Hughes has argued that past technological revolutions, such as the second industrial revolution that came with large-scale electrification in the early twentieth century, have had associated with them utopian visions of social transformations that were thought by some to be enabled by, or consequences of, the technological revolutions. These utopian visions were disappointed, in Hughes's view, largely because the new technologies became subject to existing social forces rather than instrumental in reshaping them. In Dubos's critique of medical utopias, it is not so much existing social forces as the inevitability of change in nature and society that bars the embodiment of utopian ideas. There is a pattern, nevertheless: in each case, a major technological innovation is the occasion of a vision of a more perfect society that cannot be realized in practice.[37]

Dubos's *The Dreams of Reason* (1961) followed just two years after Moser's *Diseases of Medical Progress* (1959) and coincided with the thalidomide disaster and with Congressional hearings on medicinal drugs, the pharmaceutical industry, and the FDA. It preceded by one year Rachel Carson's *Silent Spring*, which opened more than a decade of what Hughes has termed countercultural critiques of modern technology in general and large technological systems in particular.[38]

In this context, it is not surprising to find even partisans of the therapeutic revolution sounding defensive notes. Writing on the hazards of new drugs in 1963, Walter Modell, a pharmacologist at Cornell University Medical College, acknowledged the potential for disaster from multiple sources, including adverse reactions, disturbance of the ecology of disease (he cites Dubos), resistance, and the marketing of dangerous drugs or failure to market effective drugs due to inadequate screening procedures. In the face of these difficulties, he sensed "indications of movement toward therapeutic nihilism" and felt compelled to warn that while

> there might have been some justification for such an attitude 50 years ago . . . it would be an unforgivable disaster today, for never before has our ecologic balance been so dependent on drugs; never before in its history has medicine had so many useful, effective drugs on hand, and never before has there been such promise of even better ones to come.[39]

A similar mix of defensiveness, sober criticism, and optimism is evident in an essay published a decade and a half later by Colin Dollery, a professor of clinical pharmacology at the University of London. Dollery's title, *The End of an Age of Optimism: Medical Science in Retrospect and Prospect* (1978), set the tone. Dollery recalled the scientific revolution in medicine set in motion by the first antibacterial chemotherapies in about 1938: "science appeared to have the salvation of the world in its hand and mankind could look forward to an era of healthy ease and modest luxury." The scientific revolution in medicine had continued over the intervening four decades, Dollery pointed out, but the mood had changed. Medical research budgets had stopped growing.

> Problems seem larger and solutions to them more elusive. Crash programs on cancer and stroke have made only a modest impact on their targets. The

validity of claims made about past successes are being questioned. Both the morality and the cost-effectiveness of scientific medicine have been challenged. Care in the community seems more readily attainable and comfortable than the chance of high technology care in a modern hospital. The age of optimism has ended.

The paradox, in Dollery's view, was that "serious criticism of scientific medicine has arisen when its achievements are at a peak and show no signs of a decline." His explanation was that while the decisive achievements of bacterial chemotherapy had raised optimism and expectations of medicine to high levels among doctors, politicians, and the public, no subsequent innovation was ever as decisive. "Unreasonable expectations were fed by uncritical claims and a reaction was bound to come."[40]

Whatever doubts, criticisms, or difficulties beset it, the therapeutic revolution continued in the last decades of the twentieth century and the early years of the twenty-first. Billions of research dollars flowed annually into a network of academic, government, and industrial laboratories. New, powerful drugs continued to reach the marketplace and medical practice. Biotechnology, the human genome project, and stem cell research seemed to open indefinite horizons of progress. Here and there, the voices of Dollery's age of optimism could still be heard. Writing in 1987, Richard M. Weinshilboum, a clinical pharmacologist at the Mayo Clinic, recalled the "astonishing" progress made in drug therapy in the half century since the introduction of the sulfa drugs. He ventured that not even the glamour of new medical technologies such as nuclear magnetic resonance (NMR) could eclipse the cumulative achievements of medicinal drugs. "I doubt that any medical practitioner in the United States in the latter part of the twentieth century would be willing to trade the PDR [*Physician's Desk Reference*, a compendium of current medicinal drugs] for NMR," he concluded. "We are living in the golden age of pharmacologic therapy, and we are only standing on the threshold of that age."[41]

There is a sense in which Weinshilboum's celebration of the pharmaceutical revolution and its future cannot be faulted. By 1987, however, and, in light of the above discussion, for a long time before that, such a narrowly focused view had come to be regarded by some not so much as wrong as insufficient as a means of grasping the complex problems of medicine and their potential solutions. As Charles Rosenberg has argued, by the late twentieth century a number of critics had come to question a model of medicine based solely on "ability to understand and manipulate discrete biological mechanisms" in the name of a more holistic understanding of medicine as an aggregate of technical, political, economic, cultural, and demographic realities. In such a view, drug therapies and the related sciences figure as one element within a larger picture of health and disease. The need for more comprehensive and multifaceted modes of understanding has been powerfully reinforced by the AIDS pandemic, which from the beginning has defied analysis in narrow biomedical terms and has demanded instead a global and multidisciplinary approach to understanding and political, cultural, and economic responses as well as basic scientific knowledge of its mechanisms and the development of drug therapies or vaccines.[42]

"The Sulfonamide Grouping Had a Rather Exalted Position"

Among the claims made by Weinshilboum in 1987 was his contention that the sulfa drugs "were a focal point in the therapeutic revolution, and change radiated from the sulfa drugs to influence pharmacologic science . . . and the development of the discipline of clinical pharmacology." To these claims may be added the assertions that attempts to understand the mode of action of the sulfa drugs resulted in theoretical perspectives on chemotherapy that were extended to the understanding and development of other classes of medicinal drugs, and that observation of unanticipated effects of the sulfa drugs led in several instances to the development of other classes of medicines, and even of nonmedicinal compounds of practical significance. Each of these claims deserves a study in its own right. The following discussion does not substitute for such an effort but begins to suggest ways in which each claim can be given substance.[43]

Early efforts to determine the fate of sulfa drugs in the host organism led to important methodological innovations in pharmacology, especially through the work of Marshall at Johns Hopkins. Marshall, who already enjoyed an established reputation as a physiologist and pharmacologist, dropped his other projects in 1936 to devote his research to the new bacterial chemotherapy. His development of a colorimetric analytical method for measurement of concentrations of sulfonamides, improved by A. Calvin Bratton, was widely adopted by pharmacologists as an assay procedure that was especially valuable for determining low concentrations of drugs in biological materials. His emphasis in studies of sulfanilamide on drug concentration in the blood and on blood concentration versus time curves helped to establish a rational basis for therapeutic dosages, and his research on the distribution of sulfanilamide in the body became a model study of drug distribution. Marshall's introduction of sulfaguanidine, and his demonstration that its distribution and action were mainly in the intestinal tract and that it was effective in the treatment of bacillary dysentery, represented an important application of pharmacological knowledge. Sulfaguanidine's solubility in water also departed from previous patterns of intestinal disinfectants and thus widened pharmacologists' sense of what was possible.[44]

During World War II, Marshall served as chairman of the U.S. government–organized malaria program's pharmacology panel. In this context, the ideas and methods he had developed in study of the sulfa drugs were brought to bear on research on antimalarial drugs. James Shannon and B.B. Brodie, investigators at Goldwater Hospital in New York City, made use of Marshall's principles in antimalarials research during the war and after the war brought those principles to the National Institutes of Health, where they were passed on to a new generation of clinical pharmacologists. In this way, Marshall's work on bacterial chemotherapy contributed substantially to the development of both pharmacokinetics and the field of clinical pharmacology.[45]

Early work with the sulfa drugs yielded other insights and methods to pharmacology and related fields. The transformation of Prontosil to sulfanilamide in the human or animal organism was an early example of bioactivation (the conversion in the living organism to a bioactive form) of an organic compound. Sulfanilamide became, in Marcel Bickel's words, "the model substrate used to unravel the mechanism of metabolic acetylation," a key process in biochemistry. Study of the sulfa drugs led to recognition of the need to consider binding of drugs to nondiffusible body constituents when investigating their diffusion in the body. Use of sulfa drugs also led to realization that intestinal antisepsis could lead to discovery of new food factors essential to mammals.[46]

Along more practical lines, experience with sulfa drugs contributed in at least two ways to the initial recognition by Mayo Clinic researchers William H. Feldman and H. Corwin Hinshaw that streptomycin was effective in treatment of tuberculosis in animals. Limited success with sulfa drugs and the related sulfones had convinced Feldman and Hinshaw that tuberculosis could be treated with drugs. They then applied practical methods developed in work with sulfa drugs and sulfones for determining the ability of a drug to slow the course of tuberculosis in guinea pigs to establish the effectiveness of streptomycin, samples of which they had obtained from Selman Waksman.[47]

Antimetabolite theory, developed as an extension and generalization of the Woods-Fildes theory of the mode of action of sulfa drugs, was applied in the 1940s and 1950s to the development of other kinds of medicinal drugs. Noteworthy among these were p-aminosalicylic acid, used in treatment of tuberculosis; 6-mercaptopurine, a chemotherapy for leukemia; and the antibacterial trimethoprim, which in combination with sulfamethoxazole became the first important rationally designed bacterial chemotherapy, still used under the trade name Septra. Other successful drugs would follow from research programs based on the antimetabolite concept, which also made possible improved screening methods especially for receptor antagonists such as antihistamines and beta-blockers. The antimetabolite concept also clarified a variety of research findings from the 1930s and became a tool of fundamental biochemistry as well as chemotherapy in the 1940s and 1950s.[48]

One consequence of the emergence of research programs based on the antimetabolite concept in the 1940s and 1950s was a transfer of methods and language from the chemotherapy of infectious diseases to the chemotherapy of noninfectious diseases, including cancers. Chemotherapy as originally defined by Ehrlich meant treatment of systemic microbial infections with well-defined (usually synthetic organic) compounds. In contrast to earlier use of chemical agents in symptomatic treatment, chemotherapy was to attack disease at its source by disinfecting the host organism.

By 1950, a broader meaning was taking hold. Roblin, director of American Cyanamid's Chemotherapy Division, wrote that "since [chemotherapy] is essentially a field of applied research, a precise definition is less important than an operational point of view. In our laboratories we prefer to apply the concept of experimental chemotherapy to the search for new substances for the specific treatment of either infectious or noninfectious diseases." Part of the motive for adopting a more inclusive meaning was the existence of shared concepts and tools. "We believe," Roblin continued, "that such a perspective enables us to take greater advantage of the principles and methods emerging from any phase of the activities which this broader approach implies."[49]

In later decades, the shift in meaning proceeded so far that, at least in every-day speech, "chemotherapy" came to denote primarily chemical treatments for cancers. Such a shift might be accounted for, at least in part, by a perception of in-fectious diseases as relatively unproblematic in an age of antibiotics and by the increasing prominence (partly as a result of control of infectious disease) of can-cers and their therapies.[50]

The impact of the sulfa drugs on the therapeutic revolution may also be seen in the role played by sulfonamides in the development of new drugs or new classes of drugs in the 1940s, 1950s, and 1960s. In some cases, such as new drugs introduced to treat tuberculosis or leprosy (Hansen's disease), the diseases in question were infectious. In others, such as the new medicines introduced to treat hyperthyroidism, diabetes, gout, and cardiovascular disease, the conditions were noninfectious and, indeed, bore little or no relation to one another. Still other sul-fonamide or sulfonamide-related compounds made their way into veterinary medicine as anti-infective agents or into agriculture as herbicides. Circumstances varied, but the common denominator in all cases was the use of molecular modi-fication by medicinal chemists, often in industrial research settings, in pursuit of better drugs and improved understanding of the relationships between chemical structure and biological activity.[51]

A noteworthy example is the development of the important tuberculosis drug isoniazid, first introduced into medical practice in 1952. Early promising results with sulfones in treatment of tuberculosis, and the more definite success of aminos-alicylic acid, had encouraged a search for other tuberculosis medicines. In Ger-many, Domagk began with sulfonamides, especially sulfathiazole, and in 1946 reported that a related compound of the thiosemicarbazone series was active against tubercle bacilli both in the test tube and in animals. By 1949, German doctors had treated some 7,000 tuberculosis patients with the new compound, to which Bayer had given the trade name Conteben. Although never marketed in the United States because of its adverse reactions, Conteben provoked two other research groups, at Squibb and Hoffman-LaRoche in the United States, to enter the quest for a better tuberculosis drug. Bayer, Squibb, and Hoffman-LaRoche researchers all pursued systematic studies of the thiosemicarbazone series. All three came to focus, as a logical development, on the isomers of nicotinic acid, and, in a case of independent and nearly simultaneous discovery, all three concluded by the spring of 1951 that the hydrazide of nicotinic acid, or isoniazid, possessed antituberculous activity. Each company made separate arrangements for clinical studies in 1951, and the re-sults were published in 1952. Isoniazid (often called INH) joined streptomycin and aminosalicylic acid as part of standard drug therapy for tuberculosis.[52]

The early promise of the sulfones in experimental work on tuberculosis, and the close chemical relationship between these compounds and the sulfa drugs, prompted the first clinical trials of sulfones in treatment of leprosy (Hansen's dis-ease). These were undertaken in 1941 at the U.S. Public Health Service's lep-rosarium in Carville, Louisiana, at the initiative of its director, Guy Faget. Prior to his arrival at Carville, Faget had experimented with sulfa drugs in treatment of malaria and had also done work on tuberculosis. At Carville, he first attempted to treat volunteers among the patients with sulfa drugs, but soon turned to sulfones after reading Mayo Clinic reports of trials of these compounds in tuberculosis in guinea pigs. With sulfone compounds supplied by Parke Davis & Company, Abbott Laboratories, and Burroughs Wellcome, Faget and other investigators by the late 1940s were able to establish the value of sulfone therapy in leprosy. The result was a revolution in management of the disease, with effective drug treatment and outpatient care replacing the isolation of patients from society.[53]

Observations of the physiological effects of sulfa drugs or closely related compounds in the course of investigations undertaken for other purposes prompted research that led in several cases to important new drugs or classes of drugs. One such case was the work that led to the introduction of thiourea, thiouracil, and related compounds for treatment of hyperthyroidism. In 1941, Johns Hopkins biochemists C.G. Mackenzie and Julia B. Mackenzie reported that they had found in the course of nutritional experiments that sulfaguanidine, given in large doses to rats, produced a significant enlargement of the thyroid gland. The Mackenzies established that the effect was not altered by the presence or absence of p-aminobenzoic acid and so was distinct from the bacteriostatic effect of sulfaguanidine. Given the rapidly expanding medical use of the sulfa drugs, and the possibility that the newly observed physiological activity of a sulfonamide might lead to new therapeutic uses, the Mackenzies decided that their observation "demanded an immediate and detailed investigation of this effect on the thyroid gland (and possibly on the basal metabolic rate) of the rat and other experimental animals to provide a basis for the search of a similar reaction in man." In the research that followed, the Mackenzies and others demonstrated that not only sulfaguanidine but also thiourea, thiouracil, and other thio (sulfur-containing) compounds unrelated to the sulfa drugs inhibited thyroxine synthesis and that their activity could be overcome by thyroxine. One outcome was the introduction of thiourea, thiouracil, and related compounds into the therapeutics of hyperthyroidism, as complements or substitutes for surgery.[54]

The first oral hypoglycemic agents to be used in treatment of diabetes also emerged from studies prompted by observations of physiological activity of sulfonamides in the course of clinical trials in bacterial infections. For all its virtues and dramatic successes, insulin was not a cure for diabetes, and since it was not active when given by mouth, it required repeated injections. The search for diabetes treatments that would be active when given by mouth began in 1925–1930 with studies of synthalines and their derivatives by German investigators. These studies were abandoned when the compounds' efficacy proved unreliable and their toxicity too great.[55]

Early in World War II, doctors in Montpellier, France, found themselves treating many cases of typhoid fever apparently due to the contaminated wartime food supply. Investigators at Montpellier Medical School, using sulfa drugs to treat typhoid fever, found that one of them, supplied by Rhône-Poulenc and given the reference number 2254 RP, produced pronounced hypoglycemia in patients. One of the investigators, Auguste Loubatières, showed that the hypoglycemic effect of 2254 RP was due to its action on the pancreas, and he further hypothesized that the compound stimulated cells in the Islets of Langerhans, which released increased quantities of insulin into the bloodstream. The clinical observations were published in 1942 by Marcel Janbon, and Loubatières published his physiological work in 1946, but the latter was unable to interest others in the possible clinical applications of his findings.[56]

Work on hypoglycemic sulfonamides was resumed in 1954 in Germany, again as a result of observations made in the course of trials of a sulfonamide in bacterial chemotherapy. Hans Franke and Karl Joachim Fuchs, physicians at a Berlin hospital, received from Boehringer Söhne GmbH of Mannheim a sulfon-amide compound to be tried in treatment of pneumonia. The compound, called BZ 55 or carbutamide, produced a variety of symptoms. One of its effects was the production of hypoglycemia, and the doctors decided to make an extensive investigation of its possible uses in treatment of diabetes. Further studies by various German investigators, in the course of which Loubatières's earlier work was brought into the discussion, resulted in publications in 1955 showing that carbutamide was an effective medicine in the treatment of adult-onset dia-betes.[57]

As sulfonamides, both 2254 RP and carbutamide had antibacterial properties that were unnecessary in diabetes therapy. In 1956, another group of German in-vestigators published experimental and clinical findings showing that a compound identical to carbutamide, except for substitution of a methyl group for the amino group in the *para*-position of the molecule, was free of antibacterial activity while preserving the hypoglycemic and antidiabetic properties of carbutamide. This compound, called D 860 or tolbutamide, also proved to be freer of side effects than carbutamide, and it soon entered medical practice as an oral antidiabetic agent. It also became the lead compound for a whole new class of such medicines, the sulfonylureas.[58]

Another important medicine to emerge from sulfonamide-related research was probenecid, the first effective treatment for gout, a painful and debilitating condition that in the 1950s afflicted some 360,000 people in the United States alone. Probenecid was the product of a renal research program launched by Sharp & Dohme Research Laboratories in 1943 originally to study the problem of crys-tal formation in the urine by sulfa drugs. At that time, the company was supplying Homer W. Smith, a physiologist at New York University engaged in studies of re-nal function, with a compound called *p*-aminohippuric acid (PAH). In 1944, it oc-curred to Karl H. Beyer, who had joined Sharp & Dohme in 1943 and directed its renal research program, that PAH might reduce the rate of excretion of penicillin from the body by competitive inhibition of a transport mechanism involved in tu-bular secretion in the kidney. The problem was of practical importance because penicillin was in short supply, was poorly absorbed orally, and was rapidly ex-creted. Any means of retaining it in the system would have both medical and eco-nomic importance.[59]

Experiments confirmed that PAH depressed secretion of penicillin but also showed that large quantities of the compound, which was poorly absorbed when administered by mouth, were required to do so. Sharp & Dohme chemists, di-rected by James M. Sprague, supplied Beyer with other newly synthesized com-pounds. One of these, a sulfonamide called carinamide, also slowed excretion of penicillin but, like PAH, required large daily oral doses. Finally, a closely related sulfonamide, probenecid, proved equally effective while showing better oral absorption and requiring much lower daily intake.[60]

The medical and commercial value of probenecid, which was released in 1952 under the trade name Benemid, was reduced in penicillin therapy by the advent of the orally active penicillins and by the falling cost of penicillin. Its value increased in another direction, however, when Sharp & Dohme researchers observed that it reduced blood levels of uric acid by interfering with its reabsorption through the renal tubular membrane, thereby increasing its excretion in the urine. Since the pain and stiffness in gout are due to deposits of uric acid crystals in the joints, probenecid's action made it an important tool in control of this disease. The research program that led to probenecid, and the compound itself, also contributed to new fundamental knowledge of renal physiology.[61]

Sharp & Dohme's renal research program took a new direction in 1949 after publication of a clinical paper by Boston physician William Schwartz reporting that administration of sulfanilamide increased water and sodium excretion in a patient with congestive heart failure. Schwartz had been acting on an earlier finding by physiologists that sulfanilamide inhibited carbonic anhydrase, an enzyme that controlled the exchange reaction between carbon dioxide and bicarbonate ion in the kidney. His reasoning was that by inhibiting this exchange, sulfanilamide caused an excretion of bicarbonate, and with it sodium and water, into the urine. Schwartz's finding prompted researchers at American Cyanamid, led by Roblin, to begin a search for other sulfonamides that would be more efficient carbonic anhydrase inhibitors. The goal was to develop a diuretic that could be used in treatment of cardiac edema.[62]

At Sharp & Dohme, Beyer was not entirely persuaded by the carbonic anhydrase theory. In addition, he felt that if an anion was to be removed from the kidney with sodium, it should be chloride rather than bicarbonate so as to better maintain the body's acid–base balance. Sharp & Dohme investigators therefore redefined the diuretic research program as a search for a salt-removing, or saluretic, compound that would focus not on carbonic anhydrase inhibition but on kidney output. Beyer set up appropriate urine tests, and the chemists under Sprague brought to bear extensive knowledge of sulfonamide chemistry and a collection of thousands of sulfonamide compounds carried over from earlier investigations.[63]

A first success of the Sharp & Dohme team came with identification of a simple sulfonamide compound that increased excretion of both sodium and chloride. The effect proved too weak in humans, but gave Beyer, Sprague, and their colleagues the assurance that they were headed in the right direction. American Cyanamid's effort yielded acetazolamide, a carbonic anhydrase inhibitor active enough as a diuretic to be marketed under the trade name Diamox and to be used in the treatment of congestive heart failure. Continuing their search for a saluretic sulfonamide, the Beyer-Sprague team moved from aromatic to heterocyclic compounds, and then back to the aromatic series, trying different kinds of substitutions. Success came in 1955 with their synthesis and testing of the first thiazide compounds. Among these, chlorothiazide proved to be a potent saluretic and diuretic with nearly ideal pharmacological characteristics.[64]

Chlorothiazide underwent clinical trials in 1956–1957 and was released in 1958 by Merck (which had merged with Sharp & Dohme in 1953) under the trade name Diuril. Quickly embraced by doctors and patients, Diuril became a major moneymaker for Merck and revolutionized the treatment of diseases such as congestive heart failure and hypertension. Its success provoked a large-scale research effort by the international pharmaceutical industry to seek other diuretically active compounds containing the sulfonamide group. This effort resulted in turn in major new diuretics, including chlorthalidone from Geigy (after 1970, Ciba-Geigy Ltd.) and furseminide from Hoechst AG. Max Tishler, writing in 1965 as president of Merck, Sharp & Dohme Research Laboratories, was not merely praising his own establishment when he remarked of the thiazides that "as a class, they probably represent the greatest therapeutic advance in cardiovascular diseases."[65]

The reach of the sulfa drugs was not confined to human medicine. In the case of Merck, for example, it was a sulfa drug that brought about the company's move into veterinary medicine in the 1940s. Sulfaquinoxaline, a compound under study as an antimalarial, was found to produce kidney stones in dogs and never reached clinical trial. Testing it in other animals, Merck researchers found that it was effective in prevention and treatment of coccidiosis, an infection of chickens that caused significant financial losses to agriculture. Marketed as S.Q., sulfaquinoxaline was the first medicine permitted by the U.S. government to be mixed in animal food and lifted Merck to a leading position in the market for poultry drugs.[66]

In England, sulfaquinoxaline was manufactured by May & Baker under license from Merck. In the late 1950s, one of May & Baker's chemists, E.W. Parnell, began looking for other sulfonamide compounds that would be effective against avian coccidiosis. One of those he synthesized, though inactive as a coccidiostat, proved to have weed-killing properties when subjected to the company's herbicidal screening. Further modification of the molecule and field trials yielded a sulfonamide compound with selective herbicidal action against weeds afflicting a variety of crops, including sugar cane, grassland, linseed (flax seed), and oilseed poppy. Marketed by May & Baker in 1965 with the trade name Asulam, this compound became a major product for the company, with sales in Europe, Africa, the Americas, and Asia.[67]

Among those who most clearly perceived the multiple ramifications of the sulfa drugs in pharmaceutical innovation was Tishler. Looking back from the vantage point of the mid-1960s, Tishler recalled that "as time went on, it became apparent to chemists and pharmacologists that the sulfonamide grouping had a rather exalted position, since new and unexpected biological effects were being uncovered, occasionally by accident." Tishler regarded the process of drug development set in motion by the sulfa drugs as a classical instance of "one of the greatest virtues of molecular modification. The medicinal chemists following Domagk's discovery have broadened the usefulness of the [sulfonamides] and have created new drugs for conditions entirely unrelated to bacterial infections." Although clear in retrospect, this development could not be foreseen. "Who in the early forties," Tishler asked, "could have predicted that the sulfonamide grouping would have had so great an impact on the practice of medicine?"[68]

Trajectory of Change

Viewed from the time of their introduction in 1935 on, the sulfa drugs helped to initiate a therapeutic revolution and opened the era of miracle drugs. Viewed in the longer arc of their history, as presented in this volume, they were both constitutive and exemplary of a larger historical process that reaches back into the late nineteenth century and that spans the twentieth century. This is the industrialization of innovation in medicinal drugs. It is a process with many facets. In their origins, the sulfa drugs exemplify the increasing location of pharmaceutical research in industry in the twentieth century and the associated efforts to organize and routinize invention under corporate executive management.

After the breakthrough introduction of Prontosil, and recognition of sulfanilamide as its effective part, the subsequent development of the sulfa drugs may also be seen as an instance of what Hughes has called conservative invention. In this view, a successful technology, itself the product of a fundamental innovation, or what Hughes calls radical invention, serves as the starting point for research and development leading to its modification and improvement. Often, according to Hughes, radical inventions come from individual inventors or outsiders to industry not bound by its established thinking and practice, while conservative inventions involving systematic efforts to modify and improve are most effectively carried out by industrial research organizations. The development of the sulfa drugs from 1935 through the 1940s, in the course of which thousands of compounds were synthesized and screened, mostly by industrial laboratories, in an effort to expand therapeutic spectrum or reduce toxicity, appears to conform well to the notion of conservative invention. By contrast, penicillin, which may be regarded as a radical invention in the early 1940s, had its origins in academic research. I.G. Farben pharmaceutical researchers, heavily committed to the synthetic organic chemistry model of bacterial chemotherapy represented by the sulfa drugs, failed to seize the new opportunities opened by penicillin.[69]

A different status must be assigned to the initial invention of Prontosil, and to the later initiation of new kinds of medicines or classes of medicines as a result of research or practice related to the sulfa drugs. As the first successful bacterial chemotherapy, Prontosil was a fundamental innovation yet one that emerged from a highly organized industrial research program that drew extensively on earlier industrial chemotherapeutic and chemical research. Diuretics, blood-sugar-lowering drugs, and other medicines indebted directly or indirectly to work on the sulfa drugs and to the exalted position of the sulfonamide group were also fundamental innovations, and not improvements on the antibacterial activity of the sulfa drugs. Yet in most cases their development, too, was heavily indebted to industrial research.

The award of the 1939 Nobel Prize in Physiology or Medicine to Domagk for his recognition of the antibacterial activity of Prontosil placed the spotlight squarely on the individual researcher. In so doing, it exposed the lack of congruence between the industrialized system of invention examined in this volume, on the one hand, and the individualized system of credits carried over from earlier patterns of invention and from academic science, and embodied in the Nobel Prizes, on the other.

In its allotment of credits to individuals, the Nobel Prize tends to efface the roles of colleagues and supporting institutions. This distortion is especially egregious in a case such as Domagk's in which the roles of these factors were significant.

It would be a mistake, of course, to lose sight of the role of the individual, even in a setting like I.G. Farben. If Domagk had not insisted on animal tests in addition to *in vitro* ones, the antibacterial activity of Prontosil might not have been discovered. To that degree, Domagk contributed the crucial differentia between success and failure, and his Nobel award was appropriate.

Yet there is evidence that Domagk's Nobel award led to tension among the research staff of the company, especially between Domagk and the chemists who perceived Domagk's disproportionate honors as a slight to themselves. In 1945, Domagk wrote an angry letter to the company's directors complaining that other researchers were downplaying the importance of the sulfa drugs and that "various interest groups" were trying to break up his collaboration with the chemists Fritz Mietzsch and Joseph Klarer. Domagk's negotiations with the University of Heidelberg in 1946 may reflect in part tensions with the chemists over credit for the sulfa drugs. Domagk did not leave for an academic post, but tension persisted, perhaps aggravated by Domagk's collection of his Nobel Prize in 1947 and the attendant publicity. A letter of 1953 from Mietzsch to Domagk, to take only one example, complained of a press article in which Domagk was wrongly described as a chemist. In this letter and in several publications of the 1950s, Mietzsch emphasized that he and other company chemists were exclusively responsible for the chemical part of the work on the sulfa drugs.[70]

The biochemist Paul György looked beyond the roles of medical researchers and chemists and drew a logical, if far-fetched, conclusion when he stated in a 1947 affidavit submitted to the Nuremberg trials that Heinrich Hörlein should have received the Nobel Prize for the sulfa drugs rather than Domagk, because these medicines were the product of an organized, collaborative effort, of which Hörlein had been the architect, and Domagk himself had been one part.[71]

The sulfa drugs, and later medicines related to them, were products of research in medicinal chemistry, which may be defined in simplest terms as the synthesis of organic compounds and the screening of these compounds for medicinal effect. So defined, the origins of medicinal chemistry may be traced to the German chemical industry of the 1880s, and in its specifically chemotherapeutic form to Ehrlich's research program initiated in 1906. The sulfa drugs may be regarded as the most important single success of medicinal chemistry, and their introduction and example ushered in an era in which medicinal chemistry played a prominent role in pharmaceutical research, sometimes at the expense of other kinds of investigations such as those seeking vaccines. For one of the companies that has figured in this volume, Merck, and the company with which it merged, Sharp & Dohme, medicinal chemistry dominated a three-decade cycle of research and development, from the late 1930s to the late 1960s.[72]

Typically innovation in medicinal chemistry required the synthesis and systematic screening of large numbers of organic compounds. As this volume has shown for the case of Prontosil, trial and error was involved, but the process was far from random. On the contrary, it was controlled by collaborating teams of medical researchers and chemists, with each party to the collaboration defining the constraints and opportunities of the research by reference to prior research experience and to the known properties of organisms and chemical compounds. Chance could play a role, as illustrated in this volume by the synthesis of sulfapyridine from an old bottle of aminopyridine gathering dust on the laboratory shelf, but it did so generally within the framework of a structured research program.[73]

Discovery of the mode of action of sulfanilamide and formulation of the concept of antimetabolite in the early 1940s led to a wave of optimism about the rational design of medicinal drugs. Although the antimetabolite concept proved a useful one in drug research over the long run, its short-term results were modest. Roblin, writing in 1950 as director of American Cyanamid's Chemotherapy Division, pointed out that, although the antimetabolite concept was appealing, "in practice . . . practically all advances in chemotherapy have been based on screening techniques, on chance observation, or on a combination of both." Rational design placed unrealistic demands on the investigator's available fund of knowledge. "One of the most serious handicaps to the metabolite antagonist approach is that it presupposes a much greater background of information in cell metabolism than actually exists today," Roblin continued. "Given a more complete knowledge of the biochemistry and physiology of cells, we should be in a better position to apply more direct methods."[74]

In the following decades, a more complete knowledge did emerge, fueled in no small part by massive increases in government support for medical and biological research as well as expansion of research and development in the pharmaceutical industry. Over the three decades following the introduction of the sulfa drugs, however, screening methods assisted by chance observations continued to be the most common source of new drugs. And in spite of great advances in sciences closely related to medicinal drugs and their biological activity, rational drug design continued to prove elusive well into the late twentieth century.[75]

By the time that Domagk learned of his Nobel Prize in October 1939, Europe was already at war for the second time in the century, and German industry was nearing the end of some six decades of leadership in pharmaceutical research and production. The introduction of Prontosil and initiation of the sulfa drugs were a late and momentous example of such leadership, but this volume has provided other notable instances.

After studying in Germany, Ernest Fourneau adopted the German model of close cooperation between researchers on medicinal drugs and the chemical industry. Closely attuned to German developments, Fourneau's research unit in Paris was one of the first outside Germany to grasp the significance of Prontosil, and his researchers' rapid recognition that sulfanilamide was the active constituent of the new medicine opened the way to the next generation of sulfa drugs. Henry Hallett Dale had an early glimpse of the compound that became Prontosil during a visit to Germany and facilitated its testing in Britain. The May & Baker research establishment that eventually produced sulfapyridine was built up in response to the crisis that resulted when German imports of fine chemicals including drugs were cut off in World War I. Hugh Hampton Young's attempt to introduce research in chemotherapy at Johns Hopkins was inspired by Paul Ehrlich and derived part of its support in the 1920s from American efforts to encourage competition with German industry.[76]

Although Merck and Sharp & Dohme, like other American pharmaceutical companies, were beginning to build up their research facilities by the mid-1930s, neither entered the field of chemotherapy until prompted to do so by sulfanilamide in 1937. The great success of these companies in medicinal chemistry, before and after their merger in 1953, took its initial impetus from the sulfa drugs.[77]

By interrupting imports of fine chemicals, including pharmaceuticals, from Germany, the First World War stimulated expansion of industrial pharmaceutical research in France, Britain, and the United States in the 1920s and 1930s without producing a decisive challenge to German leadership. The German industrial pharmaceutical research establishment continued to function during the National Socialist regime, although the energies of its most prominent leader, Hörlein, were diverted by the need to struggle with ideologues hostile to the enterprise or to accommodate his organization to the regime's demands. The German chemical industry continued to open subsidiaries in the United States, Britain, and other countries, and in the late 1930s German pharmaceutical sales claimed approximately forty-three percent of the world market.[78]

What the 1914–1918 war and the early National Socialist regime had failed to accomplish was finally achieved by a second World War and its aftermath. German leadership in pharmaceutical research and production disappeared amid wartime losses and destruction, postwar occupation and political division, the breakup of I.G. Farben, and the need for economic recovery, the reconstruction of academic institutions, and the renewal of communication with the international scientific community. Leadership passed to the United States, where the war had accelerated an expansion of research, development, and production of pharmaceuticals already under way by 1939.[79]

American leadership in pharmaceutical innovation in the postwar decades is well illustrated by those drugs or classes of drugs considered above as products of research related to the sulfa drugs. Among these, the medicines for Hansen's disease (leprosy), hyperthyroidism, heart disease and hypertension, gout, and avian coccidiosis were all entirely or mainly products of U.S research and development. Isoniazid for treatment of tuberculosis was the product of work in two companies in the United States and one German company all following up on research begun by Domagk in Germany. The oral hypoglycemic agents for treatment of diabetes were developed in postwar Germany with some role played by wartime French research.

Most spectacular of all, of course, was the wartime U.S. development of penicillin from its beginnings in British academic research. Even before penicillin came on the scene, however, American leadership was visible in U.S. development of newer sulfa drugs such as sulfadiazine and sulfaguanidine, and in the U.S. role as major supplier of sulfa drugs in the Allied war effort. Penicillin was soon followed by streptomycin, a product of U.S. research and development, by other antibiotics, and by a flood of new medicinal drugs of other kinds.

As penicillin, then other antibiotics, became widely available, sulfa drugs were displaced from their position as medicines of choice in the treatment of most bacterial infections. It is true that any early expectations of their demise were exaggerated. Although relegated to a distinctly secondary position by antibiotics, sulfa drugs continued to be available to physicians treating bacterial infections and continued to be used. One example is the reliance of the U.S. Navy on sulfadiazine to treat meningococcal meningitis until 1965. In some cases, for example, certain kinds of urinary tract infections, sulfa drugs could be considered superior to antibiotics. Given the capacity of bacteria to develop resistance to any drug, physicians could not afford to dispense with any effective medicine, including the sulfa drugs. In the late 1960s, doctors were writing prescriptions for sulfa drugs at the rate of 15–20 million a year in the United States alone. As generics or under such familiar trade names as Septra, Gantrisin, Bactrin, and Orinase, sulfa drugs, alone or in combination with other compounds, continue to have a well-established place in therapeutics.[80]

All of this said, it remains the case that the postwar decades witnessed a transformation in the status of the sulfa drugs from that of revolutionary vanguard to that of yeoman worker in the world of medicinal drugs. As the brilliant success of penicillin was followed by the debuts of other new drugs, and as fewer patients encountered sulfa drugs in their own experience, they receded from the consciousness if not of doctors then of the public. To some extent, the very success of antibacterial medicines, sulfa drugs and antibiotics, rendered them less visible to the public as the cure of such infections came to be taken largely for granted and as heart disease, cancer, and chronic ailments occupied much of the space once taken by bacterial infections.

With the recession of the sulfa drugs from medical practice, and a declining proportion of the population with memories of their impact in the 1930s and 1940s, came also a diminishing sense of their historical importance. That sense must be recaptured and critically examined if we are to have an adequate account of the trajectory of medicine and science in the twentieth and twenty-first century. The sulfa drugs stand at a pivotal moment in that history, when the long process of the industrialization of pharmaceutical innovation reached a first culmination, ushering in a therapeutic revolution that is still with us.

Notes

Abbreviations Used in Notes

AC	*Angewandte Chemie*
AIM	*Annals of Internal Medicine*
AMCMA	Alan Mason Chesney Medical Archives, Johns Hopkins Medical Institutions, Johns Hopkins University
AS	*Annals of Surgery*
BA	Bayer Archive
BHM	*Bulletin of the History of Medicine*
BJEP	*British Journal of Experimental Pathology*
BJHH	*Bulletin of the Johns Hopkins Hospital*
BMFRS	*Biographical Memoirs of Fellows of the Royal Society*
BMJ	*British Medical Journal*
DMW	*Deutsche medizinische Wochenschrift*
GD	File Prof. Dr. Gerhard Domagk
HD	Henry Hallett Dale papers
HHY	Hugh Hampton Young papers
JAMA	*Journal of the American Medical Association*
JHMAS	*Journal of the History of Medicine and Allied Sciences*
KW	*Klinische Wochenschrift*
MA	Merck Archives
MB	May & Baker Archives
MMW	*Münchener medizinische Wochenschrift*
MR	*Merck Report*
MRC	Medical Research Council Archives
MS	*Military Surgeon*
NA	U.S. National Archives

NEJM   *New England Journal of Medicine*
PH   *Pharmacy in History*
PRSM   *Proceedings of the Royal Society of Medicine*
RG   Record Group of the U.S. National Archives
RSL   Royal Society of London Archives
SGO   *Surgery, Gynecology, and Obstetrics*
TTC   Medical Research Council Therapeutic Trials Committee
WM   *War Medicine*

Introduction

1. Peter Temin, *Taking Your Medicine: Drug Regulation in the United States* (Cambridge, MA: Harvard University Press, 1980), esp. 58–87; Nicholas Wells, *Medicines: 50 Years of Progress 1930–1980* (London: Office of Health Economics, 1980), esp. 5–11, 23; Richard M. Weinshilboum, "The therapeutic revolution," *Clinical Pharmacology and Therapeutics* 42 (1987): 481–484; and Judy Slinn, "Research and development in the UK pharmaceutical industry from the nineteenth century to the 1960s," in Roy Porter and Mikulás Teich, editors, *Drugs and Narcotics in History* (Cambridge: Cambridge University Press, 1995), 168–186, esp. 180–183. David L. Cowen has captured the same historical shift in an alternative phrase, "pharmaceutical revolution." See his "The on-going pharmaceutical revolution: the role of the industry," in *Farmacia e Industrializacion: Libro homenaje al Doctor Guillermo Folch Jou* (Madrid: Sociedad Española de Historia de la Farmacia, 1985), 95–104. A different sense of therapeutic revolution, centered on nineteenth-century changes, is explored in Morris J. Vogel and Charles E. Rosenberg, editors, *The Therapeutic Revolution: Essays in the Social History of American Medicine* (Philadelphia, PA: University of Pennsylvania Press, 1979).

2. John E. Lesch, "Conceptual change in an empirical science: the discovery of the first alkaloids," *Historical Studies in the Physical Sciences* 11: 2 (1981): 305–328; and B. Holmstedt and G. Liljestrand, *Readings in Pharmacology* (Oxford: Pergamon Press, 1963). For a broad survey of drug therapy since the mid-nineteenth century, see John Parascandola, "From germs to genes: trends in drug therapy, 1852–2002," *PH* 44 (2002): 3–11.

3. Ronald D. Mann, *Modern Drug Use: An Enquiry on Historical Principles* (Lancaster, UK: MTP Press Ltd., 1984), 480–481; Jan R. McTavish, "What did Bayer do before aspirin? Early pharmaceutical marketing practices in America," *PH* 41 (1999): 3–15; and chapter 2.

4. See chapters 1, 3, and 4.

5. Slinn, "Research and development in the UK pharmaceutical industry" (note 1); Jonathan M. Liebenau, "Scientific ambitions: the pharmaceutical industry, 1900–1920," *PH* 27 (1985): 3–11; John Parascandola, "Charles Holmes Herty and the effort to establish an institute for drug research in post World War I America," in John Parascandola and James C. Whorton, editors, *Chemistry and Modern Society* (Washington, DC: American Chemical Society, 1983), 85–103; Parascandola, "Industrial research comes of age: the American pharmaceutical industry, 1920–1940," *PH* 27 (1985): 12–21; Andrea Frances Balis, *Miracle Medicine: The Impact of Sulfa Drugs on Medicine, the Pharmaceutical Industry and Government Regulation in the U.S. in the 1930s* (Ann Arbor, MI: University Microfilms, 2000), 27–75; John P. Swann, *Academic Scientists and the Pharmaceutical Industry: Cooperative Research in Twentieth-Century America* (Baltimore, MD: Johns Hopkins University Press, 1988); Swann, "The evolution of the American pharmaceutical industry," *PH* 37 (1995): 76–86; Nicolas Rasmussen, "The drug industry and clinical research in interwar America: Three types of physician collaborator," *BHM* 79 (2005): 50–80; Michael Bliss, *The Discovery of Insulin* (Chicago: University of Chicago Press,

1982); Nelly Oudshoorn, *Beyond the Natural Body: An Archeology of Sex Hormones* (London: Routledge, 1994), esp. 65–111; Rima D. Apple, *Vitamania: Vitamins in American Culture* (New Brunswick, NJ: Rutgers University Press, 1996), 33–53; and Robert G. Denkewalter and Max Tishler, "Drug research—whence and whither," *Fortschritte der Arzneimittelforschung* 10 (1966): 11–31, on 16. On France, see chapter 6. On Britain and the United States, see chapters 6–8.

6. R. Slack and A.W. Nineham, *Medical and Veterinary Chemicals*, vol. 1 (Oxford: Pergamon Press, 1968), 3–29, on 7, 9–10.

7. F. Sherwood Taylor, *The Conquest of Bacteria: From Salvarsan to Sulphapyridine* (New York: Philosophical Library, 1942); Iago Galdston, *Behind the Sulfa Drugs: A Short History of Chemotherapy* (New York: D. Appleton-Century Co., 1943).

8. Boris Sokoloff, *The Miracle Drugs* (Chicago: Ziff-Davis Publishing Co., 1949).

9. See, e.g., Max Tishler, "Molecular modification in drug research," paper presented at the Symposium on Influence of Molecular Modification in Drug Design, Division of Medical Chemistry, American Chemical Society, September 9, 1963, MA, box R4-1.8.5; Tishler, "Perspectives in pharmaceutical research," *TVF* 36 (1965): 37–47; and Denkewalter and Tishler, "Drug research—whence and whither" (note 5). See also chapter 12.

10. A concise survey that captures some aspects of the discontinuity is Harry F. Dowling, *Fighting Infection: Conquests of the Twentieth Century* (Cambridge, MA: Harvard University Press, 1977), 105–124.

11. Daniel Bovet, *Une chimie qui guérit: histoire de la découverte des sulfamides* (Paris: Éditions Payot, 1988). My review of this book is in *BHM*: 64 (1990): 338–339.

12. Marcel H. Bickel, "The development of sulfonamides (1932–1938) as a focal point in the history of chemotherapy," *Gesnerus* 45 (1998): 67–86; Bickel, "Eli K. Marshall, Jr. (1889–1966): from biochemistry and physiology to pharmacology and pharmacokinetics," *Drug Metabolism Reviews* 28(3) (1996): 311–344.

13. Harry M. Marks, *The Progress of Experiment: Science and Therapeutic Reform in the United States, 1900–1990* (Cambridge: Cambridge University Press, 1997), 71–97; John P. Swann, "The 1941 sulfathiazole disaster and the birth of good manufacturing practices," *PH* 40 (1999): 16–25; Dale E. Cooper, "Adequate controls for new drugs: good manufacturing practice and the 1938 Federal Food, Drug and Cosmetic Act," *PH* 44 (2002): 12–23; Balis, *Miracle Medicine* (note 5).

14. John Harley Warner, *The Therapeutic Perspective: Medical Practice, Knowledge, and Identity in America, 1820–1885* (Cambridge, MA: Harvard University Press, 1986).

15. Robert H. Moser, *Diseases of Medical Progress: A Contemporary Analysis of Illness Produced by Drugs and Other Therapeutic Procedures* (Springfield, IL: Charles C. Thomas, 1959); Rene Dubos, *The Dreams of Reason: Science and Utopias* (New York: Columbia University Press, 1961).

16. Charles E. Rosenberg, "Holism in twentieth-century medicine," in Christopher Lawrence and George Weisz, editors, *Greater Than the Parts: Holism in Biomedicine, 1920–1950* (New York: Oxford University Press, 1998), 335–355, esp. 346–348.

17. Steven Epstein, *Impure Science: AIDS, Activism, and the Politics of Knowledge* (Berkeley: University of California Press, 1996).

Chapter 1

1. Paul Ehrlich, "Chemotherapy," in F. Himmelweit, editor, *The Collected Papers of Paul Ehrlich*, vol. 3, *Chemotherapy* (London: Pergamon Press, 1960), 505–518, on 517–518.

2. Paul Ehrlich, "Ansprache bei Einweihung des Georg-Speyer Hauses," in F. Himmelweit, editor, *The Collected Papers of Paul Ehrlich* (note 1), 42–52. On the early chemotherapy of protozoal diseases, see the same volume and H.J. Barber, "Antibacterial

dawn and antiprotozoal noon," in H.J. Barber, editor, *Historical Aspects of Chemotherapy: Six Essays* (Dagenham, UK: May & Baker Ltd., 1976), 24–32.

3. Erwin H. Ackerknecht, *A Short History of Medicine* (Baltimore, MD: Johns Hopkins University Press, 1982), 175–185.

4. Harry F. Dowling, *Fighting Infection: Conquests of the Twentieth Century* (Cambridge, MA: Harvard University Press, 1977), 6–7; and Gerald N. Grob, *The Deadly Truth: A History of Disease in America* (Cambridge, MA: Harvard University Press, 2002), 192.

5. William Osler, *The Principles and Practice of Medicine, Designed for the Use of Practitioners and Students of Medicine*, 3rd ed (New York: D. Appleton & Co., 1899), 108–137 (quotes on 108, 131).

6. Osler, *The Principles and Practice of Medicine* (note 5), 134–137.

7. Ackerknecht, *A Short History of Medicine* (note 3), 175–193, 210–217.

8. Anthony Travis, *The Rainbow Makers: The Origins of the Synthetic Dyestuffs Industry* (Bethlehem, PA: Lehigh University Press, 1993).

9. Hubert A. Lechevalier and Morris Solotorovsky, *Three Centuries of Microbiology* (New York: Dover Publications Inc., 1974; first published 1965), 437–439; and Carola Throm, *Das Diphtherieserum: Ein neues Therapieprinzip, seine Entwicklung und Markteinführung*, Heidelberger Schriften zur Pharmazie- und Naturwissenschaftsgeschichte (Stuttgart: Wissenschaftliche Verlagsgesellschaft, 1995).

10. Lechevalier and Solotorovsky, *Three Centuries of Microbiology* (note 9), 439. On the institutional setting of Ehrlich's work and his links to industry, see Jonathan Liebenau, "Paul Ehrlich as a commercial scientist and research administrator," *Medical History* 34 (1990): 65–78.

11. Lechevalier and Solotorovsky, *Three Centuries of Microbiology* (note 9), 231.

12. Ibid., 448–449; and Paul Ehrlich, "Ansprache bei Einweihung des Georg-Speyer-Hauses" (note 2), 42–52 (an English translation follows on 53–63). For a more detailed discussion of Ehrlich's views, see John Parascandola, "The theoretical basis of Paul Ehrlich's chemotherapy," *JHMAS* 36 (1981): 19–43.

13. Lechevalier and Solotorovsky, *Three Centuries of Microbiology* (note 9), 451–454; Sir Henry Dale, "Introduction," in F. Himmelweit, editor, *The Collected Papers of Paul Ehrlich* (note 1), 1–8 (quote on 2).

14. Ronald D. Mann, *Modern Drug Use: An Enquiry on Historical Principles* (Lancaster, UK: MTP Press Ltd., 1984), 553; Lechevalier and Solotorovsky, *Three Centuries of Microbiology* (note 9), 454–455.

15. Mann, *Modern Drug Use* (note 14), 554–555; Lechevalier and Solotorovsky, *Three Centuries of Microbiology* (note 9), 454–455.

16. Mann, *Modern Drug Use* (note 14), 555; Lechevalier and Solotorovsky, *Three Centuries of Microbiology* (note 9), 455; Dale, "Introduction" (note 13), 6–7.

17. Ehrlich, "Chemotherapy" (note 1), 515–518 (quotes on these pages).

18. Hugh Young, *A Surgeon's Autobiography* (New York: Harcourt, Brace & Co., 1940), 76, 252 (quote).

19. "Statement of Dr. Hugh H. Young," July 2, 1919, pp. 1–2, AMCMA, HHY, 24/4 [Note: Here and in subsequent citations, a/b = box a, file b]; Young, *A Surgeon's Autobiography* (note 18), 216–218.

20. Hugh H. Young, "The organization of the institute," and Griswold (first name not given in document), speech at opening ceremonies of the Brady Urological Institute (with quote from Brady letter), May 4, 1915, AMCMA, HHY, 24/8. The final cost of the institute building, equipped, came to about $275,000 in 1915 dollars. See Hugh H. Young, "The organization of a special hospital surgical unit—the James Buchanan Brady Urological Institute," AMCMA, HHY, 25/4, p. 5.

21. "The James Buchanan Brady Urological Institute" (printed article with illustrations, undated, c. 1915), AMCMA, HHY, 24/13, figure 8; Young, "The organization of a special surgical hospital unit" (note 20), 5.

22. Young, "The organization of a special surgical hospital unit" (note 20), 4, 6–7, 10. On the early staff and activities of the Brady Institute's research division, see "The James Buchanan Brady Urological Institute" (note 21); Young, *A Surgeon's Autobiography* (note 18), 233–234; bibliographies of staff members William C. Quinby, Ernest O. Swartz, and Edwin C. White, in Brady Urological Institute, Staff bibliographies, AMCMA, HHY, 31/12 and 31/14; Henry Wade, "The clinic of Dr. Hugh Hampton Young: the Buchanan Brady Institute of the Johns Hopkins Hospital, Baltimore, Maryland, U.S.A.," *British Journal of Surgery* 9 (1921): reprint 1–9, on 6.

23. Letters of John W. Churchman to Hugh H. Young, October 15 and 21, 1929, and November 9, 1929, and of Young to Churchman, October 17, 1929, AMCMA, HHY, 4/8; Young, *A Surgeon's Autobiography* (note 18), 252.

24. Young, *A Surgeon's Autobiography* (note 18), 264–339; Marjorie Winslow Kehoe, Nancy McCall, and Lisa A. Mix, *The Legacy of Hugh Hampton Young, Pioneer in Urology: A Guide to the Papers of Hugh Hampton Young in the Alan Mason Chesney Medical Archives, the Johns Hopkins Medical Institutes* (Baltimore, MD: AMCMA, 1991), 18; Leonard Keene Hirshberg, "The war service of our American doctors," *Munsey's Magazine* 64 (1918): 249–261.

25. Young, *A Surgeon's Autobiography* (note 18), 253. On venereal disease and the American Expeditionary Force, see also Allan M. Brandt, *No Magic Bullet: A Social History of Venereal Disease in the United States since 1880* (New York: Oxford University Press, 1987), 96–121. On the germicide work, see Hugh H. Young, Edwin C. White, and Ernest O. Swartz, "A new germicide for use in the genito-urinary tract: 'mercurachrome-220'," *JAMA* 73 (1919): 1483–1491; T.A. Storey to Frank N. Goodnow (president of Johns Hopkins University), June 7, 1920, AMCMA, HHY, 27/15; Hugh H. Young, handwritten notes for report on Social Hygiene Board grant activities through June 30, 1920, AMCMA, HHY, 27/15.

26. Young, handwritten notes for report (note 25).

27. Ibid., 1483–1484.

28. Ibid.

29. Ibid.

30. Ibid.; Young, *A Surgeon's Autobiography* (note 18), 235, 254–255; Edwin C. White, "Mercury derivatives of phthaleins," *Journal of the American Chemical Society* 42 (1920): 2355–2366. The substance used in practice was a water-soluble sodium salt of the original compound, prepared by the chemist H.A.B. Dunning. In this form, mercurachrome was less irritating and easier to prepare for clinical use (Young, *A Surgeon's Autobiography*, 255).

31. Young et al., "A new germicide" (note 25), 1485–1491; Young, *A Surgeon's Autobiography* (note 18), 256–257. The research staff continued to investigate other organic mercurial compounds. See "Statement from the Brady Urological Institute," December 20, 1922, AMCMA, HHY, 27/15.

32. Hugh H. Young, "Intravenous mercurachrome in the treatment of urological infections," *Journal of Urology* 13 (1925): 633–672, on 634.

33. Young, *A Surgeon's Autobiography* (note 18), 257–258; Hugh H. Young and Justina H. Hill, "The treatment of septicemia and local infections by intravenous injections of mercurachrome-220 soluble and of gentian violet," *JAMA* 82 (1924): 669–675; and Hugh H. Young, "The treatment of infections—general, local, and urinary with the intravenous injection of mercurachrome," *SGO* 40 (1925): 97–104.

34. Young, "The treatment of infections" (note 33), 103–104; Young, "Intravenous mercurachrome" (note 32), 669.

35. Young, *A Surgeon's Autobiography* (note 18), 260–261.

36. Ibid.; Young, "The treatment of infections" (note 33), 103–104; H.H. Young to Hynson, Westcott, and Dunning, May 26, 1942, AMCMA, HHY, 7/18.

37. *Journal of Urology: Experimental, Medical, Surgical* 1 (1917), Hugh Hampton Young, editor. On the *Journal of Urology*, see Young, *A Surgeon's Autobiography* (note 18), 248–251.

38. "Statement of Dr. Hugh H. Young" (note 19), 3–5; Young, *A Surgeon's Autobiography* (note 18), 231–233, 265–266; Hugh H. Young to Herbert H. Scheier, September 25, 1934, AMCMA, HHY, 27/6. On the holdings, value, and income of the Hugh H. Young Research Fund in 1927, see the business manager's report, S. Page Nelson to H.H. Young, June 1, 1927, AMCMA, HHY, 27/2.

39. "Francis P. Garvan, millionaire, injected life into dye industry," *Boston Herald*, January 27, 1930, p. 9; Richard Woods Edmunds, "Where did the suit against the Chemical Foundation originate?" *Manufacturers' Record* 88 (July 9, 1925): 83–84; "German I.G. and European dye cartel only beneficiaries of any change in present coal tar tariff," AMCMA, HHY, 27/11. No name is attached to this document, but Garvan's authorship is indicated by letters of H.H. Young to F.P. Garvan of February 6, 7, and 14, 1930, AMCMA, HHY, 27/11.

40. Edmunds, "Where did the suit against the Chemical Foundation originate?" (note 39); "Francis P. Garvan, millionaire" (note 39).

41. Hugh H. Young to Francis P Garvan, February 12, 1925; William Buffum to Young, August 6, 1925; Buffum to Young, October 1, 1925; Young to Buffum, October 2, 1925. AMCMA, HHY, 27/9.

42. Hugh H. Young to William Buffum, March 27, 1929, and "Report of the Director of the James Buchanan Brady Urological Institute, Johns Hopkins Hospital, to the Members of the Chemical Foundation," March 27, 1929, AMCMA, HHY, 27/10; Chas. H. Herty to Hugh H. Young, December 1, 1925, AMCMA, HHY, 27/9; M.L. Crossley (as Chairman, Dye Division, American Chemical Society) to Young, January 6, 1927, AMCMA, HHY, 4/1. On Herty, see John Parascandola, "Charles Holmes Herty and the effort to establish an institute for drug research in post World War I America," in John Parascandola and James C. Whorton, editors, *Chemistry and Modern Society* (Washington, DC: American Chemical Society, 1983), 85–103.

43. Hugh H. Young to William W. Buffum, August 10, 1927, AMCMA, HHY, 27/9. In a later letter to Buffum, Young confessed that the institute was "sadly in need of help" before it received Chemical Foundation support (Young to Buffum, April 12, 1929, AMCMA, HHY, 27/9).

44. See, e.g., Frederick L. Hoffman to Hugh H. Young, December 8, 1927; Young to Hoffman, December 19, 1927; Charles J. White to Young, February 20, 1928; Young to White, February 27, 1928; L.K. Mathews to Young, June 15, 1929; Young to Mathews, June 22, 1929; Young to Messrs. Hynson, Westcott, and Dunning, December 22, 1927, December 28, 1927, February 16, 1928, February 27, 1928, November 1, 1928, February 19, 1929, June 22, 1929, August 26, 1930, October 20, 1930, December 16, 1930; H.A.B. Dunning to Young, December 19, 1927, December 28, 1927, January 25, 1928, August 25, 1930. AMCMA, HHY, 7/18. See also Hugh H. Young to Harry Welday Mayes, December 3, 1927, AMCMA, HHY, 10/11.

45. Hugh H. Young to H.A.B. Dunning, December 30, 1927, AMCMA, HHY, 7/18; L.C. Shepherd to Dunning, June 6, 1928; W. Dandridge Reddish to Dunning, June 8, 1928;

Dunning to Young, June 11, 1928; Young to Dunning, June 15, 1928. AMCMA, HHY, 5/10. The article critical of mercurochrome, this time of its effectiveness as a topical antiseptic, was James Stevens Simmons, "Bactericidal action of mercurochrome-220 soluble and iodine solutions in skin disinfection," *JAMA* 91 (September 8, 1928): 704–708. The response was G.F. Reddish and W.E. Drake, "Mercurochrome-220 soluble and U.S.P. tincture of iodine: a comparison of germicidal efficiency in skin disinfection," *JAMA* 91 (September 8, 1928): 712–716. See also "The investigation of germicides" (editorial), *JAMA* 91 (September 8, 1928): 728–729.

46. Hugh H. Young to William duPont, March 12, 1929, AMCMA, HHY, 5/9; Young to H.A.B. Dunning, March 14, 1929, AMCMA, HHY, 5/10; unsigned letter (probably Dunning) to John F. Ward, November 20, 1929, AMCMA, HHY, 4/18; John W. Churchman to Young, May 20, 1927, September 30, 1929, October 15, 1929, October 21, 1929, November 9, 1929, and Young to Churchman, June 3, 1927, October 2, 1929, October 17, 1929, November 5, 1929, November 13, 1929, AMCMA, HHY, 4/8.

47. Hugh H. Young, bibliography 1895–1934, AMCMA, HHY, 31/1; Hugh H. Young to S. Bayne-Jones, November 23, 1939, with attached bibliography, AMCMA, HHY, 27/7; to Hynson, Westcott, and Dunning, May 26, 1942, AMCMA, HHY, 7/18; Young, *A Surgeon's Autobiography* (note 18), 261–262.

48. George W. Raiziss, M. Severac, and John C. Moetsch, "Bacterial chemotherapy with special reference to mercury dyestuffs," *Journal of Pharmacology and Experimental Therapeutics* 26 (1926): 447–459 (quotes on 447).

49. Ibid., 451–453.

50. Ibid., 458–459.

51. Ernest Linwood Walker and Marion A. Sweeney, "Chemotherapy of bacterial infections. I. Action of acriflavine, gentian-violet and mercurochrome in experimental bacterial infections," *Journal of Pharmacology and Experimental Therapeutics* 26 (1926): 461–467, on 461–462.

52. Ibid., 461–466.

53. Ibid., 464–466.

54. Ernest Linwood Walker and Marion A. Sweeney, "Chemotherapy of bacterial infections. II. The relation between chemical constitution and chemotherapeutic action in staphylococcic infections," *Journal of Pharmacology and Experimental Therapeutics* 31 (1927): 87–121, on 87–88, 121. For background, see John Parascandola, "The controversy over structure-activity relationships in the early twentieth century," *PH* 16 (1974): 54–63.

55. Walker and Sweeney, "Chemotherapy of bacterial infections. II" (note 54), 87–89.

56. Ibid., 90, 106–107.

57. Ibid., 107–116.

58. Ibid., 116–119.

59. John A. Kolmer, *Principles and Practice of Chemotherapy, with Special Reference to the Specific and General Treatment of Syphilis* (Philadelphia, PA: W.B. Saunders Co., 1926), 10.

60. Carl Voegtlin, "A hope of mankind—chemotherapy," in Julius Stieglitz, editor, *Chemistry in Medicine: A Cooperative Treatise Intended to Give Examples of Progress Made in Medicine with the Aid of Chemistry* (New York: Chemical Foundation Inc., 1928), 701–720, on 713. He also mentioned proflavine and hexyl-resorcinol as urinary antiseptics.

61. Hans Zinsser and Stanhope Bayne-Jones, *A Textbook of Bacteriology*, 7th ed. (New York: D. Appleton-Century Co., 1934), 120.

62. G.M. Findlay, *Recent Advances in Chemotherapy*, 2nd ed. (Philadelphia, PA: P. Blakiston's Sons, 1939), 479–481.

63. Lawrence P. Garrod, "Chemicals vs. bacteria," president's address, Section of Pathology, October 19, 1954, *PRSM* 48 (1955): 21–28, on 26. Garrod was an early and sharp critic of mercurachrome. See Lawrence P. Garrod, "The efficiency of antiseptics used in midwifery," *BMJ* (1931): 572–575.

64. See, e.g., Iago Galdston, *Behind the Sulfa Drugs: A Short History of Chemotherapy* (New York: D. Appleton-Century Co., 1943), 128–141; Daniel Bovet, *Une chimie qui guérit: histoire de la découverte des sulfamides* (Paris: Éditions Payot, 1988), 103–105; Harry F. Dowling, *Fighting Infection* (note 4), 106–107; and Fritz Mietzsch, "Chemie und wirtschaftliche Bedeutung der Sulfonamide," *Arbeitsgemeinschaft für Forschung des Landes Nordrhein-Westfalen* 31 (1954): 7–32, on 25.

65. Henry H. Dale, "Progress and prospects in chemotherapy," *Science* 60 (1924): 185–191 (quotes on 191).

66. Kolmer, *Principles and Practice of Chemotherapy* (note 59), title page, 48.

67. Ibid., 2 (quote), 48, 62–63 (quote).

68. Ibid., preface, 48–49, 62–63.

69. Voegtlin, "A hope of mankind—chemotherapy" (note 60), 701, 709, 712–713, 714, 716.

70. G.M. Findlay, *Recent Advances in Chemotherapy*, 1st ed. (Philadelphia, PA: P. Blakiston's Son & Co. Inc., 1930), 4.

71. Ibid., 480–481, 504–507.

72. Ibid., 480–481.

73. Ibid., 3–5 (quote on 3).

74. Ibid., 5, 8. Findlay recommended especially R.A. Fisher's *Statistical Methods for Research Workers*, 2nd ed. (Edinburgh: Oliver & Boyd, 1928), as an invaluable guide for working with small groups of animals.

75. Zinsser and Bayne-Jones, *A Textbook of Bacteriology*, 7th ed. (note 61), vii–x, 107–125. It is revealing that in the two chapters on streptococci and streptococcal infections (chapters 22 and 23, pp. 313–350), there are no references to chemotherapy or even to its desirability or possibility.

76. Max Gundel, *Die ansteckenden Krankheiten: ihre Epidemiologie, Bekämpfung, und spezifische Therapie* (Leipzig: Georg Thieme Verlag, 1935), v–vi, 31–38 (quote on 38; my translation).

77. Dowling, *Fighting Infection* (note 4), 23, 54; Gilbert B. Forbes and Grace M. Forbes, "An historical note on chemotherapy of bacterial infections," *American Journal of Diseases of Children* 119 (1970): 6–11, on 7; F. Sherwood Taylor, *The Conquest of Bacteria: From Salvarsan to Sulphapyridine* (New York: Philosophical Library and Alliance Book Corp., 1942), 107, 122. Max Gundel, *Die ansteckenden Krankheiten* (note 76), has no separate section on chemotherapy but two (560–569, 570–586) on sera and vaccines. The section on disinfection and sterilization (599–613) makes no mention of chemotherapy of systemic infections.

78. Gundel, *Die ansteckenden Krankheiten* (note 76), 38; Kolmer, *Principles and Practice of Chemotherapy* (note 59), 62–63.

79. Voegtlin, "A hope of mankind—chemotherapy" (note 60), 711–712.

80. Ibid., 719–720. On the last point, Voegtlin's charge was not entirely fair, since by the 1920s U.S. pharmaceutical companies were beginning to incorporate research into their activities and to set up cooperative arrangements with various kinds of academic researchers. See John P. Swann, *Academic Scientists and the Pharmaceutical Industry: Cooperative Research in Twentieth-Century America* (Baltimore, MD: Johns Hopkins Uni-

versity Press, 1988). The National Research Council was also beginning to recognize the need for more organized efforts toward the discovery of new medicinal drugs. See Caroline Jean Acker, "Addiction and the laboratory: the work of the National Research Council's Committee on Drug Addiction," *Isis* 86 (1995): 167–193.

Chapter 2

1. Georg Meyer-Thurow, "The industrialization of invention: a case study from the German chemical industry," *Isis* 73 (1982): 363–381. On the broader trends, see Timothy Lenoir, "A magic bullet: research for profit and the growth of knowledge in Germany around 1900," *Minerva* 26 (1988): 66–88; and Jeffrey Allan Johnson, "The academic-industrial symbiosis in German chemical research, 1905–1939," in John E. Lesch, editor, *The German Chemical Industry in the Twentieth Century* (Dordrecht: Kluwer Academic Publishers, 2000), 15–56. On I.G. Farben, see Gottfried Plumpe, *Die I.G. Farbenindustrie AG: Wirtschaft, Technik und Politik 1904–1945* (Berlin: Duncker & Humblot GmbH, 1990); and Peter Hayes, *Industry and Ideology: I.G. Farben in the Nazi Era* (Cambridge: Cambridge University Press, 1987).

2. "Aufgaben und Organisation der pharmazeutischen Abteilung 'Bayer-Meister Lucius' der I.G. Farbenindustrie Aktiengesellschaft," 2-vol. typescript, Verkaufszentrale, Leverkusen, 1930, BA, 166/3, vol. 1, pp. 2–4.

3. Ibid., vol. 2, 194–200.

4. Ibid., 201–202. The authors may have had in mind especially the contemporary developments in hormone or organotherapy and vitamins, which they later in the same report (p. 204) call "typical representatives for the practical use of ongoing theoretical work."

5. Ibid., 202. The exact arrangements denoted by the term *Aussendienst* need further definition. It appears to indicate a consulting arrangement between the company and individuals who are not its employees.

6. Ibid., 202–203. The report does not give details of any single step in the procedure. In particular, it does not make clear who conducted preliminary clinical trials, on whom they were conducted, or the nature of the relationship between the company and those who conducted clinical trials outside the company on its behalf. These questions require further investigation.

7. Ibid., 203–204.

8. Ibid., 378–427 (quotes on 426, 427).

9. Ibid., 431–432.

10. Curt Duisberg, "Heinrich Hörlein," typescript dated October 1955, paginated 18–34, BA, Personalia, H. Hörlein, 271/2, 18–19; Carl Duisberg, "Heinrich Hörlein zum 25 jahrigen Dienstjubiläum," *Medizin und Chemie* 2 (1934): 7–15 (quote on 11); Heinrich Hörlein, "Lebenslauf," statement prepared c. 1947 as part of testimony at Nuremburg trials, 9-pp. typescript, BA, Personalia, H. Hörlein, 271/2; and Fritz Mietzsch, "Zur Entwicklung der Pharmakotherapie in Deutschland: Heinrich Hörlein zum 70. Geburtstag," *AC* 64 (1952): 294–295.

11. Hörlein, "Lebenslauf " (note 10); Curt Duisberg, "Heinrich Hörlein" (note 10), 19–20.

12. Carl Duisberg, "Heinrich Hörlein" (note 10), 12–15; Heinrich Hörlein, "Nie ohne Forschung!," undated 5-pp. typescript, c. 1951, BA, Personalia, H. Hörlein, 271/2; "Gliederung der pharmazeutischen Abteilung 'Bayer-Meister Lucius,' " 1927, BA, 166/2, pp. 1, 25–29.

13. Hörlein, "Lebenslauf " (note 10); Curt Duisberg, "Heinrich Hörlein" (note 10), 20; career summary titled "Hörlein, Philipp Heinrich" (1959), BA, Personalia, H. Hörlein, 271/2. Hörlein thus exemplified the rise of degree-holding engineers to managerial positions

in German industry after 1900. See Jurgen Kocka, "The rise of the modern industrial enterprise in Germany," in Alfred D. Chandler, Jr., and Herman Daems, editors, *Managerial Hierarchies: Comparative Perspectives on the Modern Industrial Enterprise* (Cambridge, MA: Harvard University Press, 1980), 77–116, esp. 95.

14. Walther Wolff, "Besuch bei Heinrich Hörlein am 3 März 1930," BA, Personalia, H. Hörlein, 271/2 (my translation). The complete poem is in fifteen stanzas.

15. Hörlein, "Lebenslauf " (note 10), 2; career summary, "Hörlein, Philipp Heinrich" (note 13), 3.

16. Heinrich Hörlein, "Ueber die wissenschaftlichen Grundlagen der Arzneimittelsynthese," talk given to a gathering of Munich physicians in March 1927, *MMW* 74 (1927): 801–805 (my copy is a reprint paginated 1–15); Hörlein, "Medizin und Chemie," lecture given at the meeting of the Gesellschaft deutscher Naturforscher und Aertze, Wiesbaden, September 28, 1932, *Medizin und Chemie*, 1933 (my copy is a reprint paginated 1–19, in BA, Personalia, H. Hörlein, 271/2). For a full summary of these talks, see John E. Lesch, "Chemistry and biomedicine in an industrial setting: the invention of the sulfa drugs," in Seymour H. Mauskopf, editor, *Chemical Sciences in the Modern World* (Philadelphia, PA: University of Pennsylvania Press, 1993), 158–215.

17. On Edison, see Thomas P. Hughes, *Networks of Power: Electrification in Western Society 1880–1930* (Baltimore, MD: Johns Hopkins University Press, 1983), 18–46.

18. Ibid; and Thomas P. Hughes, "The evolution of large technological systems," in Wiebe E. Bijker, Thomas P. Hughes, and Trevor Pinch, editors, *The Social Construction of Technological Systems* (Cambridge, MA: The MIT Press, 1987), 51–83.

Chapter 3

1. Heinrich Hörlein, "Medizin und Chemie," lecture given at the meeting of the Gesellschaft deutscher Naturforscher und Aertze, Wiesbaden, September 28, 1932, *Medizin und Chemie*, 1933 (my copy is a reprint paginated 1–19, in BA, Personalia, H. Hörlein, 271/2), 10–11.

2. "60 Geburtstag, Direktor Professor Dr. ing. Dr. med. e.h. Fritz Mietzsch," stamped July 9, 1956, 4-pp. typescript, BA, Personalia, 271/2 (hereafter "Fritz Mietzsch"); "Wer ist's," *Der Chemiemarkt* (April 12, 1956). The following summary of Mietzsch's biography is based on these sources.

3. Joseph Klarer, "Lebenslauf," BA, Personalia, Klarer, Joseph 271/2.

4. "Nobelpreisträger und Inhaber des Ordens Pour le Mérite Prof. Dr. med. Dr. med. h.c. Dr. phil. h.c. Dr. med. vet. h.c. Gerhard Domagk," 8-pp. typescript, BA, Personalia, Domagk, 1938–31.12.1952, 271/2—this document, for which no author is named, is marked March 1959 (acceptable to Prof. Dr. Domagk) (p. 8); Leonard Colebrook, "Gerhard Domagk 1895–1964," *BMFRS* 10 (1964): 39–50; Ralph E. Oesper, "Gerhard Domagk and chemotherapy," *Journal of Chemical Education* 31 (1954): 188–191; Erich Posner, "Domagk, Gerhard," *Dictionary of Scientific Biography*, vol. 4 (New York: Charles Scribner's Sons, 1971), 153–156; Daniel Bovet, *Une chimie qui guérit: histoire de la découverte des sulfamides* (Paris: Éditions Payot, 1988), 137, 139.

5. "Nobelpreisträger . . . Gerhard Domagk" (note 4); Oesper, "Gerhard Domagk" (note 4), 188–189.

6. Gerhard Domagk, "Untersuchungen über die Bedeutung des retikuloendothelialen Systems für die Vernichtung von Infektionserregern und für die Entstehung des Amyloids," *Virchows Archiv für pathologische Anatomie und Physiologie und für Klinische Medizin* 235 (1924): 594–638; Bovet, *Une chimie qui guérit* (note 4), 138.

7. Posner, "Domagk" (note 4), 154; H. Weese, "Gerhard Domagk's wissenschaftliches Werk," BA, Personalia, Domagk, 1938–31.12.1952, 271/2, p. 1. Domagk's employment

was effective September 15, 1927. See H. Hörlein to G. Domagk, August 29, 1927, BA, file GD. File GD contains I.G. Farben/Bayer personnel records on Domagk from his hiring to the early 1950s.

8. Domagk refers to his "two-year furlough" from the university in a letter to Hörlein of June 10, 1928, BA, GD.

9. Document dated June 5, 1928 and signed by Hörlein, Bonhoeffer, and Domagk; G. Domagk to H. Hörlein, June 10, 1928; BA, GD.

10. Document dated July 31, 1928, and signed by Hörlein and Bonhoeffer, BA, GD.

11. Document of August 12, 1929, signed by Bonhoeffer and Hörlein, and by Domagk to indicate agreement, BA, GD.

12. See also chapter 4.

13. Weese, "Gerhard Domagk's wissenschaftliches Werk" (note 7), 1–2; "Nobelpreisträger . . . Gerhard Domagk" (note 4), 2–3; Bovet, *Une chimie qui guérit* (note 4), 138–139.

14. Gerhard Domagk, "Chemotherapie der bakteriellen Infektionen," *AC* 46 (1935): 657–667, quote on 657; Domagk, "Chemotherapie der Streptokokkeninfektionen," *KW* 15 (1936): 1585–1590, on 1585.

15. *From Germanin to Acylureidopenicillin* (Leverkusen, Germany: Bayer AG, 1980), 13, 21; Bovet, *Une chimie qui guérit* (note 4) 114, 140–141.

16. Domagk, "Chemotherapie der bakteriellen Infektionen" (note 14), 659; Domagk, "Ein Beitrag zur Chemotherapie der bakteriellen Infektionen," *DMW* 61 (1935): 250–253.

17. Domagk, "Chemotherapie der bakteriellen Infektionen" (note 14), 659; Bovet, *Une chimie qui guérit* (note 4), 105. In breaking with Wesenberg's practice, Domagk embraced a recognition of the need for animal experiment that had become fairly common in chemotherapeutic research by the 1920s.

18. Domagk, "Ein Beitrag" (note 16), 251; Domagk, "Chemotherapie der bakteriellen Infektionen" (note 16), 658–659.

19.Domagk, "Ein Beitrag" (note 16), 251; Domagk, "Chemotherapie der bakteriellen Infektionen" (note 16), 658–659; Bovet, *Une chimie qui guérit* (note 4), 106–107.

20. Domagk, "Ein Beitrag" (note 16), 250; Domagk, "Chemotherapie der bakteriellen Infektionen" (note 16), 660.

21. Hörlein, "Medizin und Chemie" (note 1); Fritz Mietzsch, "Entwicklungslinien der Chemotherapie (Vom chemischen Standpunkt gesehen)," *KW* 29 (1951): 125–134; Mietzsch, "Beiträge zur Entwicklung der Chemotherapie aus den Laboratorien der Farbenfabriken Bayer," *Arzneimittel-Forschung* (September 1956): 503–508; Mietzsch, "Neuere Entwicklung der synthetischen Chemotherapeutika," *Österreichische Chemiker-Zeitung* 53 (1952): 177–187.

22. Mietzsch, "Neuere Entwicklung" (note 21), 178; Mietzsch, "Entwicklungslinien" (note 21), 125–126, 127.

23. Mietzsch, "Beiträge" (note 21), 505–506; Mietzsch, "Entwicklungslinien" (note 21), 127.

24. Mietzsch, "Beiträge" (note 21), 505–506. Atabrine played a crucial role in World War II, after Allied supplies of quinine were cut off early in the war by the Japanese occupation of the Dutch East Indies. Its story, with that of other synthetic antimalarials, deserves a much fuller historical treatment than it has yet received.

25. Domagk, "Ein Beitrag" (note 16) 250; Mietzsch, "Entwicklungslinien" (note 21), 129; Mietzsch, "Beiträge" (note 21), 507; Bovet, *Une chimie qui guérit* (note 4), 106, 108–109.

26. Fritz Mietzsch, "Chemie und wirtschaftliche Bedeutung der Sulfonamide," *Arbeitsgemeinschaft für Forschung des Landes Nordrhein-Westfalen* 31 (1954): 7–32 (quote

on 10–11); Bovet, *Une chimie qui guérit* (note 4), 109; and John E. Lesch, "Chemistry and biomedicine in an industrial setting: the invention of the sulfa drugs," in Seymour H. Mauskopf, editor, *Chemical Sciences in the Modern World* (Philadelphia, PA: University of Pennsylvania Press, 1993), 158–215, on 198–200.

27. Bovet, *Une chimie qui guérit* (note 4), 109–110.

28. Ibid., 110.

29. Klarer, "Lebenslauf " (note 3), 2.

30. Mietzsch, "Chemie und wirtschaftliche Bedeutung der Sulfonamide" (note 26), 11–12; Mietzsch, "Entwicklungslinien" (note 21), 129.

31. Mietzsch, "Chemie und wirtschaftliche Bedeutung der Sulfonamide" (note 26), 11–12; Mietzsch, "Entwicklungslinien" (note 21), 129; Bovet, *Une chimie qui guérit* (note 4), 111.

32. Klarer, "Lebenslauf " (note 3), 2; Mietzsch, "Entwicklungslinien" (note 21), 129; Klarer, "Chemie und wirtschaftliche Bedeutung der Sulfonamide" (note 26), 12–13; Domagk, "Ein Beitrag" (note 16), 251; Bovet, *Une chimie qui guérit* (note 4), 111–112.

33. For the subsequent history of Prontosil, see chapters 4–6.

34. For Domagk's views, see Gerhard Domagk, "Weitere Untersuchungen über die chemotherapeutische Wirkung sulfonamidhaltiger Verbindungen bei bakterieller Infektionen," *KW* 16 (1937): 1412–1418; Domagk, "Ein Beitrag" (note 16); Domagk, "Chemotherapie der bakteriellen Infektionen" (note 14); Domagk, "Chemotherapie der Streptokokkeninfektionen" (note 14); and Lesch, "Chemistry and biomedicine in an industrial setting" (note 26), 177–193.

35. For Mietzsch's views on chemotherapy, see especially Fritz Mietzsch, "Neuere Entwicklung der synthetischen Chemotherapeutika," *Österreichische Chemiker-Zeitung* 53 (1952): 177–187; Mietzsch, "Entwicklungslinien" (note 21); Mietzsch, "Beiträge" (note 21); and Lesch, "Chemistry and biomedicine in an industrial setting" (note 26), 193–204.

36. Bovet, who tends to analyze the research from the chemists' point of view, credits Mietzsch with the initiative that led to Prontosil. See *Une chimie qui guérit* (note 4), 137–143.

37. Georg Meyer-Thurow, "The industrialization of invention: A case study from the German chemical industry," *Isis* 73 (1982): 363–381.

38. Scc chapter 1.

39. On Hugh Hampton Young and his institute, see chapter 1.

40. On Voegtlin's views, see chapter 1.

Chapter 4

1. Studies that address several of these questions include Michael H. Kater, *Doctors under Hitler* (Chapel Hill, NC: University of North Carolina Press, 1989); Robert N. Proctor, *Racial Hygiene: Medicine under the Nazis* (Cambridge, MA: Harvard University Press, 1988); and Proctor, *The Nazi War on Cancer* (Princeton, NJ: Princeton University Press, 1999).

2. "Tagesgeschichtliche Notizen," *MMW* 80 (1933): 204; "New regulations concerning vivisection," *JAMA* 101 (1933): 1087. On the nineteenth-century background to the German antivivisection movement, see Ulrich Tröhler and Andreas-Holger Maehle, "Antivivisection in nineteenth-century Germany and Switzerland: motives and methods," in Nicolaas A. Rupke, editor, *Vivisection in Historical Perspective* (London: Croom Helm, 1987), 149–187.

3. Heinrich Hörlein, "Lebenslauf," statement prepared as testimony at Nuremberg trials, 1947. BA, Personalia, H. Hörlein, 271/2, pp. 4–5; Peter Hayes, *Industry and Ideology:*

IG Farben in the Nazi Era (Cambridge: Cambridge University Press, 1987), 93. On the centrality of animal experiment in Hörlein's conception of medical research, see, e.g., Heinrich Hörlein, "Ueber die wissenschaftlichen Grundlagen der Arzneimittelsynthese," *MMW* 74 (1927): 801–805 (my copy is a reprint paginated 1–15); and chapter 2. On the relationship of I.G. Farbenindustrie to the Nazi regime, see Peter Hayes, *Industry and Ideology*; and Gottfried Plumpe, *Die I.G. Farbenindustrie AG: Wirtschaft, Technik und Politik 1904–1945* (Berlin: Duncker & Humblot GmbH, 1990).

4. Hayes, *Industry and Ideology* (note 3), 91–93.

5. "New regulations concerning vivisection" (note 2).

6. Hörlein, "Lebenslauf " (note 3), 5–6. On continuing links between I.G. Farben and the U.S. firms Sterling Products, Winthrop Chemical Co., and Vick Chemical Co., see, e.g., Hörlein 26/68, affidavit of Mrs. Irene Claasen Young, October 14, 1947, 3.II.48. The latter citation is to material offered in evidence at the trial of I.G. Farben executives at Nuremberg after World War II. It is part of the NA Collection of World War II War Crimes Records gathered in RG 238. The microfilm records of the I.G. Farben case, *United States of America v. Karl Krauch et al.* (case VI), August 14, 1947–July 30, 1948 (numbered M892 under RG 238) comprise 113 rolls. The 144 defense exhibits directly related to Hörlein are on roll 68. The form of citation of this material is as follows: name of defendant, document number/roll number, descriptive name of document with page numbers if needed, and date offered in evidence (day.month [Roman numeral].year). For a summary of the trial and its records, see *Records of the United States Nuernberg War Crimes Trials: United States of America v. Karl Krauch et al. (Case VI), August 14, 1947–July 30, 1948*, NA Microfilm Publications, Pamphlet Describing M892 (Washington, DC: National Archives Trust Fund Board, National Archives and Records Service, General Services Administration, 1977).

7. Hörlein 54/68, Dr. med. Eckhard, "Zur Vivisektionsfrage," *Tierrecht und Tierschutz*, Nr. 9, 1933, pp. 131–132, 30.I.48; and Hörlein 53/68, "Niederschrift der ausserordentlichen Hauptversammlung des 'Weltbundes zum Schutze der Tiere und gegen die Vivisektion,' " *Tierrecht und Tierschutz*, Nr. 9, 1933, p. 130, 30.I.48; Hörlein 52/68, "Was ist's mit dem Germanin'?" *Deutsche Volksgesundheit aus Blut und Boden!*, October 1933, 30.I.48.

8. Hörlein 54/68, Eckhard, "Zur Vivisektionsfrage" (note 7), pp. 131–132, 22.I.48; and Hörlein 53/68, "Niederschrift" (note 7), p. 130, 22.I.48.

9. Hörlein 54/68, "Niederschrift" (note 7), p. 130, 22.I.48.

10. Hörlein 54/68, Eckhard, "Zur Vivisektionsfrage" (note 7), pp. 131–132, 22.I.48; and Hörlein 53/68, "Niederschrift" (note 7), p. 130, 22.I.48.

11. "Temporary regulations for animal experimentation," *JAMA* 101 (1933): 1404; Hörlein 52/68, "Das preussische vivisektionsverbot vom 5. Sept. 1933," in excerpts from *Deutsche Volksgesundheit aus Blut und Boden!*, nos. 3–6, October–December 1933, 30.I.48.

12. Hörlein 52/68, "Das preussische Vivisektionsverbot vom 5. Sept. 1933," 30.I.48; Hörlein 16/68, affidavit of Dr. Clemens Giese, July 31, 1947, 30.I.48; Hayes, *Industry and Ideology* (note 3), 108–109.

13. Hörlein 52/68, "Was ist's mit dem 'Germanin'?" in excerpts from *Deutsche Volksgesundheit aus Blut und Boden!*, nos. 3–6, October–December 1933, 30.I.48.

14. Ibid. The cartoon last described is reproduced in Proctor, *Racial Hygiene* (note 1), opposite p. 228.

15. Hörlein 55/68, article headed "Schach den Massen-Tierversuchen bei der I.G. Farbenindustrie!" in *Der Deutsche Tierfreund* 4, no. 1, December 1933–January 1934, pp. 20–22, 30.I.48.

16. Ibid.

17. Hörlein, "Lebenslauf " (note 3), 6–7.

18. "The law pertaining to the protection of animals," *JAMA* 102 (1934): 551–552; "Experiments on animals," *JAMA* 103 (1934): 1005.

19. Hörlein 52/68, excerpts from *Deutsche Volksgesundheit aus Blut und Boden!*, 1935, 30.I.48.

20. Kater, *Doctors under Hitler* (note 1), 25, 119–120 (quote); Proctor, *Racial Hygiene* (note 1), 164–165, 223–250.

21. Kater, *Doctors under Hitler* (note 1), 111–126, 177–183; Proctor, *Racial Hygiene* (note 1), passim, esp. 162–166, 226–227. On blood purity and antisemitism, see also Jay Geller, "Blood sin: syphilis and the construction of Jewish identity," *Faultline* 1 (1992): 21–48.

22. Proctor, *Racial Hygiene* (note 1), 228.

23. On membership of the supervisory board in 1933, see Hayes, *Industry and Ideology* (note 3), 27–28. One Jewish staff member at Elberfeld was the chemist Erich Danziger. Danziger joined the company in 1916, eventually became head of the Analytical Department at Elberfeld, and left Germany in 1937 to join the Winthrop Chemical Co. in the United States. Hörlein 12/68, affidavit of Dr. Erich Danziger dated June 25, 1947, 30.I.48.

24. Curt Duisberg, "Heinrich Hörlein," BA, Personalia, H. Hörlein 271/2; Hörlein 30/68, affidavit of Adelheid Schulte dated October 27, 1947, 3.II.48; Daniel Bovet, *Une chimie qui guérit: histoire de la découverte des sulfamides* (Paris: Éditions Payot, 1988), 161–162; Hayes, *Industry and Ideology* (note 3), 102.

25. The German patent number was 607537. The patent was given for "processes for the production of azo compounds," and Fritz Mietzsch and Joseph Klarer were listed as the inventors. BA, Pharma (Prolongal-Proponal), 166/8. On early responses to Prontosil in France, Britain, and the United States, see chapter 6.

26. Jacques Tréfouël, Thérèse Tréfouël, Frédéric Nitti, and Daniel Bovet, "Activité du p. aminophenylsulfamide sur l'infection streptococcique expérimentale de la souris et du lapin," *Comptes Rendus de la Société de Biologie* 120 (November 23, 1935): 756; Harry F. Dowling, *Fighting Infection: Conquests of the Twentieth Century* (Cambridge, MA: Harvard University Press, 1977), 107–108. On Gelmo and his original publication, see Paul Gelmo, "Über Sulfamide der p-Amidobenzosulfonsäure," *Journal für praktische Chemie* 77 (1908): 369–382; and Waldemar Kaempffert, "News of Dr. Paul Gelmo, discoverer of sulfanilamide," *JHMAS* 5 (1950): 213–214. The Pasteur Institute work leading to recognition of sulfanilamide as the active constituent of Prontosil is discussed in Bovet, *Une chimie qui guérit* (note 24), 37–53, and is examined in chapter 6. Development of sulfanilamide derivatives in Germany is discussed below, and in other countries in chapters 7 and 8.

27. Ronald Hare, *The Birth of Penicillin and the Disarming of Microbes* (London: George Allen & Unwin Ltd., 1970), 145–161. Others' suspicions of I.G. Farben's motives and behavior on this point are cited by Bovet, *Une chimie qui guérit* (note 24), 135.

28. Hare, *The Birth of Penicillin* (note 27), 157–160. Hare mistakenly places the synthesis of the precursor of Prontosil in 1931. On the background and timing of its preparation, see chapter 3. I.G. Farben officially made known its intention to use Prontosil as trade name for Streptozon on September 26, 1934. BA, Pharma (Prolongal-Proponal) 166/8.

29. Bovet, *Une chimie qui guérit* (note 24), 132–133.

30. Ibid., 133–134.

31. Gerhard Domagk, "Jahresbericht 1934," submitted January 31, 1935, BA, Pathologisches Labor. 1934–1943, Betriebsberichte: Abt. für experimentelle Pathologie u. Bakteriologie, 103/11; Heinrich Hörlein, "The development of chemotherapy for bacterial diseases," paper read at the Chemistry Section of the British Association, Nottingham, September 2, 1937, *The Practitioner* 139 (1937): 635–649, on 637.

32. Domagk, "Jahresbericht 1934" (note 31), 1–29, 30–98, 100–128; personnel record in BA, Laboratorien, Pathologisches Laboratorium, Allgemeines, 103/11.

33. Philipp Klee and Herbert Römer, "Prontosil bei Streptokokkeninfektionen," *DMW* 61 (1935): 253–255; H.T. Schreus, "Chemotherapie des Erysipels und anderer Infektionen mit Prontosil," *DMW* 61 (1935): 255–256; Eugen Anselm, "Unsere Erfahrungen mit Prontosil bei Puerperalfieber," *DMW* 61 (1935): 264; and Kurt Fuge, "Die Behandlung der Puerperalsepsis mit Prontosil," *DMW* 61 (1935): 1672–1674. Schreus's assistant, Richard Foerster, had reported in May 1933 to a meeting of the Union of Dermatologists in Düsseldorf on the successful treatment of an infant with staphylococcal septicemia with Prontosil. See Bovet, *Une chimie qui guérit* (note 24), 117–118; and Schreus's paper described in text, 87–88.

34. Klee and Römer, "Prontosil bei Streptokokkeninfektionen" (note 33), 253–254.

35. Ibid., 254.

36. Ibid., 255.

37. Ibid.

38. Schreus, "Chemotherapie des Erysipels" (note 33), 255–256.

39. Ibid.

40. Anselm, "Prontosil bei Puerperalfieber" (note 33), 264 (emphasis original).

41. Fuge, "Die Behandlung der Puerperalsepsis mit Prontosil" (note 33), 1672–1674.

42. On I.G. Farben's expectations for the time required for clinical testing of a new medicine, see chapter 2 and "Aufgaben und Organisation der pharmazeutischen Abteilung 'Bayer-Meister Lucius' der I.G. Farbenindustrie Aktiengesellschaft," 2-vol. typescript, Verkaufszentrale, Leverkusen, 1930, BA, 166/3, vol. 1, 203. Bovet refers to an I.G. Farben internal document indicating that by 1934 the company knew enough of Streptozon (Prontosil) to say that it was tolerated by mouth or intravenously, that its principal indications were angina, puerperal fever, and erysipelas, and that it had failed in chronic streptococcal endocarditis. *Une chimie qui guérit* (note 24), 119.

43. Gerhard Domagk, "La chimiothérapie des maladies infectieuses par les azoiques sulfamidés," lecture delivered in German to the Société Francaises de Chimiothérapie et Sérologie, copy registered in BA July 3, 1961, BA, Personalia, Domagk 1938–31.12.1952, 271/2.

44. The compound in question, "the dye obtained from p-aminobenzene-sulfonamide," is described in Walter A. Jacobs and Michael Heidelberger, "Synthesis in the cinchona series. I-III," *Journal of the American Chemical Society* 41 (1919): 817–833, 2090–2120, 2131–2147 (on 2145). Hare, *The Birth of Penicillin*, 152, wrote that Heidelberger and Jacobs had shown that "sulfanilamide coupled with a derivative of quinine could kill microbes in the test tube. Although the chemotherapeutic potentialities of the compound were never tested, this suggested that sulfanilamide might have properties not hitherto suspected." This gives a prominence and significance to the substance that it did not have for Heidelberger and Jacobs. The compound containing p-aminobenzene sulfonamide—later called sulfanilamide—was only one of some forty azo-cinchona compounds prepared by the two chemists. The azo-cinchona compounds were only a part of their much larger study of cinchona alkaloids. And since their colleague Martha Wollstein's work on the biological activity of the compounds was never published, we do not even know if the sulfonamide-containing compound was among those found to have bactericidal action in vitro. Bovet, *Une chimie qui guérit*, 176, quotes Heidelberger as writing later that "the possibility that a substance as simple as sulfanilamide could cure bacterial infections never occurred to us." On the importance of analogical thinking in the research that led to Prontosol, see chapter 3.

45. On skepticism about bacterial chemotherapy, see chapter 1. On Hörlein's caution, see chapter 2 and Hörlein 18/68, affidavit of Dr. Helmut Weese, August 21, 1947, 3.II.48. Weese, who headed a pharmacological laboratory at Elberfeld from 1931, recalled that all compounds prepared by his unit and thought to be promising were carefully reviewed by Hörlein before being sent to Leverkusen for clinical testing. Weese was especially impressed by Hörlein's strong sense of responsibility and his commitment to a medical ethos although not himself a physician.

46. Gerhard Hecht, "Gesetzmässigkeiten in der Verteilung von Arzneimitteln und anderen Stoffen im Organismus" (lecture given September 18, 1934), *AC* 48 (1935): 14–17; Hecht, "Synthetische Farbstoffe und ihre Bedeutung in der medizinischbiologischen Forschung" (lecture given November 25, 1934), *AC* 48 (1935): 169–171. On sulfanilamide as fragment, see, e.g., Gerhard Domagk, "Chemotherapie der Streptokokkeninfektionen" *KW* 15 (1936): 1585–1590; and Domagk, "Weitere sulfonamidhaltiger Verbindungen bei bakteriellen Infektionen" *KW* 16 (1937): 1412–1418. For Domagk's reference to French and British authors, see his, "Weitere Untersuchungen über die chemotherapeutische Wirkung sulfonamidhaltiger Verbindungen bei bakterieller Infektionen," *KW* 16 (1937): 1412–1418, on 1418. Later, Mietzsch called for awarding of increased patent protection for known compounds for which pharmacological effects were subsequently discovered. Citing as prime example sulfanilamide, Mietzsch ventured that numerous such compounds already existed but that companies and other researchers lacked incentives to seek them out. Since Mietzsch did not say who had first recognized the action of sulfanilamide, the statement does not contribute to evaluation of the Hare thesis. It does show that after the fact the nonpatentability of sulfanilamide was seen by Mietzsch, who was by this time director of pharmaceutical research at Bayer, as one example of a general problem of patentability of compounds as pharmaceutical agents. Fritz Mietzsch, "Anwendungsschutz für pharmazeutische Produkte?" 6-pp. typescript in BA, Personalia, Meyer, Emil-Mittler, Oskar, 271/2. This item is not dated, but on internal evidence was probably written in 1952 or 1953.

Chapter 5

1. On the situation of German pharmaceutical patents and products in France in the 1930s, see Peter Hayes, *Industry and Ideology: IG Farben in the Nazi Era* (Cambridge: Cambridge University Press, 1987), 278–279. Heinrich Hörlein underlined the pharmaceutical industry's need of patent and trademark protection in "Arzneimittelfabriken und persönliche Behandlung," *Gesundheitslehre* (1929; my copy is an unpaginated reprint in BA, Personalia, H. Hörlein, 271/2), and complained of the fate of Prontosil in particular in "Mangelhafter Schutz deutschen geistigen Eigentums auf therapeutischen Gebiet," *DMW* 61 (1935): 1090.

2. Heinrich Hörlein, "Zur Chemotherapie der durch Protozoen und Bakterien bedingten Infektionskrankheiten" *Medizin und Chemie* 3 (1936; my copy is an offprint paginated 1–19, on 18–19).

3. Gerhard Domagk, "Weitere Untersuchungen über die chemotherapeutischen Wirkung sulfonamidhaltiger Verbindungen bei bakteriellen Infektionen," *KW* 16 (1937): 1412–1418; Domagk, "Die Sulfonamidtherapie bakterieller Infektionen," *Hoppe-Seyler's Zeitschrift für Physiologische Chemie* 274 (1942): 55–65, on 57–59.

4. Hörlein 22/68, affidavit of Dr. Werner Knauff, September 15, 1947, 3.II.48. Knauff worked in the I.G. Farben patent office from late 1934 to early 1943 and was responsible for preparing secret patent applications. On the form of citation used here and in subsequent notes, see chapter 4, note 6. On Hörlein's confrontation with a party official and on press attacks, see chapter 4.

5. Heinrich Hörlein, "Lebenslauf," statement prepared as testimony at Nuremberg trials, 1947. BA, Personalia, H. Hörlein, 271/2, p. 7; Hörlein 42/68, affidavit of Heinrich Hörlein, January 14, 1948, 2.II.48.

6. Hörlein 42/68, affidavit of Heinrich Hörlein, January 14, 1948, 2.II.48. Reference is made in the affidavit to Waldmann's letter as a separate document.

7. Heinrich Hörlein to Richard Kuhn, July 21, 1937, BA, file GD.

8. Joseph Klarer and Fritz Mietzsch, affidavit dated May 27, 1947, in BA, Personalia H. Hörlein, 271/2; Domagk, "Die Sulfonamidtherapie bakterieller Infektionen" (note 3), 58–59.

9. Klarer and Mietzsch, affidavit dated May 27, 1947; H. Löhe and R. Wawersig, "Vergleichende Untersuchungen über die Wirksamkeit der verschiedenen Diseptale bei der Behandlung der Gonorrhoe," DMW 66 (1940): 283–286; and Joseph Klarer, "Über die chemische Konstitution des Marfanil (Mesudin)," KW 20 (1941): 1250.

10. Personnel record, BA, Pathologisches Laboratorium, Allgemeines, 103/11; Gerhard Domagk, "Jahresbericht 1939," BA, Betriebsberichte: Abt. für experimentelle Pathologie u. Bakteriologie, 103/11; I.G. Farben press release, January 10, 1940, BA, Personalia, Domagk, 1938–31.12.1952, 271/2; Gerhard Domagk, "Der derzeitige Stand der Chemotherapie der bakteriellen Infektionen," Zeitschrift für Klinische Medizin 136 (1939): 167–199; Domagk, "Die Chemotherapie der bakteriellen Infektionen mit Prontosil und seinen Derivaten, unter besonderer Berücksichtigung der Grenzen dieser Therapie," Zentralblatt für Bakteriologie, Parasitenkunde und Infektionskrankheiten 144 (1939): 206–223. On sulfapyridine, see chapters 7 and 8.

11. Domagk, "Jahresbericht 1939" (note 10), 1–3.

12. Gerhard Domagk, "Jahresbericht 1942," dated January 1943, BA, Betriebsberichte: Abt. für experimentelle Pathologie und Bakteriologie, 103/11, pp. 1–20.

13. Domagk, "Jahresbericht 1942" (note 12), 21–27.

14. Gerhard Domagk to the management of I.G. Farbenindustrie, May 26, 1943, BA, file GD.

15. Gerhard Domagk, "Jahresbericht 1943," dated January 30, 1944, BA, Betriebsberichte: Abt. für experimentelle Pathologie und Bakteriologie, 103/11, part I, pp. 1–4.

16. Domagk, "Jahresbericht 1943" (note 15), part I, pp. 5–10, 45, 75–76, 77–91; part II, pp. 47, 54, 59.

17. Ibid., part II, pp. 1–34.

18. Ibid., pp. 44–46.

19. Domagk to management of I.G. Farbenindustrie, May 26, 1943; Gerhard Domagk, "Zehn Jahre Sulfamidotherapie," Deutsche Ärzblatt 73 (May 1943), 118; Gerhard Domagk, Joseph Klarer, and Fritz Mietzsch, "Noch einmal: Zehn Jahre Sulfamidotherapie," Deutsche Ärzblatt 73 (November 1943), 190. On the roles of Domagk, Klarer, and Mietzsch in the invention of Prontosil, see chapter 3. On credits and rewards for the sulfonamides, see chapter 12.

20. Daniel Bovet, Une chimie qui guérit: histoire de la découverte des sulfamides (Paris: Éditions Payot, 1988), 143–145; letter of P. Maré to Nobel Committee on Medicine, January 29, 1938, Nobel archives. On the context of this incident, see the Nobel Foundation, editor, Nobel: The Man and His Prizes (Stockholm: Sohlmans Förlag, 1950), 170–178; and Elisabeth Crawford, "German scientists and Hitler's vendetta against the Nobel Prizes," Historical Studies in the Physical and Biological Sciences 31, part 1 (2000): 37–53.

21. "Nobelpreis mit achtjähriger Verzögerung: nachträgliche Ehrung des Wupperthaler Professors Dr. Gerhard Domagk," Westdeutsche Rundschau, December 20, 1947; "Geschichte eines Nobelpreises: Gespräch mit Professor Gerhard Domagk," Die Neue Zeitung, December 19, 1947; Bovet, Une chimie qui guérit (note 20), 145.

22. Hörlein 109/68, affidavit of Dr. Gerhard Domagk, January 20, 1948, 3.II.48; "Geschichte eines Nobelpreises" (note 21); Bovet, *Une chimie qui guérit* (note 20), 145; G. Domagk to Gunnar Holmgren, November 3, 1939, Nobel archives (my translation).

23. "Nobelpreis war 'unerwunscht': warum Gerhard Domagk von der Gestapo verhaftet wurde," *Die Welt*, December 6, 1950; "Nobelpreis mit achtjähriger Verzögerung" (note 21); Hörlein 109/68, affidavit of Dr. Gerhard Domagk, January 20, 1948, 3.II.48; Bovet, *Une chimie qui guérit* (note 20), 146.

24. "Nobelpreis war enerwunscht" (note 23); "Nobelpreis mit achtjähriger Verzögerung" (note 21); G. Domagk to Caroline Institute, Stockholm, November 23, 1939, Nobel archives (my translation); Bovet, *Une chimie qui guérit* (note 20), 146–147.

25. "Geschichte eines Nobelpreises" (note 21).

26. Bovet, *Une chimie qui guérit* (note 20), 124.

27. *KW* 1935–1943. Bovet, citing lists prepared by I.G. Farben, gives the numbers of publications on Prontosil in the German-language medical press as about twenty in 1935, forty-seven in 1936, and thirty-three in 1937. *Une chimie qui guérit* (note 20), 121.

28. A. Roth, "Heilung eines Falles von Streptokokkensepsis unter Prontosilbehauptung," *DMW* 61 (1935): 1734; L. Gmelin, "Zur Chemotherapie des Erysipels im Kindesalter," *MMW* 82 (1935): 221–222.

29. Domagk, "Chemotherapie der Streptokokkeninfektionen," *KW* 15 (1936): 1585–1590, on 1588–1589.

30. Gerhard Domagk, "Grundlagen der modernen Chemotherapie der bakteriellen Infektionen," in Max Gundel, editor, *Die ansteckenden Krankheiten*, 2nd ed. (Leipzig: Georg Thieme Verlag, 1942), 667–691; and G. Säker, "Sulfamidwirkung auf die bakteriotoxische Entzündung," *KW* 20 (1941): 1121–1124. Säker was a physician at the *Allgemeinen Krankenhaus St Georg* in Hamburg. On Gundel's views in 1935, see chapter 1.

31. Gerhard Domagk, "Sulfonamidtherapie bakterieller Infektionen im Experiment und in der Praxis," *Deutsche Tierärztliche Wochenschrift* 50 (1942): 301–311 (Götze's introduction, p. 301); and three articles following Domagk's in the same volume: P. Henkels, "Über chirurgisch-klinische Ehrfahrungen mit einer Kombinierten Prontosil-Omnadin Therapie," 312–313; R. Völker, "Die Sulfonamide in der Kleintierpraxis," 313–314; and R. Götze, "Die Sulfonamide in der Buiatrik und in der Geburtshilfe," 314–316. For a panegyric of Koch as German hero, see Max Gundel, "Zur 25. Wiederkehr des Todestages von Robert Koch," *DMW* 61 (1935): 822. For a list of Domagk's publications in chronological order, see Leonard Colebrook, "Gerhard Domagk 1895–1964," *BMFRS* 10 (1964): 39–50, on 44–50.

32. Table of sales figures for 1940–1950, on Prontosil, Uliron, Conteben, Marfanil-Prontalbin (a combination product), and Marfanil, in BA, file GD; Hörlein, "Lebenslauf" (note 5), 7; Hörlein 42/68, affidavit of Heinrich Hörlein, January 14, 1948, 2.II.48.

33. Robert Proctor, *Racial Hygiene: Medicine under the Nazis* (Cambridge, MA: Harvard University Press, 1988), 76, 315–326. Proctor's remarks on the apolitical character of much of the German medical press are the more notable for their location in a study of the most heavily politicized area of German science and medicine: eugenics and racial hygiene.

34. Cortez F. Enloe, "The war and the German drug industry," *Chemical and Engineering News* 24 (1946): 3046–3048. Enloe served on an American intelligence team in Germany immediately after the war.

35. H. Hörlein and C. Lutter to Military Government, Wuppertal, May 16, 1945; letter of CIOS Team, Group 3, To Whom It May Concern, May 30, 1945; Lt. Col. Joseph W. Hensel to I.G. Farbenindustrie Aktiengesellschaft, May 24, 1945; Capt. John F. Sweeney to Production Control Agency, G-4 Division, SHAEF (Supreme Headquarters, Allied

Expeditionary Force), May 31, 1945; Major C.J. Wilson to Office of the Chief Surgeon, May 31, 1945. All items in BA, Elberfeld Allgemein 1866–1949, 7/B.1.

36. Hörlein 29/68, affidavit of Dr. Paul Loth, October 27, 1947, 3.II.48; *Records of the United States Nuernberg War Crimes Trials. United States of America v. Carl Krauch et al. (Case VI). August 14, 1947–July 30, 1948*, pamphlet describing National Archives RG 238, M 892 (Washington, DC: National Archives and Records Service, 1977), 1–8.

37. *Records of the United States Nuernberg War Crimes Trials. United States of America v. Carl Krauch et al. (Case VI)* (note 36), 1–2.

38. Hörlein 30/68, affidavit of Adelheid Schulte, October 27, 1947, 3.II.48; Hörlein 15/68, affidavit of Heinrich Rembold, July 24, 1947, 3.II.48.

39. Hörlein 57/68, affidavit of 32 employees of Bayer at Wuppertal-Elberfeld, January 13, 1948, 30.I.48; Hörlein 19/68, affidavit of twelve former antifascists, September 1, 1947, 30.I.48.

40. Hörlein 16/68, affidavit of Dr. Clemens Giese, July 31, 1947, 30.I.48.

41. Hörlein 26/68, affidavit of Mrs. Irene Claasen Young (U.S.), October 14, 1947, 3.II.48.

42. Hörlein 13/68, affidavit of Paul György, July 9, 1947, 30.I.48.

43. Hörlein 8/68, affidavit of Marcel Bô, June 27, 1947, 2.II.48. Another case was that of Fritz Kögl, a German physiological chemist whose work on plant hormones and cancer had been known to Hörlein since 1931. Hörlein, affidavit of Fritz Kögl, June 20, 1947, 2.II.48.

44. Hörlein 12/68, affidavit of Dr. Erich Danziger, June 25, 1947, 30.I.48; Hörlein 11/68, affidavit of Dr. S.J. Thannhauser, June 24, 1947, 30.I.48; Hörlein 41/68, affidavit of Dr. Gerhard Hecht, December 2, 1947, 30.I.48; Hörlein 110/68, affidavit of Dr. Ludwig Taub, October 29, 1947, 3.II.48. On Thannhauser's circumstances, see Frederic Lawrence Holmes, *Hans Krebs: Architect of Intermediary Metabolism 1933–1937*, vol. 2 (New York: Oxford University Press, 1993), 54–55, 68, 130–131.

45. Hörlein 4/68, affidavit of Benno Reifenberg, May 23, 1947, 3.II.48.

46. For Windaus's testimony, see Hörlein 5/68, affidavit of Dr. Adolf Windaus, May 27, 1947, 3.I.48. For that of Hahn, Wieland, and Butenandt, see below at note 49.

47. Hörlein 33/68, affidavit of Dr. Karl Freudenberg, November 6, 1947, 3.II.48. On Mentzel, see Kristie Macrakis, *Surviving the Swastika: Scientific Research in Nazi Germany* (New York: Oxford University Press, 1993), esp. 64, 78–80, 94–96.

48. Hörlein 7/68, affidavit of Dr. Otto Hahn, June 9, 1947, 30.I.48.

49. Hörlein 32/68, affidavit of Dr. Otto Hahn and Dr. Adolf Windaus, December 8, 1947, 30.I.48; Hörlein 37/68, affidavit of Dr. Heinrich Wieland, December 9, 1947, 30.I.48. Hörlein's efforts on behalf of science had been recognized during the war by the dedication to him of a volume of a leading German scientific journal. See *Hoppe-Seyler's Zeitschrift für physiologische Chemie* 274 (1942), dedication following title page.

50. Hörlein 10/68, affidavit of Adolf Butenandt, July 5, 1947, 30.I.48.

51. Ibid.

52. Ibid. On virus research at Berlin-Dahlem, see Macrakis, *Surviving the Swastika* (note 47), 118–120. For other examples of Hörlein's continuing commitment to basic research throughout the National Socialist period, see Hörlein 6/68, affidavit of Dr. Alfred Kühn, May 28, 1947, 30.I.48; and Hörlein 35/68, affidavit of Rudolf Höber, August 4, 1946, 30.I.48. Höber was chairman of the German Physiological Society in 1929 when Hörlein made available to the Society 10,000 marks to subsidize travel of younger German physiologists to the Nineteenth International Congress of Physiology in Boston. One of the beneficiaries of the 1929 travel grant was probably Hans Krebs (later a Nobel laureate for his work on the citric acid (Krebs) cycle), who received funds from the German Physiological

Society to attend the Boston Congress. Frederic Lawrence Holmes, *Hans Krebs: The Formation of a Scientific Life 1900–1933*, vol. 1 (New York: Oxford University Press, 1991), 202.

53. Hörlein 20/68, affidavit of Dr. Eberhard Gross, September 1, 1947, 3.II.48; Hörlein 29/68, affidavit of Dr. Paul Loth, October 27, 1947, 3.II.48.

54. Hörlein 18/68, affidavit of Dr. Helmut Weese, August 21, 1947, 3.II.48; Hörlein 28/68, affidavit of Dr. Helmut Thielicke, October 23, 1947, 3.II.48.

55. Curt Duisberg, "Heinrich Hörlein," typescript dated October 1955, paginated 18–34, BA, Personalia, H. Hörlein, 271/2, pp. 31–33.

56. Hörlein 74/68, affidavit of Dr. Karl Koenig, January 10, 1948, 3.II.48; Hörlein 79/68, affidavit of Dr. Karl Koenig, January 9, 1948, 3.II.48; Curt Duisberg, "Heinrich Hörlein" (note 55), 31–33. On Vetter, see also International Auschwitz Committee, *Nazi Medicine: Doctors, Victims, and Medicine in Auschwitz* (New York: Howard Fertig, 1986), 13–45, 201. On the importance of the typhus problem to the Nazi authorities and on the role of SS doctors in typhus experiments in the concentration camps, see Paul Weindling, "Medicine and the Holocaust: the case of typhus," in Ilana Löwy, editor, *Medicine and Change: Historical and Sociological Studies of Medical Innovation* (Montrouge, France: Éditions John Libbey Eurotext, 1993), 447–464.

57. Hörlein 74/68, affidavit of Dr. Karl Koenig, January 10, 1948, 3.II.48 (quote, p. 4); Hörlein 79/68, affidavit of Dr. Karl Koenig, January 9, 1948, 3.II.48; Hörlein 97/68, affidavit of Dr. Karl Koenig, December 11, 1947, 3.II.48; Hörlein 113/68, affidavit of Dr. Ludwig Heilmeyer, January 20, 1948, 3.II.48; Hörlein 108/68, affidavit of Dr. Karl Koenig and Dr. Otto Lücker, January 22, 1948, 3.II.48; Hörlein 94/68, affidavit of Dr. Karl Koenig, January 20, 1948, 3.II.48; Hörlein 150/68, report of Dr. Vetter, Auschwitz, December 8, 1943, 23.IV.48.; Hörlein 114/68, memo of Scientific Department, Pharma II, December 14, 1943, 23.IV.48; Hörlein 76/68, affidavit of Dr. Otto Lücker, January 9, 1948, 5.II.48; Curt Duisberg, "Heinrich Hörlein" (note 55), 33. For a statement by the Elberfeld research staff on the meaning of *Versuch*, see, e.g., Hörlein 40/68, affidavit by Drs. Domagk, Kikuth, and Weese, November 28, 1947, 3.II.48. On comparable cases of deliberate infection of concentration camp inmates at Buchenwald and Nutzweiler, see George J. Annas and Michael A. Grodin, editors, *The Nazi Doctors and the Nuremberg Code: Human Rights in Human Experimentation* (New York: Oxford University Press, 1992), 81–83. On the status of human subjects in American medical research prior to the Nuremberg Code of 1946, see Susan Lederer, *Subjected to Science: Human Experimentation in America before the Second World War* (Baltimore, MD: Johns Hopkins University Press, 1995).

58. Hayes, *Industry and Ideology* (note 1), 361–367; Joseph Borkin, *The Crime and Punishment of I.G. Farben* (New York: Free Press, 1978), 122–123; Curt Duisberg, "Heinrich Hörlein" (note 55), 30–31; Hörlein 43/68, affidavit of Heinrich Hörlein, January 10, 1948, 30.I.48, p. 8.

59. Hörlein 34/68, affidavit of Dr. Clemens Lutter, November 28, 1947, 3.II.48; Hörlein 49/68, copy of report in the *Pharmaceutical Journal*, August 1939, and letter from the editor to Heinrich Hörlein dated July 29, 1939, 30.I.48; Hörlein 43/68, affidavit of Heinrich Hörlein, January 10, 1948, 30.I.48, p. 6; Hörlein 31/68, affidavit of Otto Schoerger and Carl Lupp, November 3, 1947, 3.II.48; Curt Duisberg, "Heinrich Hörlein" (note 55), 27–28.

60. Curt Duisberg, "Heinrich Hörlein" (note 55), 28–29; Hörlein 64/68, affidavit of Eberhard Gross, n.d., 2.II.48; Hörlein 38/68, affidavit of Dr. Leopold von Sicherer, December 16, 1947, 2.II.48; and Borkin, *The Crime and Punishment of I.G. Farben* (note 58), 131–133.

61. Curt Duisberg, "Heinrich Hörlein" (note 55), 28–29; Hörlein 38/68, affidavit of Dr. Wolfgang Wirth, November 4, 1947, 2.II.48; Hörlein 64/68, affidavit of Eberhard Gross, n.d., 2.II.48; Hörlein, "Lebenslauf " (note 5), 7–9.

62. Hörlein 3/68, affidavit of Amandus Hoffman, May 27, 1947, 30.I.48. On Hitler's plans for destruction of German industry at the end of the war, see Albert Speer, *Inside the Third Reich* (New York: Macmillan Co., 1970), 475–480, 512–545.

63. Alan D. Beyerchen, *Scientists under Hitler: Politics and the Physics Community in the Third Reich* (New Haven, CT: Yale University Press, 1977), 69.

64. Ibid., 63–64; J.L. Heilbron, *The Dilemmas of an Upright Man: Max Planck as Spokesman for German Science* (Berkeley: University of California Press, 1986), esp. 149, 150, 152, 201 (quote).

65. Macrakis, *Surviving the Swastika* (note 47), esp. 6, 58–59, 110–130, 146, 199–205.

66. On the reception of the sulfa drugs by German physicians, see pages 85–90 and 104–108. On the continuity of the German medical press, see Proctor, *Racial Hygiene* (note 33), 74–79, 315–326. On the German medical profession, see Michael Kater, *Doctors under Hitler* (Chapel Hill, NC: University of North Carolina Press, 1989).

Chapter 6

1. Daniel Bovet, *Une chimie qui guérit: histoire de la découverte des sulfamides* (Paris: Éditions Payot, 1988), 51 n.1, 67–68, 75 n.1; Constantin Levaditi and Aron Vaisman, "Action curative et préventive du chlorhydrate de 4'-sulfamido-2,4-diaminobenzène dans l'infection streptococcique expérimentale," *Comptes Rendus de l'Académie des Sciences* 200 (1935): 1694. Bovet, *Une chimie qui guérit*, 75–76 n.1, gives several references to early French clinical reports. For a more extended listing, see G. Bickel, *La sulfamide et ses dérivés en therapeutique* (Lausanne: Payot, 1940). The section of this chapter covering France draws extensively on Bovet, *Une chimie qui guérit*, chapters 1–6.

2. Bovet, *Une chimie qui guérit* (note 1), 37, 60.

3. Ibid., 24–25.

4. Ibid., 25.

5. Ibid., 24–27

6. Ibid., 27.

7. Ibid.

8. Ibid., 15–16, 25–26, 57, 59. In 1935, the total budget of the Pasteur Institute was seven million francs, of which 600,000 went to the service of therapeutic chemistry, one of some thirty services in the institute. Of that amount, 250,000 francs, or forty-two percent, came from Rhône-Poulenc. See ibid., 23, 25–26.

9. Ibid., 37, 60. Bovet traces the friendship between Fourneau, Blaise, and Delépine to their student days, when all had been members of a group of young chemists called "the molecule." Their ties had continued during Fourneau's tenure as secretary of the Société chimique de France from 1919 to 1932.

10. Ibid., 17–19, 38–39.

11. Ibid., 39–40.

12. Ibid., 40–41.

13. Ibid., 42–43.

14. Ibid., 43–45.

15. J. and T. Tréfouël, F. Nitti, and D. Bovet, "Activité du p-aminophénylsulfamide sur l'infection streptococcique expérimentale de la souris et du lapin" *Comptes Rendus des Séances de la Société de Biologie* 120 (1935): 756; Bovet, *Une chimie qui guérit* (note 1), 45–47. On the early *Société de biologie*, see E. Gley, "La Société de Biologie et l'évolution des sciences biologiques en France de 1849 à 1900," in Gley, *Essais de philosophie et*

d'histoire de la biologie (Paris: Masson, 1900); and John E. Lesch, *Science and Medicine in France: The Emergence of Experimental Physiology, 1790–1855* (Cambridge, MA: Harvard University Press, 1984), 222–224.

16. Tréfouël et al., "Activité du p-aminophénylsulfamide" (note 15); Bovet, *Une chimie qui guérit* (note 1), 47.

17. See, e.g., Frederic Lawrence Holmes, *Hans Krebs: The Formation of a Scientific Life 1900–1933*, vol. 1 (New York: Oxford University Press, 1991); and Holmes, *Hans Krebs: Architect of Intermediary Metabolism, 1933–1937*, vol. 2 (New York: Oxford University Press, 1993).

18. On the Hare thesis, see chapter 4.

19. Bovet, *Une chimie qui guérit* (note 1), 30–32.

20. Ibid., 30–32.

21. Ibid., 68–69.

22. Ibid., 69.

23. Ibid., 79–81.

24. H.H. Dale to F.H.K. Green, March 18, 1935; L. Colebrook to Green, March 19, 1935. MRC file 1523/33, vol. 1.

25. Correspondence connected with Dale's January 1933 visit to Düsseldorf and Elberfeld is in RSL 93 HD, 73.6. The dates of Dale's talk and visit are in a letter of Dale to Professor U.G. Bijlsma, December 23, 1932, in this file. Dale's recollections of his visit to Elberfeld are in Dale to D.W. Adamson, August 6, 1962, RSL 93 HD, 35.21.14; and in a 7-pp. document Dale drew up on February 17, 1967, RSL 93 HD, 55.8.8. See also related correspondence between Dale and Landsborough Thomson, in RSL 93 HD, 47.5.151, and RSL 93 HD, 55.8.

26. On Dale's later claims, see the February 17, 1967, document, RSL 93 HD, 55.8.8. This document, written when Dale was ninety-two years of age and in a nursing home, is unreliable on at least some points of chronology. E.g., Dale has Colebrook testing both Prontosil and sulfanilamide in early 1935 and reporting his first positive results within three or four weeks. Neither assertion is correct. L. Colebrook to F.H.K. Green, March 19, 1935, and Green to Colebrook, March 20, 1935, MRC 1523/33, vol. 1.

27. A. Landsborough Thomson, *Half a Century of Medical Research*, vol. 2, *The Programme of the Medical Research Council (UK)* (London: Her Majesty's Stationary Office, 1975), 237–238. See also minutes of the first meeting of the TTC, July 8, 1931, MRC, MB 55. On similar suspicion of the pharmaceutical industry by American physicians, see John Parascandola, "The 'preposterous provision': the American Society for Pharmacology and Experimental Therapeutics' ban on industrial pharmacologists, 1908–1941," in Jonathan Liebenau, Gregory H. Higby, and Elaine C. Stroud, editors, *Pill Peddlers: Essays on the History of the Pharmaceutical Industry* (Madison, WI: American Institute of the History of Pharmacy, 1990), 29–47.

28. Correspondence in MRC 1523/33, vol. 1. Quotation is from T.R. Elliott to F.H.K. Green, May 8, 1935.

29. Correspondence in MRC 1523/33, vol. 1.

30. Ibid. On the company's concern to remain within the bounds of TTC procedure, see esp. H.F. Kotthof to F.H.K. Green, September 5, 1935.

31. Heinrich Hörlein, "The chemotherapy of infectious diseases caused by protozoa and bacteria," *PRSM* 29 (1936): 313–324; "Chemotherapy in streptococcal infections," *Lancet* 2 (1936): 840.

32. "Chemotherapy in streptococcal infections" (note 31).

33. A.H. Douthwaite to F.H.K. Green, October 4, 1935; Green to Douthwaite, October 11, 1935; and Green to Colebrook, October 17, 1935. MRC 1523/33, vol. 1.

34. L. Colebrook to F.H.K. Green, October 18, 1935; C.H. Browning to Green, October 28, 1935; Green to H.H. Dale, October 30, 1935. For an example of Green's warnings to physicians, see Dale to J.A. Cruickshank, October 28, 1935; Dale to Green, October 28, 1935; and Green memo of meeting with J.A. Cruickshank, November 4, 1935. All correspondence in MRC 1523/33, vol. 1.

35. L. Colebrook to F.H.K. Green, November 20, 1935; Green memo of visit by Colebrook, November 20, 1935. MRC 1523/33, vol. 1.

36. F.H.K. Green to C.H. Browning, January 8, 1936; Green to L. Colebrook, January 8, 1936; Colebrook to Green, January 9, 1936. For an example of Green's more upbeat tone, see John Gibbens to Green, December 10, 1935; Green to Gibbens, December 11, 1935. All correspondence in MRC 1523/33, vol. 1.

37. L. Colebrook to F.H.K. Green, February 3, 1936; Green to H.H. Dale, February 4, 1936; Dale to Green, February 6, 1936. MRC 1523/33, vol. 1.

38. *Lancet* 1 (1936): 269–270; Hörlein, "The chemotherapy of infectious diseases" (note 31).

39. T.W.P. Thompson to F.H.K. Green, February 24, 1936, with handwritten memo by Green. MRC 1523/33, vol. 1.

40. L. Colebrook to F.H.K. Green, February 27, 1936; Green to Colebrook, March 3, 1936. MRC 1523/33, vol. 1; minutes of TTC meeting of February 28, 1936. MRC Minute Book MB 55.

41. F.W. Eurich to F.H.K. Green, March 3, 1936. MRC 1523/33, vol. 1.

42. F.H.K. Green memo of conversation with T.W.P. Thompson, March 7, 1936. MRC 1523/33, vol. 1.

43. F.H.K. Green to C.H. Browning, March 16, 1936; Browning to Green, March 23, 1936; Green to W.R. Snodgrass, March 30, 1936; Green to A.W.M. Ellis, March 19, 1936; Green to J.W.P. Thompson, March 24, 1936; Green to Sir David Wilkie, March 21, 1936; Wilkie to Green, March 24, 1936; E. M[ellanby] to J.H. Brincker, March 21, 1936; Brincker to Mellanby, March 30, 1936; Brincker to Green, April 1, 1936. MRC 1523/33, vol. 1. W.J. Coughlan and C.R.M. Greenfield, "Prontosil treatment in scarlet fever and measles" 3-pp. typescript, undated, MRC 1523/33, vol. 2.

44. Bayer Products application dated March 16, 1936, in MRC 1523/33, vol. 1. J.W.P. Thompson to F.H.K. Green, April 3, 1936; Green to Thompson, April 4, 1936. MRC 1523/33, vol. 2.

45. J.W.P. Thompson to F.H.K. Green, March 26, 1936; MRC 1523/33, vol. 1. Bayer Products leaflet, and Thompson to Green April 3, 1936, April 8, 1936, and April 21, 1936; A.F. Cameron to Green, April 6, 1936; Green to Thompson, April 7, 1936. MRC 1523/33, vol. 2.

46. L. Colebrook to F.H.K. Green, April 7, 1936; Green memo dated May 15, 1936. MRC 1523/33, vol. 2. On Colebrook's cooperation with Buttle, see G.A.H. Buttle, W.H. Gray, and Dora Stephenson, "Protection of mice against streptococcal and other infections by p-aminobenzenesulphonamide and related substances," *Lancet* 1 (1936): 1286–1290.

47. H.H. Dale to F.H.K. Green, May 21, 1936; T.R. Elliott to Green, May 25, 1936; L. Green to Colebrook, May 26, 1936. MRC 1523/33, vol. 2. Leonard Colebrook and Meave Kenny, "Treatment of human puerperal infections, and of experimental infections in mice with Prontosil," *Lancet* 1 (1936): 1279–1286.

48. Colebrook and Kenny, "Treatment of human puerperal infections" (note 47), 1279.

49. Ibid., 1279–1280.

50. Ibid., 1280.

51. Ibid., 1281–1283. On mode of action theories, see chapter 11.

52. Ibid., 1282–1284.

53. Ibid., 1284.
54. Ibid., 1282, 1284.
55. Ibid., 1284–1285.
56. Ibid., 1285.
57. Buttle et al., "Protection of mice" (note 46).
58. Ibid., 1287–1288.
59. Ibid., 1289–1290.
60. "The chemotherapy of streptococcal infections," *Lancet* 1 (1936): 1303–1304.
61. "Childbed fever: good results of a new drug," *The Times*, June 6, 1936.
62. Report on meeting of the Section of Public Medicine, British Medical Association, in *Lancet* 1 (1936): 432–433; report on meeting of the Section of Obstetrics, Royal Academy of Medicine in Ireland, October 16, 1936, in *Lancet* 2 (1936): 1273–1274.
63. F.H.K. Green to W.R. Snodgrass, June 5, 1936; Snodgrass to Green, June 8, 1936, July 8, 1936, and September 28, 1936. All letters in MRC 1523/33, vol. 2.
64. J.S. Anderson, "The use of 'Prontosil' in certain acute infections," 13-pp. typescript, dated July 18, 1936; J.S. Anderson to F.H.K. Green, July 18, 1936; E. Mellanby to Green, July 22, 1936; J.H. Brincker to Mellanby, July 29, 1936; Mellanby to Green, October 8, 1936; J.S. Anderson to Green, October 30, 1936; Green to Anderson, November 2, 1936. MRC 1523/33, vol. 2.
65. L. Colebrook to F.H.K. Green, July 8, 1936; Green to Colebrook, July 11, 1936; Green to J.W.P. Thompson, July 11, 1936; Thompson to Green, July 18, 1936. MRC 1523/33, vol. 2.
66. L. Colebrook to F.H.K. Green, July 8, 1936; Green to W.R. Snodgrass, October 21, 1936; MRC 1523/33, vol. 2. "Editorial," *Clinical Excerpts* 2 (1936), 165–167.
67. F.H.K. Green to W.R. Snodgrass, October 28, 1936; Green to J.S. Anderson, November 2, 1936; Ripley Oddie to Green, November 9, 1936; Green to Oddie, November 12, 1936; Oddie to Green, November 16, 1936. MRC 1523/33, vol. 2.
68. Leonard Colebrook and Meave Kenny, "Treatment with Prontosil of puerperal infections due to hemolytic streptococci," *Lancet* 2 (1936): 1319–1322.
69. Ibid., 1320–1321.
70. Ibid., 1321, 1322.
71. Leonard Colebrook, G.A.H. Buttle, and R.A.Q. O'Meara, "The mode of action of p-aminobenzenesulphonamide and Prontosil in haemolytic streptococcal infections," *Lancet* 2 (1936): 1323–1326.
72. Ibid.; A.T. Fuller, "Is p-aminobenzenesulphonamide the active agent in Prontosil therapy?" *Lancet* 1 (1937): 194–198.
73. "Chemotherapy of streptococcal infections" (editorial), *Lancet* 2 (1936): 1339; *Clinical Excerpts* 11 (12) (December 1936): 233.
74. "Treatment of puerperal infections," and "Protection against experimental infections," *JAMA* 107 (September 12, 1936): 914; Waldemar Kaempffert, "New control for infections: the chemical given to F.D. Roosevelt, Jr. for streptococcus hailed as important discovery," *New York Times*, December 20, 1936; "Prontosil," *Time*, December 28, 1936.
75. Arthur B. Musgrave, "Medical science conquers a foe," *Baltimore Sun*, June 6, 1937; "International Society of Microbiologists," *JAMA* 107 (1936): 723; "International Congress of Microbiology," *JAMA* 107 (1936): 976; "E.K. Marshall, Jr.'s assessment of his own scientific work," 6-pp. typescript in E.K. Marshall biographical file, AMCMA; and Perrin H. Long and Eleanor A. Bliss, "Para-amino-benzene-sulfonamide and its derivatives: experimental and clinical observations on their use in the treatment of beta-hemolytic streptococcal infection: a preliminary report," *JAMA* 108 (1937): 32–37.

76. Long and Bliss, "Para-amino-benzene-sulfonamide and its derivatives" (note 75), quotes on 36, 37; "Chemotherapy in streptococcal infections" (editorial), *JAMA* 108 (1937): 48.

77. John E. Dees and J.A.C. Colston, "The use of sulfanilamide in gonococcic infections," *JAMA* 108 (1937): 1855–1858; E.K. Marshall, Jr., Kendall Emerson, and W.C. Cutting, "Para-aminobenzenesulfonamide: absorption and excretion: method of determination in urine and blood," *JAMA* 108 (1937): 953–957. Other studies appearing in the first half of 1937 included Francis F. Schwentker, Sidney Gelman, and Perrin H. Long, "The treatment of meningococcic meningitis with sulfanilamide: a preliminary report," *JAMA* 108 (1937): 1407–1408; Edward Dyer Anderson, "Hemolytic streptococcus meningitis: a report of case with recovery after the use of Prontosil and sulfanilamide," *JAMA* 108 (1937): 1591–1592; and Ralph R. Mellon, Paul Gross, and Frank B. Cooper, "Experimental studies with sulfanilamide and with Prontosil in hemolytic streptococcus infections," *JAMA* 108 (1937): 1858–1861.

78. " 'Sulfanilamide' (the council name for para-aminobenzenesulfonamide)," *JAMA* 108 (1937): 1340. I have not yet located an earlier use of the term outside the United States.

79. "Report of the council: sulfanilamide and related compounds," *JAMA* 108 (1937): 1888–1890.

80. Jane Stafford, "Prontosil," *Science* 85 (suppl., 1937): 9–10.

81. "Prontosil," *Time*, December 28, 1936, p. 21; J.D. Ratcliff, "Magic dye," *Colliers*, April 3, 1937, pp. 62, 79–80.

82. Arthur B. Musgrave, "Medical science conquers a foe," *Baltimore Sun*, June 6, 1937.

83. On the U.S. connections, see John P. Swann, *American Scientists and the Pharmaceutical Industry: Cooperative Research in Twentieth-Century America* (Baltimore, MD: Johns Hopkins University Press, 1988).

84. Hörlein 66/68, German translation of lecture by Ernest Fourneau, "Über die Industrie der pharmazeutischen Produkte und über die Mittel, ihre Entwicklung in Frankreich sicherzustellen," April 17, 1915, 2.II.48. I have not yet been able to consult the French original, which is in *Bulletin des sciences pharmacologiques* 22 (1915): 129–159. Heinrich Hörlein, "Mangelhafter Schutz deutschen geistigen Eigentums auf therapeutischen Gebiet," *DMW*, Nr. 27 (1935): 1090; and Peter Hayes, *Industry and Ideology: I.G. Farben in the Nazi Era* (Cambridge: Cambridge University Press, 1987), 278–279.

85. On the negative climate of opinion among some American physicians regarding German research in 1935, see Walsh McDermott, "The story of INH," *Journal of Infectious Diseases* 119 (1969): 678–685, on 682–683. These comparisons are based on examination of best practice by leading medical researchers and do not address the apparently wide variations in the way new medicines were evaluated within each country.

86. On the lingering effects of the failure of mercurachrome, see, e.g., Wesley W. Spink, *Infectious Diseases: Prevention and Treatment in the Nineteenth and Twentieth Centuries* (Minneapolis: University of Minnesota Press, 1978), 81–82.

Chapter 7

1. Martin Gilbert, *Road to Victory: Winston S. Churchill 1941–1945* (London: Heinemann, 1986), 603–604; Richard Lovell, *Churchill's Doctor: A Biography of Lord Moran* (London: Royal Society of Medicine, 1992), 228–235.

2. Gilbert, *Road to Victory* (note 1), 603–654; Lovell, *Churchill's Doctor* (note 1), 228–235.

318   NOTES TO PAGES 159–163

3. See, e.g., "Mr. Churchill's own bulletin," *Yorkshire Post*, December 30, 1943; "Premier off to convalescence," *East Anglian Times*, December 30, 1943; and "Premier goes to convalescence: 'destination unknown'," *Newcastle Journal*, December 30, 1943.

4. Montague A. Phillips, a chemist who had contributed to the development of M&B 693, guessed that Churchill had been treated with M&B 760 (*Northern Daily Telegraph*, December 30, 1943). So did the writer of an unsigned article in the *Wolverhampton Express & Star* for December 30, 1943. On Pulvertaft and penicillin, see *News Chronicle*, December 17, 1943. Examples of the more representative focus on M&B 693 are "New drugs can defeat pneumonia," *News Chronicle*, December 17, 1943; and "M&B Churchill version," *Norwich Eastern Daily Press*, December 30, 1943.

5. For surveys of the history of the sulfonamides, see Daniel Bovet, *Une chimie qui guérit: histoire de la découverte des sulfamides* (Paris: Éditions Payot, 1988); and Marcel H. Bickel, "The development of sulfonamides (1932–1938) as a focal point in the history of chemotherapy," *Gesnerus* 45 (1988): 67–86.

6. Ronald D. Mann, *Modern Drug Use: An Enquiry on Historical Principles* (Boston, MA: MTP Press Ltd., 1984), 556–557; Bickel, "The development of sulfonamides" (note 5), 75–76; Elmore H. Northey, *The Sulfonamides and Allied Compounds* (New York: Reinhold Publishing Corp., 1948), v. On the sulfas in World War II, see chapters 9 and 10.

7. H.E. Ungerleider, H.W. Steinhaus, and R.S. Gubner, "Public health and economic aspects of pneumonia: a comparison with pre-sulfonamide years," *American Journal of Public Health* 33 (1943): 1093–1102.

8. Bovet, *Une chimie qui guérit* (note 5), 167–201; see also chapter 6.

9. M&B Test Register, compound nos. 1–606, and M&B Test Register, compound nos. 607–1358, MB. Prontosil was entered as compound 576 on January 17, 1936. See also H.J. Barber, "Antibacterial dawn and antiprotozoal noon," in Barber, *Historical Aspects of Chemotherapy: Six Essays* (Dagenham: May & Baker Ltd., 1976), 24–32. On the research establishment at May & Baker, see Judy Slinn, *A History of May & Baker 1834–1984* (Cambridge: Hobsons Ltd., 1984), esp. 95–126.

10. Henry H. Dale, "Arthur James Ewins, 1882–1958," *BMFRS* 4 (1958): 81–91; H.J. Barber, "Obituary: Dr. A.J. Ewins, F.R.S.," *Chemistry and Industry* (February 22, 1958): 224–225. Dale errs on the year of death, since Barker reports Ewins's date of death as December 24, 1957.

11. Dale, "Arthur James Ewins" (note 10), 86–87; Barker, "Dr. A.J. Ewins" (note 10), 224; Slinn, *A History of May & Baker* (note 9), 91–94.

12. Dale, "Arthur James Ewins" (note 10), 87–88; Barker, "Dr. A.J. Ewins" (note 10), 224.

13. Dale, "Arthur James Ewins" (note 10), 88–90; Barker, "Dr. A.J. Ewins" (note 10), 224–225.

14. On Rhône-Poulenc's ownership of May & Baker, and on Grillet's influence, see Slinn, *A History of May & Baker* (note 9), 95–99, 113, 121; and Fred Aftalion, *A History of the International Chemical Industry*, translated by Otto Theodor Benfey (Philadelphia, PA: University of Pennsylvania Press, 1991), 196. The argument for a division of labor is made by Jean-Pierre Billon, "La découverte des sulfamides: implication et contribution de l'industrie" (Paris-La Défense: Rhône-Poulenc Santé, n.d.), 11 pp. and 4 tables, MB. On the chemical possibilities as perceived at the time, see Barber, "Antibacterial dawn" (note 9), 27.

15. Bovet, *Une chimie qui guérit* (note 1), 205.

16. G.A.H. Buttle, W.H. Gary, and Dora Stephenson, "Protection of mice against streptococcal and other infections by p-aminobenzenesulphonamide and related substances," *Lancet* 1 (1936): 1286–1290; A.J. Ewins, "British achievements in sulphonamide

research and production," *Pharmaceutical Journal* (April 28, 1951): 312–314. On the work of Buttle and his colleagues, see chapter 6.

17. "Transcription of a tape recording made at a meeting on the discovery of M&B 693 held 2.6.61," file 270, MB, pp. 5–6, 8. Present at this meeting were H.J. Barber, L.E. Hart, E.J. Baines, and a Mrs. Wragg. Barber, Hart, and Baines, all of whom had worked in May & Baker's pharmaceutical research division, were attempting to reconstruct the discovery of M&B 693 for an exhibition then being planned at the Science Museum in London. In one of the cited passages, Hart was drawing upon memories of another colleague, F.W. Bampton.

18. M&B Test Register, compound nos. 1–606, and M&B Test Register, compound nos. 607–1358; "Transcription" (note 17), 8–11.

19. "Sir Lionel Whitby" (obituary), *BMJ* (December 1, 1956): 1306–1309; "Lionel Ernest Howard Whitby" (obituary), *Lancet* (December 1, 1956): 1165–1167.

20. "Sir Lionel Whitby" (note 19); "Lionel Ernest Howard Whitby" (note 19).

21. "Sir Lionel Whitby" (note 19); "Lionel Ernest Howard Whitby" (note 19).

22. "Transcription" (note 17), 4–13 (quotes on 4, 5).

23. Ibid., 11–13; and M&B Test Register, compounds nos. 607–1358.

24. R.F.B. Welford, personal communication, February 21, 1994; J.F. Hodgson, personal communication, February 11, 1994; M&B Test Register, compound nos. 607–1358; Lionel E.H. Whitby, "Chemotherapy of pneumococcal and other infections with 2-(p-aminobenzenesulphonamide) pyridine," *Lancet* (May 28, 1938): 1210–1212.

25. R. Wien to A.J. Ewins, December 3, 1937, and A.J. Ewins to R. Wien, December 28, 1937, both in file 269, MB; "Transcription" (note 17), 14; M.A.F. Lake, "25 years of sulfapyridine," nonpaginated reprint from *Chemist and Druggist*, October 26, 1963.

26. "Transcription" (note 17), 14.

27. R.F.B. Welford, personal communication, February 21, 1994.

28. Ibid.; M.A.F. Lake, "25 years of sulfapyridine" (note 25).

29. R.F.B. Welford, personal communication, February 21, 1994; J.F. Hodgson, personal communication, February 11, 1994.

30. R.F.B. Welford, personal communication, February 21, 1994.

31. Ibid.

32. Ibid.; J.F. Hodgson, personal communication, February 11, 1994.

33. J.F. Hodgson, personal communication, February 11, 1994.

34. G.M. Evans and Wilfrid F. Gaisford, "Treatment of pneumonia with 2-(p-aminobenzenesulphonamide) pyridine," *Lancet* (July 2, 1938): 14–19.

35. Whitby, "Chemotherapy of pneumococcal and other infections" (note 24), 1212.

36. Evans and Gaisford, "Treatment of pneumonia" (note 34).

37. A.J. Ewins to R. Wien, January 5, 1939 [letter is dated 5th January 1938 but internal evidence clearly indicates that the year is 1939], file 269, MB; Merck & Co. Inc., Report to Stockholders, 1939; Slinn, *A History of May & Baker* (note 9), 124; R.F.B. Welford, personal communication, February 21, 1994.

38. Harry F. Dowling, *Fighting Infection: Conquests of the Twentieth Century* (Cambridge, MA: Harvard University Press, 1977), 45.

39. Ibid., 34–35; Rufus Cole, "The treatment of pneumonia," *AIM* 10 (1936): 1–12, on 5–6.

40. Dowling, *Fighting Infection* (note 38), 47–48.

41. Ibid., 47–49 (quote on 47); Harry F. Dowling, "Frustration and foundation: management of pneumonia before antibiotics," *JAMA* 220 (June 5, 1972): 1341–1345; Harry M. Marks, *The Progress of Experiment: Science and Therapeutic Reform in the United States, 1900–1990* (Cambridge: Cambridge University Press, 1997), 60. On the early

development of serum therapy and passive immunization, see Carola Throm, *Das Diphtherieserum. Ein neues Therapieprinzip, seine Entwicklung und Markteinführung* (Stuttgart: Wissenschaftliche Verlagsgesellschaft, 1995).

42. Dowling, *Fighting Infection* (note 38), 48–49; Dowling, "Frustration and foundation" (note 41), 1342; Marks, *Progress of Experiment* (note 41), 60–62; Daniel T. Davies, H. Graham Hodgson, and Lionel E.H. Whitby, "A study of pneumococcal pneumonia," *Lancet* (April 6, 1935): 791–796, 849–853, 919–924; Benjamin White, *The Biology of Pneumococcus: The Bacteriological, Biochemical, and Immunological Characters and Activities of Diplococcus Pneumoniae* (New York: Commonwealth Fund, 1938), 598–612.

43. Lewis Thomas, *The Youngest Science: Notes of a Medicine Watcher* (New York: Viking Press, 1983), 41–44 (quote on 44); Dowling, "Frustration and foundation" (note 41), 1342–1344. On early cooperative studies of serum treatment in pneumonia, see Marks, *Progress of Experiment* (note 41), 62–70, and below. For a more extensive analysis of antipneumococcal serums in the United States before and after the introduction of the sulfa drugs, see Scott Podolsky, *Pneumonia Before Antibiotics: Therapeutic Evolution and Evaluation in Twentieth-Century America* (Baltimore: Johns Hopkins University Press, forthcoming). On Britain, see Michael Worboys, "Treatments for pneumonia in Britain, 1910–1940," in Ilana Löwy, editor, *Medicine and Change: Historical and Sociological Studies of Medical Innovation* (Montrouge, France: Éditions John Libbey Eurotext, 1993), 317–336.

44. Cole, "The treatment of pneumonia" (note 39), 5–6; White, *The Biology of Pneumococcus* (note 42), 507–521.

45. Cole, "The treatment of pneumonia" (note 39), 6–12.

46. Ibid., 12; White, *The Biology of Pneumococcus* (note 42), 520–521.

47. "Chemotherapy in gonorrhea" (editorial), *BMJ* (August 6, 1938): 294–295; G.L.M. McElligott and A.J. Cokkinis, "Sulphonamide chemotherapy in gonorrhea," *BMJ* (August 20, 1938): 424; R.C.L. Batchelor, Robert Lees, Marjorie Murrell, and G.I.H. Braine, "2-Sulphanilyl-aminopyridine (M&B 693) in treatment of gonorrhea," *BMJ* (December 3, 1938): 1142–1145; and F.J.T. Bowie, T.E. Anderson, A. Dawson, and J.F. Mackay, "Treatment of gonorrhea by M&B 693," *BMJ* (April 8, 1939): 711–716. Two samples of press reports are "Pneumonia robbed of its terror-experiments with a wonderful new drug," *News of the World*, June 19, 1938; and "New drug cures dread disease—Wolverhampton girl's recovery—'dramatic response'," *Morning Advertiser*, September 9, 1938. For further discussion of the public reception of M&B 693 in Britain, see chapter 8.

48. W.S. Roche and C.J. McSweeney, "Treatment of cerebrospinal meningitis: a review of 103 cases," *BMJ* (June 24, 1939): 1278–1281; Wilfrid F. Gaisford, "Results of the treatment of 400 cases of lobar pneumonia with M&B 693," in "Discussion of recent advances in the treatment of pneumonia" (March 28, 1939), *PRSM* (section of medicine) 32 (1939): 1063–1076, on 1070–1075.

49. "Chemotherapy in gonorrhea" (note 47). See also W.R. Thrower, "Complications of chemotherapy" (letter), *BMJ* (September 10, 1938): 591–592.

50. Lionel E.H. Whitby, "Chemotherapy of bacterial infections," *Lancet* (November 12, 1938): 1095–1103, on 1096, 1098, 1100.

51. "Discussion of recent advances" (note 48), 1076; and "Recent advances in the treatment of pneumonia," *BMJ* (April 8, 1939): 741–743.

52. "Recent advances in the treatment of pneumonia" (note 51), 742–743.

53. Bowie et al., "Treatment of gonorrhea" (note 47), 715.

54. "Discussion of recent advances" (note 48), 1067–1075; Roche and McSweeney, "Treatment of cerebrospinal meningitis" (note 48), 1278–1281.

55. "Discussion of recent advances" (note 48), 1075–1076; Whitby, "Chemotherapy of bacterial infections" (note 50), 1096, 1100; R.C.L. Batchelor, Robert Lees, Marjorie

Murrell, and G.I.H. Braines, "2-Sulphanilyl-aminopyridine (M&B 693) in treatment of gonorrhoea," *BMJ* (December 3, 1938): 1142–1145; Bowie et al., "Treatment of gonorrhoea" (note 47), 714–715.

56. " 'Sulfapyridine' " (editorial), *BMJ* (March 25, 1939): 623–624. Therapeutic Trials Committee, meeting of March 28, 1939, Medical Research Council Minute Book, MB 55.

57. A.J. Ewins to R. Wien, January 5, 1939, February 14, 1939, and March 7, 1939. MB, file 269; "Discussion of recent advances" (note 48), 1063–1067.

58. A.J. Ewins, "Toxicity of M&B 693" (letter), *BMJ* (April 8, 1939): 749–750.

59. Paul Gross and Frank B. Cooper, "Toxicity of M&B 693" (letter), *BMJ* (May 20, 1939): 1058.

60. Marks, *The Progress of Experiment* (note 41), chapters 1–3.

61. Ibid., 23–25.

62. Ibid., 32–41.

63. Ibid., 52–53.

64. Ibid., 59–70.

65. Ibid., 73–75. On the background to the 1906 law and on efforts to enforce it, see also James Harvey Young, *The Medical Messiahs: A Social History of Health Quackery in Twentieth-Century America* (Princeton, NJ: Princeton University Press, 1992; first published 1967): 3–112.

66. David F. Cavers, "The Food, Drug, and Cosmetic Act of 1938: its legislative history and its substantive provisions," *Law and Contemporary Problems* 6 (1939): 2–42; Young, *The Medical Messiahs* (note 65), 159–190; Marks, *Progress of Experiment* (note 60), 77. The most thorough study of the legislative process is Charles O. Jackson, *Food and Drug Legislation in the New Deal* (Princeton, NJ: Princeton University Press, 1970).

67. Young, *The Medical Messiahs* (note 65), 160–163, 180–182.

68. Ibid., 161–162, 183–184.

69. James Harvey Young, "Sulfanilamide and diethylene glycol," in John Parascandola and James C. Whorton, editors, *Chemistry and Modern Society: Historical Essays in Honor of Aaron J. Ihde* (Washington, DC: American Chemical Society, 1983), 105–125, on 107–108; "Deaths due to Elixir of Sulfanilamide-Massengill. Report of Secretary of Agriculture submitted in response to House Resolution 352 of November 18, 1937 and Senate Resolution 194 of November 16, 1937," *JAMA* 109 (December 11, 1937): 1985–1988. On the early American reception of sulfanilamide, see chapter 6.

70. "Elixir of Sulfanilamide Massengill: chemical, pharmacologic, pathologic and necropsy reports; preliminary toxicity reports on diethylene glycol and sulfanilamide," *JAMA* 109 (1937): 1531–1539.

71. "Deaths due to Elixir of Sulfanilamide-Massengill" (note 69), 1985–1987; Young, "Sulfanilamide and diethylene glycol" (note 69), 115; Walter G. Campbell, "1938 Report of Food and Drug Administration," in *Federal Food, Drug and Cosmetic Law. Administrative Reports, 1907–1949* (Chicago: Commerce Clearing House Inc., 1951), 899–922, on 911.

72. "Deaths due to Elixir of Sulfanilamide-Massengill" (note 69), 1987; Young, "Sulfanilamide and diethylene glycol" (note 69), 115.

73. "Deaths due to Elixir of Sulfanilamide-Massengill" (note 69), 1985; Young, Sulfanilamide and diethylene glycol" (note 69), 108.

74. Young, "Sulfanilamide and diethylene glycol" (note 69), 109; James Harvey Young, "The 'Elixir Sulfanilamide' disaster," *Emory University Quarterly* 14 (1958): 230–237.

75. "Deaths following Elixir of Sulfanilamide-Massengill" (editorial), *JAMA* 109 (1937): 1367; "Deaths following Elixir of Sulfanilamide-Massengill—II" (editorial), *JAMA* 109 (October 30, 1937): 1456.

76. "Deaths following Elixir of Sulfanilamide-Massengill: III" (editorial), *JAMA* 109 (November 6, 1937): 1544–1545; "Food and Drug legislation" (editorial), *JAMA* 109 (November 6, 1937): 1546. On physicians' failure to follow Council on Pharmacy and Chemistry reports, see also "Deaths following Elixir of Sulfanilamide-Massengill: IV" (editorial), *JAMA* 109 (November 20, 1937): 1727.

77. "Safeguards proposed to govern distribution of dangerous drugs" (editorial), *JAMA* 109 (December 11, 1937): 1911–1912; "Deaths due to Elixir of Sulfanilamide-Massengill" (note 69), 1988.

78. Young, "Sulfanilamide and diethylene glycol" (note 69), 119–121; Cavers, "The Food, Drug, and Cosmetic Act of 1938" (note 66), 2–42, esp. 20, 40; Jackson, *Food and Drug Legislation in the New Deal* (note 66), 161–200.

79. Marks, *The Progress of Experiment* (note 41), 72, 78–81, 89; Dale E. Cooper, "Adequate controls for new drugs: good manufacturing practice and the 1938 Federal Food, Drug and Cosmetic Act," *PH* 44 (2002): 12–23; and John P. Swann, "FDA and the practice of pharmacy: prescription drug regulation before the Durham-Humphrey Amendment of 1951," *PH* 36 (1994): 55–70.

80. Marks, *The Progress of Experiment* (note 41), 83–85.

81. Ibid., 85–89; Council on Pharmacy and Chemistry, "Preliminary report of the Council," and Perrin H. Long, "Sulfapyridine," *JAMA* 112 (1939): 538–539; Council on Pharmacy and Chemistry, "Special report of the council: sulfapyridine," *JAMA* 112 (May 6, 1939): 1830; and "New and nonofficial remedies," *JAMA* 112 (1939): 1831.

82. Marks, *The Progress of Experiment* (note 41), 91–97. Although the 1938 law addressed the problem of safety, questions of the efficacy of new drugs could and did come into play. On the history of efficacy considerations in the evaluation of new drugs in the United States, see John P. Swann, "Sure cure: public policy on drug efficacy before 1962," in Gregory J. Higby and Elaine C. Stroud, editors, *The Inside Story of Medicines: A Symposium* (Madison, WI: American Institute of the History of Pharmacy, 1997), 223–261.

83. Council on Pharmacy and Chemistry, "Special report of the council" (note 81); "Sulfapyridine" (editorial), *JAMA* 112 (May 6, 1939): 1833.

84. H.L. Marriott, "Sulphapyridine (M&B 693) and pneumococcal infections," *BMJ* (November 11, 1939): 944–947. The article concluded with 122 citations to the British and overseas medical literature.

85. M.H. Hughes, "Otogenic cellular meningitis treated with M&B 693," *BMJ* (February 4, 1939): 214–215; A. Morton Gill, "Staphylococcal meningitis treated with sulphapyridine: recovery," *BMJ* (May 18, 1940): 810; D.F. Johnstone and P. Forgacs, "Cerebral symptoms occurring during sulphapyridine treatment of meningococcal meningitis," *BMJ* (May 24, 1941): 772–774; G. Marsden Roberts, "Sulphapyridine and soluseptasine in meningitis due to Pfeiffer bacillus: recovery," *BMJ* (November 25, 1939): 1041; John M. Teasdale, "Pneumococcal peritonitis with bilateral pneumococcal empyemata—treatment with M&B 693: recovery," *BMJ* (June 10, 1939): 1179; W. Bonnar, "Sulphapyridine in human anthrax," *BMJ* (March 9, 1940): 389; G.A. Richards, "Sulphapyridine in bacterial endocarditis," *BMJ* (April 13, 1940): 637; R.J. McNeill Love, "Treatment of gas gangrene with sulphapyridine," *BMJ* (June 1, 1940): 908; J.H. Jordan, J.H. Blakelock, and W.R. Johnston, "Treatment of cerebrospinal fever with sulphapyridine," *BMJ* (June 22, 1940): 1005–1008; Rudolf Reitler and Kurt Marberg, "Note on the treatment of acute bacillary dysentery with sulphapyridine," *BMJ* (February 22, 1941): 277–278; V. Ruth Sharp, "Sulphapyridine in suppurative otitis media," *BMJ* (August 9, 1941): 211; Sydney Tibbles, "Corneal ulcers cured by sulphapyridine," *BMJ* (August 23, 1941): 292; F.J.T. Bowie, "Chemotherapy in gonorrhea: a preliminary report on the use of 2-(p-aminoben-

zenesulphonamido) pyridine, M&B 693," *BMJ* (August 6, 1938): 283–284; R.M.B. MacKenna, "Recent experiences in the treatment of gonorrhea in the male," *BMJ* (June 28, 1941): 958–961; R.F.B. Welford, personal communication, February 11, 1994.

Chapter 8

1. The following discussion draws heavily on the collection of press clippings on M&B 693 housed in the MB at Rhône-Poulenc-Rorer (now Sanofi-aventis) in Dagenham, UK. I am grateful to the staff of Rhône-Poulenc-Rorer, and especially to John Salmon, for making these materials available to me.

2. *Yorkshire Evening Post*, June 17, 1938; *Everybody's*, July 25, 1938; *Glasgow Herald*, September 9, 1938.

3. " 'Miracle drug' saves life of W'ton girl—mother wishes it had been discovered before," *Midland Counties Express*, September 10, 1938. For other examples, see "Septicaemia victim cured—new drug's great success," *Belfast Telegraph*, September 16, 1938; "Miracle drug saves woman," *Daily Mirror*, October 29, 1938; "Dublin cure with remarkable drug—striking claims," *Irish Independent*; "M and B 693 is in the news again," *News Chronicle*, November 25, 1938; and "3-Weeks baby saved by new wonder drug," *Daily Express*, June 21, 1939.

4. "M and B 693," *Times*, June 7, 1938; "Germs disarmed by a new drug: success claimed in treatment of pneumonia," *Yorkshire Evening Post*, June 17, 1938; and "Dooming the germ: explaining discoveries in the modern treatment of dangerous germs," *Lancashire Daily Post*, date incomplete but probably from December 1938. In MB, file 14B.

5. "Freedom from disease in fifty years' time?" *Birmingham Gazette*, July 4, 1938; Anthony Weymouth, "Hunt for new drugs brings new cures," *Daily Express*, November 12, 1938; "New ally," *Daily Express*, January 20, 1939; "Miracle drugs start 'a new era'," *Sunday Dispatch*, January 22, 1939.

6. "Claim by Harvard professor—'no more deaths from pneumonia'," *Bristol Evening Post*, March 31, 1939; "Triumph of a new drug—'biggest discovery of our generation'— works like a charm, says expert," *Reynolds News*, May 7, 1939; "How science advances— drugs that conquer death," by a doctor, *Doncaster Gazette*, August 31, 1939.

7. "Pneumonia discovery," *Evening Standard*, July 2, 1938; "Pneumonia discovery," *Lancashire Daily Post*, July 4, 1938; "James Agate takes notes—and revises the honours list," *Daily Express*, January 9, 1939; "Thank you, Dr. Whitby," *Evening Standard*, January 30, 1939; and "Medical science passes another milestone," *Sheffield Weekly Telegraph*, March 8, 1939.

8. "The new drug for pneumococcal meningitis," *Manchester Guardian*, September 13, 1938; "The miracle workers," *Glasgow Sunday Post*, January 22, 1939; "Shy man who found wonder drug—three years' search—'It was just a job of work'—success at his 693rd attempt," *Sunday Chronicle*, February 5, 1939.

9. "The new drug for pneumococcal meningitis," *Manchester Guardian*, September 13, 1938; Ritchie Calder, "Reporting progress," *Daily Herald*, February 10, 1939. On the testing of compounds prior to T693, see chapter 7.

10. "How M and B came about," *People*, February 18, 1940; James Harpole, " 'This marvelous drug'," *Sunday Graphic*, January 2, 1944; "Workman's pennies bought drug that saved soldier," *Eastern Evening News*, February 28, 1940; "Beginning of a long series of experiments," *Limerick Leader*, April 29, 1939.

11. "Captain of the men of death," *Sunday Sun*, March 12, 1939; "M. and B. 693— the new wonder drug," *Manchester Evening Chronicle*, August 15, 1939; "Discovered M. & B. 693," *Southend Standard*, August 31, 1939; "Men who prepared drug were S. Londoners," *Sydenham Gazette*, June 30, 1939 (quote); "Luck led to this great discovery," *Sunday*

Pictorial, February 6, 1944. On Phillips' later attack on May & Baker's version of the discovery, see pages 195–196.

12. Ritchie Calder, "Reporting progress," *Daily Herald*, February 10, 1939; "Captain of the men of death," *Sunday Sun*, March 12, 1939; "Triumph of a new drug—'biggest discovery of our generation'—works like a charm, says expert," *Reynolds News*, May 7, 1939; "M. and B. 693—the new wonder drug," *Manchester Evening Chronicle*, August 15, 1939. On Rhône-Poulenc's controlling interest in May & Baker, see chapter 7.

13. "Dooming the germ," by a Doctor, *Lancashire Daily Post* (undated but grouped with articles from July 1938), MB, file 14B; John Langdon-Davies, "2-(p-Aminobenzene-sulphonamido) pyridine," *Picture Post*, January 19, 1939; "Notes of the week," *Sunday School Chronicle*, July 1, 1943.

14. "Freedom from disease in fifty years' time?—big Birmingham discovery: 'M and B 63 [*sic*]' drug for pneumonia," *Birmingham Gazette*, July 4, 1938; "Wife tells of her pneumonia cure," *Daily Express*, November 19, 1939. See also "Birmingham beats pneumonia with new drug—M and B 63 [*sic*] puts patients on road to rapid recovery," *Evening Dispatch*, November 18, 1938.

15. "Research workers' wonderful discovery—Queen Charlotte's Hospital has cure for septicaemia," *Middlesex Independent*, April 22, 1939; "Pneumonia is conquered: Crumpsall Hospital verdict after sensational twelve-months test with 'wonder drug,'" *Manchester City News*, February 24, 1940.

16. "Saved by miracle drug—Swinden man owes life to 'M&B 693'," *Swinden Evening Advertiser*, November 23, 1939; "New cure for pneumonia," *Croyden Advertiser*, November 25, 1938; "New drug saves life of Lewisham baby," *Lewisham Borough News*, June 27, 1939.

17. "Two doctors prove cure for pneumonia," *Daily Express*, November 18, 1938; "New drug is curing city pneumonia cases," *Manchester Evening Chronicle*, November 18, 1938; "Knock-out for pneumonia," *Glasgow Sunday Post*, May 7, 1939; "Miracle drug cures 'fatal' disease," *Pearson's Weekly*, December 17, 1938; "M. B. 693," *Financial Times*, March 9, 1939, and correction, March 15, 1939; and "Man saved by drug admits murders," *Daily Express*, March 30, 1939.

18. "Birmingham plea for caution in new drug 'cure' for pneumonia—'M. & B. 693' tablet research work not yet complete," *Evening Dispatch*, June 5, 1938; "Dooming the germ," *Lancashire Daily Post*, undated but grouped with articles from July 1938, MB, file 14B; and "Disease you need no longer dread—new drug conquers deadly germ," *Everybody's*, July 25, 1938. For warnings on possible toxicity in reference to the sulfonamides as a group, see, e.g., "Important drug discovery—arresting disease bacteria—the sulphonamide group," *Daily Telegraph*, November 11, 1938; and "Synthetic cure: government grant £30,000 for further sulfanilamide research," *Cavalcade*, November 12, 1938.

19. "Prontosil and its successors," *Northern Whig* (Belfast), April 4, 1939; "The care of your health," *National Welfare* (Johannesburg), April 1939.

20. "Cured pneumonia with new drug—but died of it himself," *Dundee Evening Telegraph*, April 17, 1939; "Dangers in new drug—warning by city doctor," *Star*, July 3, 1939; "The chemist says 'No!'" *Sunday Post*, February 20, 1944; "'As directed by the physician'," *Star*, August 4, 1939.

21. "A mouthful for our spelling bees," *Antivivisection Journal*, July 1938; "Review of the month," *Antivivisection Journal*, April 1939; "So soon?," *Antivivisection Journal*, February 1940.

22. On the Betty Walters case, see above at note 3.

23. "M&B 693," *Manufacturing Chemist*, August 1938; "The new drug for pneumococcal meningitis," *Manchester Guardian*, September 13, 1938 (quote); Vigilant, "Gossip," *Wolverhampton Express*, September 3, 1938.

24. "New meningitis drug now available," *Manufacturing Chemist*, October, 1938; "M&B 693," *Retail Chemist*, October, 1938; "Novelties in medicine: exhibition at Westminster," *Observer*, October 13, 1938; "New aids to nursing," *Nursing Mirror*, October 22, 1938.

25. T. Farnsworth Anderson and R.M. Dowdeswell, "Treatment of pneumonia in Kenya with M&B 693," *Lancet* i (1939): 252, reprinted in *East African Medical Journal* 16 (1939): 76–77; T. Farnsworth Anderson, "Reminiscenses" (1973), unpublished typescript, Mss. Afr. S. 1653, Rhodes House Library, Oxford. I am grateful to Patrick Malloy for making available to me copies of this item and other materials from the Rhodes House Library and the *East African Medical Journal*. The British press report is "The colonial empire's year of progress," *Glasgow Herald*, June 2, 1939.

26. "Success of new drug: combating pneumonia in South Africa," *Edinburgh Evening Dispatch*, January 14, 1939; "Drug for pneumonia treatment: experiments in Africa," *Times*, February 14, 1939; "Lives saved by 'M&B 693'," *Star*, May 5, 1939; "Mine natives' health: high standard maintained: treatment of pneumonia," *Star*, January 30, 1940; "Famous drug to be a 'poison'," *Nottingham Evening News*, August 10, 1939; "Recoveries from meningitis," *Times Weekly Edition*, April 5, 1939; R.B. Usher Somers, "M&B 693 in cerebro-spinal fever: a review of 143 cases treated under field conditions," *Lancet* 236 (April 22, 1939): 921–922; "M&B 693 and cerebro-spinal meningitis in the Sudan," *Nursing Mirror*, July 1939.

27. Philip Jordan, "250,000 aspirins for the B.E.F.," *News Chronicle*, October 25, 1939; "B.E.F.'s huge medical stores, and the Epsom salts!" *Edinburgh Evening News*, n.d., in MB; "Finland!—S.O.S. for pneumonia specific!" *Glasgow Herald*, January 24, 1940; "News in brief: M&B 693 for Finland," *Pharmaceutical Journal*, February 10, 1940.

28. Photo in *Glasgow Evening Times*, December 31, 1943; "Churchill drug saves lion too," *Glasgow Evening News*, January 7, 1944; "M&B lioness is improving," *Sunday Chronicle*, January 30, 1944; cartoon, *Yorkshire Evening Post*, January 21, 1944; cartoon, *The Wall Planet*, reproduced in Judy Slinn, *A History of May & Baker 1834–1984* (Cambridge: Hobsons Ltd., 1984), 135.

29. On the conflation of different May & Baker products, see "The development of sulphonamides," 2-pp. typescript, n.d., file 131, MB. On M&B as a source of national pride, see page 188 and "Pneumonia robbed of its terror: experiments with a wonderful new drug," *News of the World*, June 19, 1938. The article reported that "British doctors and British chemists are rejoicing in the knowledge that the drug is a product of one of our own research laboratories. The new drug is the answer to criticisms so often made that research in chemistry in this country is a long way behind that in Germany and America."

30. Henry H. Dale, "Arthur James Ewins 1882–1958," *BMFRS* 4 (1958): 81–91 (83); "Sir Lionel Whitby" (obituary) *BMJ* (December 1, 1956): 1306–1309.

31. Peter Bishop, "Why leave this genius out in the cold?" *The People*, June 21, 1964.

32. "Luck led to this great discovery," *Sunday Pictorial*, February 2, 1944. One exception to Phillips's lack of notice was "Birthplace of a new drug," *Romford Times*, September 7, 1938. Romford was Phillips's place of residence. The "inside story" is in Bishop, "Why leave this genius out in the cold?" (note 31). Phillips's later career as a chemical consultant is reported in Jo Weedon, "Fighting doctor who discovered a miracle," *Recorder Review*, October 20, 1972.

33. Jo Weedon, "Fighting doctor" (note 32).

34. Ibid.

35. Daniel Bovet's first generation is identical with mine, but he differentiates what I have called the second generation into second, third, and fourth generations. Bovet's

second generation includes sulfanilamide and its homocyclic derivatives. His third generation comprises the "first heterocyclic derivatives of sulfanilamide," namely, sulfapyridine and sulfathiazole. His fourth generation is constituted by the "new heterocyclic derivatives of sulfanilamide," e.g., sulfadiazine. I acknowledge the chemical interest of this classification but have chosen not to adopt it because it would complicate my story without illuminating the themes that I emphasize. See Daniel Bovet, *Une chimie qui guérit: histoire de la découverte des sulfamides* (Paris: Éditions Payot, 1988), 311–313.

36. On conservative invention, see Thomas P. Hughes, "The evolution of large technological systems," in Wiebe E. Bijker, Thomas P. Hughes, and Trevor J. Pinch, editors, *The Social Construction of Technological Systems: New Directions in the Sociology and History of Technology* (Cambridge, MA: MIT Press, 1987), 51–82. One exception to the industrial origins of second-generation sulfas was sulfaguanidine (originally named sulfanilguanidine), which emerged from academic research in pharmacology carried out by Eli Kennerly Marshall, Jr., and colleagues at Johns Hopkins. See E.K. Marshall, Jr., A.C. Bratton, H.J. White, and J.T. Litchfield, Jr., "Sulfanilguanidine: a chemotherapeutic agent for intestinal infections," *BJHH* 67 (1940): 163–188; and F. Hawking and J. Stewart Lawrence, *The Sulphonamides* (New York: Grune & Stratton, 1951), 26.

37. Slinn, *A History of May & Baker* (note 28), 151–153.

38. Ibid., 101, 127–144.

39. Ibid., 145–160.

40. Ibid., 157, 160–162.

41. *The Merck Institute for Therapeutic Research* (Rahway, NJ: Merck Institute for Therapeutic Research, 1942), unpaginated, MA box R4-1.5.1; *The Merck Institute for Therapeutic Research* (Rahway, NJ: Merck Institute for Therapeutic Research, 1953), 1, MA box R4-1.5.1.

42. *The Merck Institute for Therapeutic Research* (1953) (note 41), 3: C.R. Addinall, "Fifty years progress in medicinal chemistry," *MR* 50 (January 1941): 13–16; interview with Max Tishler, July 13, 1988, MA box R2-5.2.1, pp. 4–5.

43. *The Merck Institute for Therapeutic Research* (1942) (note 41); Merck & Co. Inc. "Backgrounder 5. Sulfa drugs," December 10, 1959, MA box R7-4.8.1.

44. "Another milestone attained," *MR* 48 (April 1939): 3; " 'Dagenan' (Sulfapyridine Merck) now available for the treatment of pneumococcic pneumonia," *MR* 48 (April 1939): 6; C.R. Addinall, "Sulfapyridine (2-sulfanilyl-aminopyridine Merck): the new sulfanilamide derivative," *MR* 48 (April 1939): 11–14; Merck & Co. Inc. "Report to stockholders 1939," MA.

45. Merck & Co. Inc. "Report to shareholders 1939" (note 44); Merck Institute for Therapeutic Research, "Seventh annual report (1939)," MA box R4-1.5.1, pp. 1–5.

46. Merck Institute for Therapeutic Research, "Seventh annual report (1939)" (note 45), pp. 3–8, 12–13; Wm. Antopol and H. Robinson, "Urolithiasis and renal pathology after oral administration of 2-(sulfanilamino)-pyridine (sulfapyridine)," *Proceedings of the Society for Experimental Biology and Medicine* 40 (1939): 428–430.

47. Hans Molitor, "The experimental evaluation of sulfanilamide derivatives," *MR* 48 (July 1939): 24–27. On leadership of research policy at Merck in the late 1930s and early 1940s, see "Interviews with Max Tishler," July 13, 1988, MA box R2-5.2.1, p. 5.

48. Merck Institute for Therapeutic Research, "Eighth annual report 1940," submitted March 20, 1941, MA box R4-1.5.1, pp. 1–2, 5–12.

49. Merck & Co. Inc., "Report to stockholders" for 1940, 1941, 1942, 1943, 1944, 1945, MA. Percentage increases in sales of sulfas were calculated from data in "Comparison of sales, gross profits, and research & development expenses for selected major products and all other products, January 1, 1939–September 30, 1949," MA box R12-1.9.2.

50. *The Merck Institute for Therapeutic Research* (1942) (note 41); *The Merck Institute for Therapeutic Research. Annual Report 1943* (Rahway, NJ: Merck Institute for Therapeutic Research, 1944), 3–4, 8–9, 21; Harry F. Dowling, *Fighting Infection: Conquests of the Twentieth Century* (Cambridge, MA: Harvard University Press, 1977), 105.

51. *The Merck Institute for Therapeutic Research. Annual Report 1943* (note 50), 4, 6–7, 10–11, 15–18.

52. *The Merck Institute for Therapeutic Research* (1953) (note 41), 4–7, 21; "Merck Institute dedicates new research center," *Merck Review* (May-June 1953), MA box R4-1.5.1. On the long-term growth of Merck expenditures for research and development, see also John P. Swann, "The evolution of the American pharmaceutical industry," *PH* 37 (1995): 76–86, on 82.

53. Louis Galambos and Jane Elliott Sewell, *Networks of Innovation: Vaccine Development at Merck, Sharp & Dohme, and Mulford, 1895–1995* (Cambridge: Cambridge University Press, 1995), 33–38.

54. "Interviews with James Maurice Sprague," May 23, 1990, MA box R2-5.1.1, pp. 10–11. The article in question was almost certainly Lionel E. H. Whitby, "Chemotherapy of pneumococcal and other infections with 2-(p-aminobenzenesulphonamide) pyridine," *Lancet* (May 28, 1938): 1210–1212.

55. "Interview with James Maurice Sprague" (note 54), 11–12; Merck & Co. Inc., "Backgrounder 4. Merck Research," n.d. but probably 1958 or 1959, MA, box R7-4.8.1; Merck & Co. Inc., "Backgrounder 5. Sulfa drugs" (note 43), 3.

56. Galambos and Sewell, *Networks of Innovation* (note 53), p. 38 and n. 10; "Interview with James Maurice Sprague" (note 54), 16, 24–25.

57. Peter Temin, *Taking Your Medicine: Drug Regulation in the United States* (Cambridge, MA: Harvard University Press, 1980), 5–6; David L. Cowen, "The on-going pharmaceutical revolution: the role of the industry," in F. Javier Puerto Sarmiento, editor, *Farmacia e Industrializacion: Libro homenaje al Doctor Guillermo Folch Jou* (Madrid: Sociedad Española de Historia de la Farmacia, 1985), 95–114; Marcel H. Bickel, "The development of sulfonamides (1932–1938) as a focal point in the history of chemotherapy," *Gesnerus* 45 (1988): 67–86, on 75–81; Swann "The evolution of the American pharmaceutical industry" (note 52), 82, 84. Temin includes a table of numbers of new drug introductions by year, 1941–1979.

Chapter 9

1. John J. Moorhead, "Surgical experience at Pearl Harbor," *JAMA* 118 (1942): 712–714; Walter Lord, *Day of Infamy* (New York: Henry Holt & Co., 1957), 193–194.

2. Moorhead, "Surgical experience at Pearl Harbor" (note 1), 713.

3. Ibid., 712–714.

4. Ibid., 714.

5. Ralph B. Cloward, "War injuries to the head: treatment of penetrating wounds," *JAMA* 118 (January 24, 1942): 267–270. Cloward reported at that time that he was not permitted to disclose the number of persons treated.

6. "Sulfa drugs win high praise in Pearl Harbor lives saved," *Baltimore Sun*, January 19, 1942. On Ravdin, see "Festschrift for Dr. Isidor Schwaner Ravdin," *Surgery* 56 (1964), esp. Jonathan E. Rhoads and Leonard D. Miller, "Foreword," pp. 606–608; Sidney Farber, "I.S. Ravdin—civilian activities at the national level," pp. 611–613; and John Paul North. "The 20th General Hospital—I.S. Ravdin, Commanding General," pp. 614–623.

7. Quoted in "Sulfa drugs win high praise in Pearl Harbor lives saved" (note 6). See also "Civilian cooperation at Honolulu and Pearl Harbor," *JAMA* 118 (February 7, 1942): 465.

8. "A verray parfit praktiseur," *Medical Times* (June 1966): 687–702, on 692.

9. Norman Berlinger, "From death comes life," *American Heritage of Invention & Technology* 11 (3) (Winter 1996): 22–31; and Angela N.H. Creager, "Biotechnology and blood: Edwin Cohn's plasma fractionation project, 1940–1953," in Arnold Thackray, editor, *Private Science: Biotechnology and the Rise of the Molecular Sciences* (Philadelphia, PA: University of Pennsylvania Press, 1998), 39–62.

10. See, e.g., Peter Neushul, "Science, government, and the mass production of penicillin," *JHMAS* 48 (1993): 371–395.

11. S. Dewitt Clough, "Preparedness with drugs and medicinal chemicals," *WM* 1 (1941): 102–106.

12. Ibid., 106; "Drugs and Cosmetics Branch," undated history of the Drugs and Cosmetic Branch of the War Production Board (probably from second half of 1945), paginated 319–344, NA, RG 179, 052.508, History of the Chemicals Bureau, War Production Board, 1940–1945, vol. 1, on p. 319.

13. "Drugs and Cosmetics Branch" (note 12), 319–321.

14. Ibid., 321.

15. John S. Lockwood, "War-time activities of the National Research Council and the Committee on Medical Research; with particular reference to team-work on studies of wounds and burns," *AS* 124 (1946): 314–327; Sanford V. Larkey, "The National Research Council and medical preparedness," *WM* 1 (January, 1941): 77–94.

16. Larkey, "The National Research Council and medical preparedness" (note 15), 79.

17. Ibid., 79–86; the names and membership of all committees and subcommittees are given on 80–84, and the names and committee assignments of contact officers on 85–86.

18. Lockwood, "War-time activities" (note 15), 315; Perrin H. Long, "Medicine in World War II," *Baltimore Sun* (n.d., but on internal evidence from 1948), AMCMA.

19. E.H. Cushing, "The Health and Medical Committee," *WM* 1 (1941): 66–68; "Activities of the Medical Department in augmentation of the Army: official statement from the Office of the Surgeon General of the United States Army," *WM* 1 (1941): 69–76; Rosco G. Leland, "A census of physicians for military preparedness," *WM* 1 (1941): 95–101.

20. "Editorial: war medicine," *WM* 1 (1941): 1–2; Larkey, "The National Research Council and medical preparedness" (note 15), 83; *WM* 1 (1941): title page; "War Medicine—a new publication," *JAMA* 115 (December 14, 1940): 2086–2087.

21. "Chemotherapy for infectious diseases and other infections: Circular Letter No. 81," *WM* 1 (1941): 55–65. See also "Chemotherapy in infectious diseases and other infections," Circular Letter no. 81, December 5, 1940, War Department, Office of the Surgeon General, NA, RG 112, box 11.

22. See, e.g., Donald L. Rose, H. Worley Kendell, and Walter M. Simpson, "Refractory gonococcic infections: elimination by combined artificial fever and chemotherapy as related to military medicine," *WM* 1 (1941): 470–478; and "Editorial: measures to combat gonorrhea and syphilis," *WM* 2 (1942): 132–135.

23. Eleanor A. Bliss, Perrin H. Long, and Dorothy G. Smith, "Chemotherapy of experimental gas gangrene and tetanus infections in mice," *WM* 1 (1941): 799–810. See also Benjamin Kropp and Dorothy G. Smith, "Connective tissue and phagocytes in experimental gas gangrene infection in guinea pigs: effect of sulfanilamide," *WM* 1 (1941): 682–689.

24. Lockwood, "War-time activities" (note 15), 315.

25. Ibid., 315–316.

26. Larkey, "The National Research Council and medical preparedness" (note 15), 319.

27. Ibid., 89–90; Lockwood, "War-time activities" (note 15), 319–320.

28. Lockwood, "Wartime activities of the National Research Council and the Committee on Medical Research" (note 15), 320.

29. Leonard Colebrook to Perrin Long, July 18, 1941. AMCMA, Lewis Weed Papers, box 21.

30. Lockwood, "War-time activities" (note 15), 320; Larkey, "The National Research Council and medical preparedness" (note 15), 80.

31. Lockwood, "War-time activities" (note 15), 320–321.

32. Memorandum, Surgeon General's Office to Office of the Under Secretary of War, Production Division, December 15, 1941, NA, RG 112.

33. C.F. Shook to Carson P. Frailey, January 10, 1942, NA, RG 112; C.F. Shook to Office of Production Management, January 19, 1942, NA, RG 112; L.L. Gardner to J.A.V. Hyatt, February 5, 1942, NA, RG 112.

34. "War shortage of drugs and medical appliances," report of a Subcommittee of the Committee on Public Health Relations of the New York Academy of Medicine, and cover letter, Malcolm Goodridge to Major General James C. Magee, March 18, 1942, NA, RG 112; and Carson P. Frailey to the Surgeon General, U.S. Army, February 27, 1942, NA, RG 112.

35. "A chronology of the War Production Board and predecessor agencies, August 1939 to June 1943," NA, RG 179, 033.308, p. 6; "Drugs and Cosmetics Branch" (note 12), 322.

36. "Drugs and Cosmetics Branch" (note 12), 323, 334; "History of the Chemicals Bureau of the War Production Board, June 1940–September 30, 1945" February, 1946, NA, RG 179, box 371, p. 13.

37. Statements on sulfanilamide (June 25, 1942), sulfathiazole (July 3, 1942), sulfapyridine (July 2, 1942), sulfadiazine (July 3, 1942), and sulfaguanidine (July 2, 1942), Health Supplies Section, Statistical Division, War Production Board, NA, RG 374, 533.1201. On the replacement of sulfapyridine by sulfathiazole in the United States, see also "Foreign requirements of sulfapyridine for 1942," memorandum to American Requirements Committee of War Production Board from Inter-departmental Foreign Requirements Committee of the Board of Economic Warfare, NA, RG 179, box 74, pp. 4–5. On the introduction of sulfathiazole in the United States, see John P. Swann, "The 1941 sulfathiazole disaster and the birth of good manufacturing practices," *PH* 40 (1999): 16–25, on 17.

38. C.F. Shook to the Priorities Committee, Army and Navy Munitions Board, June 8, 1942, NA, RG 112; Clifford V. Morgan to Chief, Health Supplies Branch, War Production Board, July 18, 1942, NA, RG 112.

39. Leonard Engel, *Medicine Makers of Kalamazoo* (New York: McGraw-Hill Book Co., 1961), 93–94.

40. Clifford V. Morgan to Parke, Davis & Co., July 18, 1942; Clifford V. Morgan to E.R. Squibb & Sons, July 18, 1942; and Clifford V. Morgan to Calco Chemical Division, American Cyanamid Co., July 18, 1942. All in NA, RG 112. On the increasing demand for sulfadiazine, see also C.F. Shook to Carl Bigelow, July 18, 1942, NA, RG 112. Winthrop Chemical Co. had a contract with the Army and Navy to supply 50,000 pounds of sulfathiazole in 1942. See Swann, "The 1941 sulfathiazole disaster" (note 37), 22.

41. "Drugs and Cosmetics Branch" (note 12), 324; "History of the Chemicals Bureau of the War Production Board" (note 36), 11.

42. Fred J. Stock, "Status of drug supplies," text of a talk to the American Pharmaceutical Manufacturers Association, December 12, 1944, NA, RG 179, box 73, p. 7; Memoranda: George W. Fiero to Robert P. Fischelis, November 28 and December 10, 1942, NA, RG 179, box 73; and Robert P. Fischelis, "Civilian requirements for drugs," statement to the Proprietary Drug Industry Advisory Committee, July 13, 1943, NA, RG 179, box 73. On the specter of World War I, see also "Review of literature on shortages of drugs, medical

supplies, and food during World War I," War Production Board, Office of Civilian Supply, Consumers Programs Branch, Medical and Health Supplies Section, Research and Planning Study no. 3, October 28, 1942, NA, RG 374, 533.1017.

43. "Production of important therapeutic agents during the period 1940 through 1944," table dated December 24, 1943, Research and Statistics Unit, Drugs and Cosmetics Section, Chemicals Division, War Production Board, NA, RG 179, box 74.

44. Ibid.

45. "Raw materials and intermediates in the production of sulfonamides," statement of November 25, 1943, Research and Statistics Unit, Drugs and Cosmetics Section, Chemicals Division, War Production Board, NA, RG 179, box 313.

46. Stock, "Status of drug supplies" (note 42), 7; "History of the Chemicals Bureau of the War Production Board" (note 36), 17–19; "Drugs and Cosmetics Branch" (note 12), 334; "Sulfaguanidine," Commodity Review no. 4, May 31, 1945, War Production Board, Office of Civilian Requirements, Chemicals, Drugs, and Health Supplies Division, NA, RG 374, 533.12, Table VI; "Production of important therapeutic agents during the period 1940 through 1944" (note 43).

47. Mickey C. Smith and Dennis Worthen, "Soldiers on the production line," *PH* 37 (1995): 183–188; "Merciful Munitions," advertisement in *MR* 52(3) (July 1943). Another "E" Award recipient, the Upjohn Co., had doubled its production between 1941 and 1945 in spite of labor shortages and management changes. See Engel, *Medicine Makers of Kalamazoo* (note 39), 100. For the context of the "E" Awards, see also Ernest Risley Eaton, "Use of industrial incentives in war production of medical materiel," *WM* 6 (1944): 236–240.

Chapter 10

1. For an overview of the role of communicable diseases in World War II, see John E. Gordon, "General considerations of modes of transmission," in Medical Department, U.S. Army, *Preventive Medicine in World War II*, vol. 4, *Communicable Diseases Transmitted Chiefly through Respiratory and Alimentary Tracts* (Washington, DC: Office of the Surgeon General, Department of the Army, 1958), 3–52.

2. On the development of penicillin, see Peter Neushul, "Science, government, and the mass production of penicillin," *JHMAS* 48 (1993): 371–395; and W.H. Helfand, H.B. Woodruff, K.M.H. Coleman, and D.L. Cowen, "Wartime industrial development of penicillin in the United States," in John Parascandola, editor, *The History of Antibiotics: A Symposium* (Madison, WI: American Institute of the History of Pharmacy, 1980), 31–56.

3. E.C. Andrus, D.W. Bronk, G.A. Carden, Jr., C.S. Keefer, J.S. Lockwood, J.T. Wearn, and M.C. Winternitz, editors, *Advances in Military Medicine Made by American Investigators under the Sponsorship of the Committee on Medical Research*, vol. 1 (Boston, MA: Little, Brown & Co., 1948), 717–719.

4. "Drugs and Cosmetics Branch," undated history of the Drugs and Cosmetics Branch of the War Production Board (probably from second half of 1945), paginated 319–344, NA, RG 179, 052.508, History of the Chemicals Bureau, War Production Board, 1940–1945, vol. 1, on 331; "Penicillin," Circular Letter no. 125, July 16, 1943, War Department, Office of the Surgeon General, NA, RG 112, box 12.

5. "Drugs and Cosmetics Branch" (note 4), 332; C.R. Addinall, "Recent advances in the chemistry of natural products," *MR* 52(4) (October 1943): 4–9; "History of the Chemicals, Drugs, and Health Supplies Division, 1942–1945," September 13, 1945, War Production Board, NA, RG 179, 035.008, p. 108. On wartime rationing of penicillin, see David P. Adams, *"The Greatest Good to the Greatest Number": Penicillin Rationing on the American Home Front, 1940–1945* (New York: Peter Lang, 1991).

6. "Meeting: Conference of Penicillin Producers," March 14–16, 1944, War Production Board, Office of Industry Advisory Committees, NA, RG 179, box 73.

7. Figures taken from "Drugs and Cosmetics Branch" (note 4), 333 (table gives production figures on a monthly basis).

8. Norman Berlinger, "From death comes life," *American Heritage of Invention & Technology* 11(3) (winter 1996): 22–31, on 25; "Drugs and Cosmetics Branch" (note 4), 332; Fred J. Stock, "Status of drug supplies," text of a talk to the American Pharmaceutical Manufacturers Association, December 12, 1944, NA, RG 179, box 73, 9.

9. Medical Department, U.S. Army, *Internal Medicine in World War II*, vol. 2, *Infectious Diseases* (Washington, DC: Office of the Surgeon General, Department of the Army, 1963), xiii; "The new drug and the war," *Baltimore Sun*, December 14, 1939; Gerald N. Grob, *The Deadly Truth: A History of Disease in America* (Cambridge, MA: Harvard University Press, 2002), 224. Grob points out that in World War I "almost as many military personnel died of influenza and pneumonia (44,000) as were killed in battle (50,000)."

10. Horace P. Marvin and Eugene P. Campbell, "The treatment of lobar pneumonia with serum and sulfanilamide," *MS* 84 (January-June 1939): 224–231.

11. E.P. Campbell to D.F. Robertson, February 7, 1939; M.E. Griffin to Merck & Co. Inc., February 13, 1939; J.M. Carlisle to Griffin, February 16, 1939; and Griffin to Merck & Co. Inc., February 25, 1939; all in NA, RG 112, box 50; Horace P. Marvin, Aubrey L. Bradford, and Walter H. Ketchum, "Sulfapyridine therapy in pneumonia" (based on a talk presented February 20, 1940), *MS* 86 (January-June 1940): 554–560 (quotes on 559).

12. Marvin et al., "Sulfapyridine therapy in pneumonia" (note 11), 559; "Chemotherapy in infectious diseases and other infections," Circular Letter no. 81, December 5, 1940, War Department, Office of the Surgeon General, NA, RG 112, box 11, p. 6; Horace P. Marvin, Franklin D. Owings, and Edward K. Edelson, "Pneumonia therapy with sulfathiazole in military practice," *MS* 91 (July-December 1942): 55–58. The transition from sulfapyridine to sulfathiazole is also visible in Henry K. Mohler, "The therapeutic use of sulfanilamide and related compounds," *MS* 88 (January-June 1941): 473–486, esp. 482–486.

13. "Dr. Long tells of new drug being studied," *Baltimore Sun*, February 11, 1941; Marvin et al., "Pneumonia therapy with sulfathiazole in military practice" (note 12), 57; "Chemotherapy in infectious diseases and other infections," Circular Letter no. 17, February 23, 1942, War Department, Office of the Surgeon General, NA, RG 112, box 666, pp. 7–9; Memorandum: George W. Fiero to Robert P. Fischelis, August 28, 1943, Division of Civilian Requirements, War Production Board, NA, RG 374, 533.1204; "Sulfathiazole," January 22, 1945, Production Digest, Office of Civilian Requirements, War Production Board, NA, RG 374, 833.12141; "Sulfadiazine," Commodity Review no. 3, June 8, 1945, Office of Civilian Requirements, War Production Board, NA, RG 374, 533.12341; "Sulfapyridine," Commodity Review no. 5, June 19, 1945, Office of Civilian Requirements, War Production Board, NA, RG 374, 533.12441.

14. "Penicillin," Circular Letter no. 125 (note 4); Herbert J. Fox, "Penicillin program at the United States Naval Hospital, Portsmouth, Va.," *WM* 7 (1945): 170–172; Medical Department, U.S. Army, *Preventive Medicine in World War II*, vol. 4 (note 1), 212; Medical Department, U.S. Army, *Internal Medicine in World War II*, vol. 2 (note 9), 30.

15. On supplies of penicillin, see pages 223–224. On Army use of sulfadiazine in pneumonia, see Medical Department, U.S. Army, *Internal Medicine in World War II*, vol. 2 (note 9), 30–32.

16. Ibid., 26–27, 29; Medical Department, U.S. Army, *Preventive Medicine in World War II*, vol. 4 (note 1), 222.

17. Medical Department, U.S. Army, *Preventive Medicine in World War II*, vol. 4 (note 1), 212, 221–222; Medical Department, U.S. Army, *Internal Medicine in World War II*, vol. 2 (note 9), 26–32.

18. Hugh J. Morgan, "Treatment of gonorrhea and syphilis in the United States Army," *MS* 96 (January-June 1945): 127–131; "Editorial: measures to combat gonorrhea and syphilis," *WM* 2 (1942): 132–135 (quote on 132). On efforts to control venereal disease among U.S. troops in World War I, see Allan M. Brandt, *No Magic Bullet: A Social History of Venereal Disease in the United States Since 1880* (New York: Oxford University Press, 1987), 52–121.

19. Sanford V. Larkey, "The National Research Council and medical preparedness," *WM* 1 (January 1941): 77–94, on 80, 89; Medical Department, U.S. Army, *Internal Medicine in World War II*, vol. 2 (note 9), 409–410.

20. Medical Department, U.S. Army, *Internal Medicine in World War II*, vol. 2 (note 9), 411–412. On the use of sulfanilamide and sulfapyridine, see Circular Letter no. 12, July 21, 1937, Circular Letter no. 13, March 31, 1938, and Circular Letter no. 35, August 3, 1939, all in NA, RG 112, box 10; Memorandum, L.L. Gardner to Colonel Gentry, December 8, 1938, War Department, Office of the Surgeon General, NA, RG 112, box 50; James C. Kimbrough, "Sulfanilamide in the treatment of gonorrhea: report of the results obtained in 100 cases," *MS* 84 (January–June 1939): 568–577; Mohler, "The therapeutic use of sulfanilamide and related compounds" (note 12), 492; and James P. Pappas, "Sulfapyridine '8-7-7-6' treatment of acute gonorrheal urethritis in the male," *MS* 90 (January-June 1942): 45–57. On early use of sulfathiazole in gonorrhea, see Harold M. Boslow, "Treatment of gonorrhea with sulfathiazole," *MS* 88 (January-June 1941): 659–660; James P. Pappas, "Sulfathiazole single-massive-dose therapy of acute gonorrheal urethritis in the male," *MS* 90 (January-June 1942): 662–667; and Harry A. Zide and Irving Davis, "Chemotherapy of gonorrheal urethritis in the male with sulfanilamide, sulfapyridine and sulfathiazole," *WM* 2 (1942): 445–449.

21. Medical Department, U.S. Army, *Internal Medicine in World War II*, vol. 2 (note 9), 410–411.

22. Ibid., 412; Circular Letter no. 74, July 25, 1942, NA, RG 112, box 12 (quote on p. 3).

23. Circular Letter no. 32, February 1, 1932, NA, RG 112, box 12; Medical Department, U.S. Army, *Internal Medicine in World War II*, vol. 2 (note 9), 413–414.

24. Circular Letter 97, May 12, 1943, NA, RG 112, box 12; Medical Department, U.S. Army, *Internal Medicine in World War II*, vol. 2 (note 9), 412–413. For an example of combined chemotherapy-fever therapy, see Earl C. Lowry and Linus W. Hewitt, "The treatment of sulfonamide resistant gonorrhea—preliminary report," *MS* 93 (July-December 1943): 449–453.

25. Medical Department, U.S. Army, *Internal Medicine in World War II*, vol. 2 (note 9), 414–415. On the low supplies of penicillin well into 1944, see, e.g., Leander W. Riba, Carl J. Schmidlapp, and Nathaniel L. Bosworth, "Use of penicillin for gonorrhea resistant to sulfonamide compounds," *WM* 6 (1944): 72–79; and Herbert M. Ill, "Treatment of gonococcus infection," *MS* 96 (January-June 1945): 78–80. On prophylaxis with sulfathiazole, see Circular Letter no. 146, August 12, 1943, NA, RG 112, box 12. On increasing dosages of sulfathiazole and sulfadiazine, see Circular Letter no. 129, July 22, 1943, NA, RG 112, box 12.

26. Medical Department, U.S. Army, *Internal Medicine in World War II*, vol. 2 (note 9), 415; W.W. Hall, "The present status of the sulfonamides," *MS* 96 (January-June 1945): 457–460, on 459.

27. Medical Department, U.S. Army, *Preventive Medicine in World War II*, vol. 4 (note 1), 26–29 (table 10), 33; Morgan, "Treatment of gonorrhea and syphilis in the United States Army" (note 18), 128.

28. Morgan, "Treatment of gonorrhea and syphilis in the United States Army" (note 18), 128, 130 (quote); Medical Department, U.S. Army, *Internal Medicine in World War II*, vol. 2 (note 9), 1416. On efforts to control venereal diseases among U.S. military personnel in World War II with other than therapeutic methods, see Brandt, *No Magic Bullet* (note 18), 161–171; and Medical Department, U.S. Army, *Preventive Medicine in World War II*, vol. 5, *Communicable Diseases Transmitted through Contact or Unknown Means* (Washington, DC: Office of the Surgeon General, Department of the Army, 1960), 139–331.

29. Medical Department, U.S. Army, *Internal Medicine in World War II*, vol. 2 (note 9), 239–273, on 239: and Medical Department, U.S. Army, *Preventive Medicine in World War II*, vol. 4 (note 1), 191–209, on 191–192. The latter volume, which includes a historical overview of meningococcal meningitis, gives its case mortality rate in World War I as approximately forty percent, on 192.

30. Francis F. Schwentker, Sidney Gelman, and Perrin H. Long, "The treatment of meningococcic meningitis with sulfanilamide: preliminary report," *JAMA* 108 (April 24, 1937): 1407; Medical Department, U.S. Army, *Preventive Medicine in World War II*, vol. 4 (note 1), 200. On the introduction of sulfanilamide in the United States, see chapter 6.

31. Circular Letter no. 52, October 31, 1939, War Department, Office of the Surgeon General, NA, RG 112, box 10; Circular Letter no. 81, December 5, 1940, War Department, Office of the Surgeon General, NA, RG 112, box 11, pp. 4–5.

32. Medical Department, U.S. Army, *Preventive Medicine in World War II*, vol. 4 (note 1), 202. On anxiety about possible meningitis epidemics in the military or civilian population, see, e.g., John H. Dingle and Maxwell Finland, "Diagnosis, treatment, and prevention of meningococcic meningitis," *WM* 2 (January 1942): 1–58, on 1.

33. Medical Department, U.S. Army, *Internal Medicine in World War II*, vol. 2 (note 9), 239–241, 244, 265; Circular Letter no. 17, February 23, 1942, War Department, Office of the Surgeon General, NA, RG 112, box 666, pp. 5–6; Circular Letter no. 119, October 9, 1942, War Department, Office of the Surgeon General, NA, RG 112, box 12. On the transition from sulfa drugs and serum to sulfa drugs alone, see, e.g., Milosh Kasich and Bernard Shulman, "Thirteen cases of meningitis treated with serum and sulfonamides at Station Hospital, Fort Dix, New Jersey," *MS* 90 (1942): 419–424.

34. Medical Department, U.S. Army, *Internal Medicine in World War II*, vol. 2 (note 9), 240–242.

35. Paul S. Strong and Joe M. Blumberg, "The treatment of fifty-six meningococcus carriers with chemotherapy," *MS* 92 (1943): 59–60; William B. Lewis, Herman Bolker, and David Klein, "Mass treatment with sulfadiazine: its effect during an outbreak of meningococcus meningitis," *MS* 93 (1943): 443–447; Joseph F. Painton, "Prophylactic use of sulfadiazine in meningococcic infections," *MS* 95 (1944): 267–269.

36. Medical Department, U.S. Army, *Internal Medicine in World War II*, vol. 2 (note 9), 242.

37. Medical Department, U.S. Army, *Preventive Medicine in World War II*, vol. 4 (note 1), 209; William B. Borden and Paul S. Strong, "Epidemic meningitis: a report of 15 cases at Fort Eustis, Virginia," *MS* 91 (1942): 517–522 (quote on 519); and Joe M. Blumberg and James M. Suter, "Diagnosis of meningococcemia: presentation of three cases," *MS* 94 (1944): 35–40.

38. Medical Department, U.S. Army, *Internal Medicine in World War II*, vol. 2 (note 9), 266–269; Hall, "The present status of the sulfonamides" (note 26), 459; and Aaron Weisberg, "Meningococcemia with four case reports," *MS* 97 (1945): 478–485.

39. Medical Department, U.S. Army, *Internal Medicine in World War II*, vol. 2 (note 9), 242–243, 263–266.

40. Medical Department, U.S. Army, *Preventive Medicine in World War II*, vol. 4 (note 1), 319–320; William Osler, *The Principles and Practice of Medicine, Designed for the Use of Practitioners and Students of Medicine*, 3rd ed. (New York: D. Appleton & Co., 1899), 193.

41. Joseph Felson, "Human convalescent serum and vaccination in the prevention and treatment of bacillary dysentery," *MS* 87 (July-December 1940): 417–423; E.K. Marshall, Jr., A. Calvin Bratton, H.J. White, and J.T. Litchfield, Jr., "Sulfanilylguanidine: a chemotherapeutic agent for intestinal infections," *BJHH* 67 (1940): 163–188 (quote on 163).

42. E.K. Marshall, Jr., A. Calvin Bratton, Lydia B. Edwards, and Ethyl Walker, "Sulfanilylguanidine in the treatment of acute bacillary dysentery in children," *BJHH* 68 (January 1941): 94–111; N. Hamilton Fairley, "Medicine in jungle warfare," *PRSM* 38 (1945): 195–198; G.A.H. Buttle to E.K. Marshall, Jr., February 15, 1941, and March 10, 1941, NA, RG 112; E.H. Cushing to Marshall, April 16, 1941, and Cushing to J.S. Simmons, April 21, 1941, NA, RG 112.

43. G.P. Grabfield to Surgeon General's Office, June 15, 1941, Surgeon General's Office (Lieberman) to Charles T. Young, October 29, 1941, Surgeon General's Office (Lieberman) to G.P. Grabfield, November 6, 1941, and Surgeon General's Office (James S. Simmons) to V.H. Cornell, March 16, 1942, all in NA, RG 112; "Sulfaguanidine," Health Supplies Section, Statistical Division, War Production Board, July 2, 1942, NA, RG 374, 533.1204. On the transition to use of sulfa drugs, see also Joseph Felson, "The prevention and control of infectious diarrheas among military forces," *MS* 91 (July-December 1942): 65–74.

44. Medical Department, U.S. Army, *Preventive Medicine in World War II*, vol. 4 (note 1), 320–335, 340–345.

45. Ibid., 412–413; Ernie Pyle, *Brave Men* (New York: Henry Holt & Co., 1944), 45; "Bacillary dysentery," War Department Technical Bulletin, TB MED 119, *WM* 7 (January 1945): 36–39.

46. Medical Department, U.S. Army, *Preventive Medicine in World War II*, vol. 4 (note 1), 319, 366, 371; Sir Sheldon F. Dudley, *Our National Ill Health Service: An Essay on the Preservation of Health* (London: Watts & Co., 1953), 145–146.

47. Fairley, "Medicine in jungle warfare" (note 42), 195–196; Dudley, *Our National Ill Health Service* (note 46), 146.

48. John W. Adams and Raymond T. Atwood, "Bacillary dysentery: a bacteriologic and clinical analysis of 251 cases occurring in an Army camp," *WM* 5 (January 1944): 14–20; V.H. Cornell, James Watt, and G.J. Dammin, "Sulfaguanidine in the control of Shigella paradysenteriae infections in troops," *MS* 92 (January-June 1943): 253–255; Hyman M. Hurevitz, "Bacillary dysentery," *WM* 6 (October 1944): 247–250; Hall, "The present status of the sulfonamides" (note 26), 459.

49. "Bacillary dysentery," War Department Technical Bulletin, TB MED 119, *WM* 7 (January 1945): 36–39 (quote on 37).

50. Alvin F. Coburn, "The control of streptococcus hemolyticus," *MS* 96 (January 1945): 17–40, on 17–19; Medical Department, U.S. Army, *Preventive Medicine in World War II*, vol. 4 (note 1), 229–230. For a monographic treatment of hemolytic streptococcal infections, see Alvin F. Coburn and Donald C. Young, *The Epidemiology of Hemolytic Streptococcus during World War II in the United States Navy* (Baltimore, MD: Williams & Wilkins Co., 1949).

51. Coburn, "The control of streptococcus hemolyticus" (note 50), 18, 22–23, 26.

52. Ibid., 23–26; Henry M. Lemon, Henry Wise, and Morton Hamburger, "Bacterial content of air in Army barracks: results of a study with especial reference to dispersion of bacteria by the air circulation system," *WM* 6 (August 1944): 92–101.

53. Coburn, "The control of streptococcus hemolyticus" (note 50), 27–28, 38–39.

54. Ibid., 39; Medical Department, U.S. Army, *Preventive Medicine in World War II*, vol. 4 (note 1), 250–251; Harry F. Dowling, *Fighting Infection: Conquests of the Twentieth Century* (Cambridge, MA: Harvard University Press, 1977), 112. On mass prophylaxis to prevent meningitis, see pages 231–232.

55. Coburn, "The control of streptococcus hemolyticus" (note 50), 29–37.

56. Ibid., 29–40 (quote on 40).

57. Medical Department, U.S. Army, *Preventive Medicine in World War II*, vol. 4 (note 1), 233–234, 252; Coburn, "The control of streptococcus hemolyticus" (note 50), 37–39; Dowling, *Fighting Infection* (note 54), 112–113.

58. Medical Department, U.S. Army, *Preventive Medicine in World War II*, vol. 4 (note 1), 229–257, esp. 232–233, 250–252.

59. Ibid., 233–234, 236–237; Herbert J. Fox, "Penicillin program at the United States Naval Hospital, Portsmouth, Va.: observations and results," *WM* 7 (March 1945): 170–172.

60. See chapter 9.

61. "The new drug and the war," *Baltimore Sun*, December 14, 1939; "The chemotherapy of infected war wounds," *JAMA* 113 (December 16, 1939): 223; "War wounds and microorganisms," *JAMA* 114 (March 9, 1940): 904.

62. "The chemotherapy of war wounds," *JAMA* 114 (April 27, 1940): 1683–1684; "The use of sulfonamide derivatives in the army," *JAMA* 115 (October 12, 1940): 1291; "The chemotherapy of war wounds," *JAMA* 115 (December 21, 1940): 2194.

63. N.K. Jensen, L.W. Johnsrud, and M.C. Nelson, "Local implantation of sulfanilamide in compound fractures," *Surgery* 6 (1939): 1–12; Edgar J. Poth, "Succinylsulfathiazole: an adjuvant in surgery of the large bowel," *JAMA* 120 (1942): 265–269, on 268; John F. Anderson to Col. Shook, "Memorandum concerning the local use of sulfonamide derivatives," November 28, 1940; and C.F. Shook to John F. Anderson (quote), December 4, 1940, both in NA, RG 112, box 50.

64. Mohler, "The therapeutic use of sulfanilamide and related compounds" (note 12), 477; Circular Letter no. 81, December 5, 1940, War Department, Office of the Surgeon General, NA, RG 112, box 11, p. 8; George R. Hazel to F.C. Tyng, January 9, 1941, Tyng to Hazel, January 14, 1941, and Hazel to Tyng, January 21, 1941, all in NA, RG 112; and memorandum, C.C. Hillmen to Walter M. Harrison, July 24, 1941, NA, RG 112; E.L. Cook, Memorandum for Finance and Supply Division, September 5, 1941, NA, RG 112.

65. See, e.g., G.B. Reed and J.H. Orr, "Local chemotherapy of experimental gas gangrene," *WM* 2 (1942): 59–78; Theodore H. Sweetser, "Treatment of war wounds based on their bacteriology," *MS* 89 (July-December 1941): 17–24; Warner F. Bowers, "Healing of wounds," *MS* 90 (January-June 1942): 140–152; Leonard Weiner, "The local use of sulfanilamide and sulfathiazole in extraction wounds: a preliminary report," *MS* 90 (January–June 1942): 157–164; and Hall G. Holder and Eaton M. Mackay, "Wound therapy," *MS* 90 (January-June 1942): 509–518. On the Subcommittee on Surgical Infections' views, and on John Moorhead, see chapter 9.

66. Circular Letter no. 10, February 9, 1942, War Department, Office of the Surgeon General, NA, RG 112, box 12; Circular Letter no. 17, February 23, 1942, War Department, Office of the Surgeon General, NA, RG 112, box 666; E.L. Cook to Commanding General, Army Air Forces, March 27, 1942, NA, RG 112.

67. "Prevention of infection in wounds and burns," *WM* 2 (1942): 488–496 (quote on 489–490).

68. M.J. Aston, "Wartime experiences aboard a naval hospital ship," *MS* 94 (January–June 1944): 157–160. Other examples of wartime reports by medical officers reflecting practices in 1942 are Merle W. Ogle, "Chemotherapy in gunshot wounds of the face, neck,

and jaws," *MS* 90 (January-June 1942): 650–655; Oscar A. Turner, "The care and treatment of wartime injuries to the head: a review of some recent literature," *MS* 92 (January-June 1943): 473–490; L.D. Heaton, "Abdominal war wounds," *MS* 93 (July-December 1943): 22–25; and Robert M. Hardaway, "Treatment of war wounds," *MS* 95 (July-December 1944): 37–42.

69. Circular Letter no. 164, November 28, 1942, War Department, Services of Supply, Office of the Surgeon General, NA, RG 112, box 12.

70. G. Ward Crampton to James C. Magee, August 10, 1942; E.L. Cook to L.L. Gardner, August 22, 1942; and Gardner to Crampton, August 29, 1942, all in NA, RG 112.

71. Circular Letter no. 17, February 23, 1942, War Department, Office of the Surgeon General, NA, RG 112, box 666, pp. 15–21.

72. E.W. Archibald to J.C. Magee, October 5, 1942; James C. Magee to E.W. Archibald, October 13, 1942, both in NA, RG 112.

73. James F. Kelly to Henry L. Stimson, October 6, 1942, NA, RG 112. On the beginnings of the NRC study, see chapter 9.

74. James F. Kelly to Henry L. Stimson, October 6, 1942, NA, RG 112.

75. Peter M. Keating and Frank M. Davis, "Prophylactic treatment of wounds in war," *MS* 86 (January-June 1940): 235–240; Warner F. Bowers, "Healing of wounds," *MS* 90 (January-June 1942): 140–152, on 150; Operations Branch, Attorney General's Office to Surgeon General's Office (draft of reply), October 20, 1942, NA, RG 112.

76. John S. Lockwood, "Definition of objectives, and the importance of controls in evaluating the local use of sulfonamides in wounds," *SGO* 79 (1944): 1–9. On the background and plan of the study, see chapter 9, section on "Preparation."

77. Frank L. Meleney, "A statistical analysis of a study of the prevention of infection in soft part wounds, compound fractures, and burns with special reference to the sulfonamides," *SGO* 80 (1945): 263–296, on 264–265, 295.

78. Frank L. Meleney, "The prevention of infection in accidental wounds," in E.C. Andrus, D.W. Bronk, G.A. Carden, C.S. Keefer, J.S. Lockwood, J.T. Wearn, and M.C. Winternitz, editors, *Advances in Military Medicine* (Boston, MA: Little, Brown & Co., 1948), 95–110, on 99.

79. Meleney, "A statistical analysis" (note 77), 295.

80. Ibid., 295; Meleney, "The prevention of infection in accidental wounds" (note 78), 102–103, 105–106, 108.

81. Meleney, "A statistical analysis" (note 77), 264, 296.

82. Ibid., 263, 264, 265, 270–271, 295.

83. John S. Lockwood, "War-time activities of the National Research Council and the Committee on Medical Research; with particular reference to teamwork on studies of wounds and burns," *AS* 124 (1946): 314–327, on 321–323; Meleney, "The prevention of infections in accidental wounds" (note 78), 108–109; and John Winslow Hirshfeld, "The application of penicillin to surgical problems," in Andrus et al., editors, *Advances in Military Medicine* (note 78), 123–133, on 124, 132. On penicillin in treatment of burns, see Oliver Cope, "The burn problems," in *Advances in Military Medicine*, 149–158, on 157–158.

84. Frank L. Meleney, "The study of the prevention of infection in contaminated accidental wounds, compound fractures and burns," *AS* 118 (1943): 171–186.

85. Lockwood, "Definition of objectives" (note 76), 1–2, 4.

86. Champ Lyons, "The re-evaluation of sulfa drugs," *MS* 95 (July–December 1944): 301–304; W.W. Hall, "The present status of the sulfonamides," *MS* 96 (January–June 1945): 457–460.

87. Lyons, "The re-evaluation of sulfa drugs" (note 86); Hall, "The present status of the sulfonamides" (note 86), 458.

88. See, e.g., Joseph Fetterman, "Factors in recovery from injuries to the head," *WM* 5 (April 1944): 232–237; James D. O'Connor, "Massive craniocerebral trauma from airplane propeller: report of a case with recovery," *WM* 5 (June 1944): 383–384; Edward Gallardo, "Sensitivity of bacteria from infected wounds to penicillin," *WM* 6 (August 1944): 86–91; R.R. Barondes and F.G. Drischel, "Treatment of war wounds with the sulfonamides," *MS* 93 (July–December 1943): 72–77; R.I. Harris, "Treatment of war fractures," *MS* 94 (January–June 1944): 246–250; and Robert M. Hardaway, "Treatment of war wounds," *MS* 95 (July–December 1944): 37–42.

89. Jerome F. Grunnagle, "Early treatment of open wounds," *WM* 8 (1945): 376–381.

90. H.A. Barnes, "Observations in frontal area surgery," *MS* 97 (July–December 1945): 285–288.

91. E.S. Groseclose, "Troop casualties aboard an attack transport," *MS* 97 (July–December 1945): 100–105.

92. M. Baldwin and C.W. Reynolds, "The treatment of battle casualties in the initial phases of the operations at Iwo Jima Island," *MS* 97 (July–December 1945): 288–297. On treatment of burns from 1943 to the end of the war, see also Lockwood, "Definition of objectives" (note 76), 8; Lockwood, "War-time activities" (note 83), 323–325; Louis H. Roddis, "Burns incident to war: measures for their prevention and for treatment," *MS* 94 (January–June 1944): 65–75; Frederic L. Conklin, "Burns," *MS* 96 (January–June 1945): 139–142; and Somers H. Sturgis, "Observations on physiology, metabolism, and treatment of a severe burn," *MS* 97 (July-December 1945): 215–224.

93. Quoted in Lockwood, "War-time activities" (note 83), 322.

94. Ibid., 326.

95. On the organization of medical services in the field see, e.g., "Medical care in the combat zones," *MR* 52(1) (January 1943): 3; James C. Magee, "An appraisal of the Medical Department at war," *MS* 92 (February 1943): 113–119; Isador Ripps, "Medical service in the combat zone," *MR* 54(3) (July 1945): 12–15; and Pyle, *Brave Men* (note 45), 51–57.

96. Pyle, *Brave Men* (note 45), 143.

97. Ernie Pyle, *Here Is Your War* (New York: Henry Holt & Co., 1943), 72–73. On the importance of early medical attention, especially by aid men, for morale, see also Ripps, "Medical service in the combat zone" (note 95), 13–14; and Bill Mauldin, *Up Front* (New York: Henry Holt & Co., 1945), 117–125.

Chapter 11

1. See, e.g., Champ Lyons, "The re-evaluation of sulfa drugs," *MS* 95 (July–December 1944): 301–304; and W.W. Hall, "The present status of the sulfonamides," *MS* 96 (January-June 1945): 457–460. On the Woods-Fildes theory, see pages 256–262.

2. Gerhard Domagk, "Ein Beitrag zur Chemotherapie der bakteriellen Infektionen," *DMW* 61 (1935): 250–253; Domagk, "Untersuchungen über die Bedeutung des retikuloendothelialen Systems für die Vernichtung von Infektionserregern und für die Entstehung des Amyloids," *Virchow's Archiv für Pathologische Anatomie und Physiologie und für Klinische Medizin* 235 (1924): 594–638. On German clinicians' views, see Daniel Bovet, *Une chimie qui guérit: histoire de la découverte des sulfamides* (Paris: Éditions Payot, 1988): 122–123; and Marcel H. Bickel, "The development of sulfonamides (1932–1938) as a focal point in the history of chemotherapy," *Gesnerus* 45 (1988): 67–86, on 77–78.

3. On the Pasteur Institute's findings, see chapter 6.

4. Bovet, *Une chimie qui guérit* (note 2), 240–241. For an early example of uncertainty and of the multiple hypotheses under consideration, see Leonard Colebrook and Meave Kenny, "Treatment of human puerperal infections, and of experimental infections in mice, with Prontosil," *Lancet* 230 (January–June 1936): 1279–1286.

5. Marcel H. Bickel, "Eli K. Marshall, Jr. (1884–1966): from biochemistry and physiology to pharmacology and pharmacokinetics," *Drug Metabolism Reviews* 28 (3) (1996): 311–344, esp. 320–323; A. McGehee Harvey, "The story of chemotherapy at Johns Hopkins: Perrin H. Long, Eleanor A. Bliss, and E. Kennerly Marshall, Jr.," *Johns Hopkins Medical Journal* 138 (1976): 54–60; and "February 8, 1953: E.K. Marshall, Jr.'s assessment of his own scientific work," in E.K. Marshall, biographical file, AMCMA, pp. 4–5.

6. Bovet, *Une chimie qui guérit* (note 2), 235–236; Colebrook and Kenny, "Treatment of human puerperal infections" (note 4); Leonard Colebrook, G.A.H. Buttle, and R.A.Q. O'Meara, "The mode of action of p-aminobenzenesulphonamide and Prontosil in hemolytic streptococcal infections," *Lancet* 231 (July-December 1936): 1323–1326; and Eleanor A. Bliss and Perrin H. Long, "Observations on the mode of action of sulfanilamide," *JAMA* (November 6, 1937): 1524–1528.

7. Perrin H. Long and Eleanor A. Bliss, *The Clinical and Experimental Use of Sulfanilamide, Sulfapyridine, and Allied Compounds* (New York: Macmillan Co., 1939), 85–115 (quotes on 85–86).

8. Ibid., 139–141. See also Philip Shaffer, "The mode of action of sulphanilamid [*sic*]," *Science* 89 (June 16, 1939): 547–550; and Arthur Locke, E.R. Main, and R.R. Mellon, "Anti-catalase and the mechanism of sulfanilamide action," *Science* 88 (December 30, 1938): 620–621.

9. Long and Bliss, *The Clinical and Experimental Use of Sulfanilamide* (note 7), 133–135.

10. Ibid., 135–136.

11. John S. Lockwood, Alvin F. Coburn, and Herbert E. Stokinger, "Studies on the mechanism of the action of sulfanilamide. I. The bearing of the character of the lesion on the effectiveness of the drug," *JAMA* 111 (1938): 2259–2264.

12. John S. Lockwood, "Studies on the mechanism of the action of sulfanilamide. III. The effect of sulfanilamide in serum and blood on hemolytic streptococci in vitro," *Journal of Immunology* 35 (1938): 155–193 (quotes on 187–188).

13. Long and Bliss, *The Clinical and Experimental Use of Sulfanilamide* (note 7), 137, 139, 141.

14. The last assertion, developed on pages 255–256 and 260–261, supports Bovet's view. See Bovet, *Une chimie qui guérit* (note 2), 236–237.

15. Lionel Whitby, "Chemotherapy of bacterial infections," *Lancet* ii (November 12, 1938): 1095–1103.

16. James McIntosh and Lionel E.H. Whitby, "The mode of action of drugs of the sulfonamide group," *Lancet* i (1939): 431–435 (quote on 435).

17. T.C. Stamp, "Bacteriostatic action of sulfanilamide in vitro," *Lancet* ii (July 1, 1939): 10–17.

18. Alexander Fleming, "Observations on the bacteriostatic action of sulphanilamide and M&B 693 and on the influence thereon of bacteria and peptone," *Journal of Pathology and Bacteriology* 50 (1940): 69–81, esp. 77–81.

19. H.N. Green, "The mode of action of sulphanilamide. With special reference to a bacterial growth-stimulating factor ("P factor") obtained from *Br. abortus* and other bacteria," *BJEP* 21 (1940): 38–64.

20. Ibid., 40–64.

21. D.D. Woods and P. Fildes, "The anti-sulphanilamide activity (in vitro) of p-aminobenzoic acid and related compounds" (abstract), *Chemistry and Industry* 18 (February 24, 1940): 133–134; and Donald D. Woods, "The biochemical mode of action of the sulphonamide drugs," *Journal of General Microbiology* 29 (1962): 687–702, on 696–697.

22. Robert E. Kohler, "Bacterial physiology: the medical context," *BHM* 59 (1985): 54–74.

23. Ernest F. Gale and Paul Fildes, "Donald Devereux Woods," *BMFRS* 11 (1965): 203–219, on 203–206. On Marjory Stephenson's school, see Robert E. Kohler, "Innovation in normal science: bacterial physiology," *Isis* 76 (1985): 162–181.

24. Woods, "The biochemical mode of action" (note 21), 691–692. On Whitby and McIntosh's work on the mode of action of the sulfonamides, see page 255.

25. Paul Fildes, "A rational approach to research in chemotherapy," *Lancet* 238 (1940): 955–957; Kohler, "Bacterial physiology" (note 22), 71.

26. Woods, "The biochemical mode of action" (note 21), 691–692. On Stamp's paper, see also pages 255–256.

27. Ibid., 691.

28. Ibid., 691–693.

29. Ibid., 688, 692.

30. Ibid., 693; D.D. Woods, "The relation of p-aminobenzoic acid to the mechanism of the action of sulphanilamide," *BJEP* 21 (1940): 74–90.

31. Woods, "The relation of p-aminobenzoic acid to the mechanism of the action of sulphanilamide" (note 30); Woods, "The biochemical mode of action" (note 21), 693–695. On Green, see page 256.

32. Woods, "The relation of p-aminobenzoic acid to the mechanism of the action of sulphanilamide" (note 30), 82–83; Woods, "The biochemical mode of action of the sulphonamide drugs" (note 21), 695.

33. Woods, "The relation of p-aminobenzoic acid to the mechanism of the action of sulphanilamide" (note 30), 83–88 (quote on 88); Woods, "The biochemical mode of action" (note 21), 695 (quote).

34. Stamp, "Bacteriostatic action of sulfanilamide in vitro" (note 17), 10. On Stamp, see also pages 255–256.

35. Kohler, "Bacterial physiology" (note 22), 72.

36. Fildes, "A rational approach to research in chemotherapy" (note 25), 955.

37. Ibid., 956–957.

38. Hans Molitor, "The experimental evaluation of sulfanilamide derivatives," *MR*, 48(3) (July 1939): 24–27 (quotes on 27). See also, e.g., Whitby, "Chemotherapy of bacterial infections" (note 15); and Long and Bliss, *The Clinical and Experimental Use of Sulfanilamide* (note 7), 86. F. Sherwood Taylor attempted to convey the urgency of achieving an understanding of the mode of action of the sulfa drugs to a lay audience in *The Conquest of Bacteria: From Salvarsan to Sulphapyridine* (New York: Philosophical Library and Alliance Book Corp., 1942), 162–163.

39. John S. Lockwood, "Sulfanilamide in surgical infections: its possibilities and limitations," *JAMA* 115 (October 5, 1940): 1190–1195; Lockwood, "Sulfonamide therapy as an aid to surgery," *SGO* 72 (1941): 307–311; Lockwood, "Progress toward an understanding of the mode of chemotherapeutic action of sulfonamide compounds," in *Chemotherapy*, University of Pennsylvania Bicentennial Conference (Philadelphia, PA: University of Pennsylvania Press, 1941), 9–28, esp. 21–26.

40. See esp. Elmore H. Northey, *The Sulfonamides and Allied Compounds* (New York: Reinhold Publishing Corp., 1948), 5, 483. See also Lyons, "The re-evaluation of sulfa drugs" (note 1): 301–304; Bernard D. Davis, "New biologic concepts derived from research on sulfonamide drugs," *NEJM* 230 (1944): 734–739, on 736; Alvin F. Coburn, "The control of streptococcus hemolyticus," *MS* 96 (January–June 1945): 17–40, on 27–28; W.W. Hall, "The present status of the sulfonamides," *MS* 96 (January–June 1945): 457–460, on 457; F. Hawking and F.H.K. Green, editors, *The Medical Use of*

Sulphonamides, Medical Research Council War Memorandum no. 10 (London: His Majesty's Stationery Office, 1945), 8–9; D.W. Woolley, "Some aspects of biochemical antagonism," in David E. Green, editor, *Currents in Biochemical Research* (New York: Interscience Publishers Inc., 1946), 357–377, on 365–367; and René Dubos, *The Bacterial Cell in Its Relation to Problems of Virulence, Immunity and Chemotherapy* (Cambridge, MA: Harvard University Press, 1947), 277, 282–286, 335–336.

41. For expressions of optimism see, e.g., E.K. Marshall, Jr., "Bacterial chemotherapy," *Annual Review of Physiology* 3 (1941): 643–670, on 661; and Sir Henry Dale, "General introductory remarks," to "Modes of drug action: a general discussion," *Transactions of the Faraday Society* 39 (1943): 319–322. On the search for new antibacterial agents, see, e.g., E.M. Lourie, "A sketch of the history of chemotherapy," *British Medical Bulletin* 4 (1946): 241–248, on 247; Dubos, *The Bacterial Cell* (note 40), 311–315, 335–336; Rollin D. Hotchkiss, "Chemotherapy: applied cytochemistry," in Green, editor, *Currents in Biochemical Research* (note 40), 379–398, on 384–386; Northey, *The Sulfonamides and Allied Compounds* (note 40), 5, 483; and D.D. Woods: "Microorganisms and vitamin research," in David E. Green and W. Eugene Knox, editors, *Research in Medical Science* (New York: Macmillan Co., 1950), 167–183, on 179.

42. Department for Research in Bacterial Chemistry, Annual Reports for 1939–1940, 1940–1941, in MRC, file 1300/1, vol. 4; and D.W. Woolley, *A Study of Antimetabolites* (New York: John Wiley & Sons Inc., 1952), 8. For a summary of Fildes's work on indoleacrylic acid and tryptophan, see Richard O. Roblin, Jr., "Metabolite antagonists," *Chemical Reviews* 38 (1946): 255–377, on 264.

43. Department for Research in Bacterial Chemistry, Annual Reports for 1941–1942, 1942–1943, 1943–1944, in MRC, file 1300/1, vol. IV; Woolley, *A Study of Antimetabolites* (note 42), 8–9.

44. Richard J. Henry, "The mode of action of sulfonamides," *Bacteriological Reviews* 7 (1943): 175–262; Northey, *The Sulfonamides and Allied Compounds* (note 40), 484, 510; F. Hawking and J. Stewart Lawrence, *The Sulphonamides* (New York: Grune & Statton, 1951), 64.

45. For a survey of theories of the mechanism of action of the sulfa drugs to 1948, see Northey, *The Sulfonamides and Allied Compounds* (note 40), 466–511. Northey's discussion of Bell and Roblin's theory is on 495–500, 511.

46. Lockwood, "Progress" (note 39), 26. On the antimetabolite concept, see Woolley, *A Study of Antimetabolites* (note 42). On antimetabolite ideas in cancer research, see pages 265–268.

47. On the biochemical uses of antimetabolites, see Richard O. Roblin, Jr., "Metabolite antagonists," *Chemical Reviews* 38 (1946): 255–377; and Woolley, *A Study of Antimetabolites* (note 42), esp. 198–211.

48. Woolley, *A Study of Antimetabolites* (note 42), esp. 1–19. See also Northey, *The Sulfonamides and Allied Compounds* (note 40), 484.

49. Jörgen Lehmann, "Para-aminosalicylic acid in the treatment of tuberculosis," *Lancet* i (January 5, 1946): 15–16; Woolley, *A Study of Antimetabolites* (note 42), 172, 194–195.

50. Therapeutic Trials Committee of the Swedish National Association against Tuberculosis, "Para-aminosalicylic acid treatment in pulmonary tuberculosis: comparison between 94 treated and 82 untreated cases," *American Review of Tuberculosis* 61 (1950): 597–612; William B. Tucker, "The evolution of the cooperative studies in the chemotherapy of tuberculosis of the Veteran's Administration and Armed forces of the U.S.A.," *Advances in Tuberculosis Research* 10 (1960): 1–68; Harry F. Dowling, *Fighting Infection: Conquests of the Twentieth Century* (Cambridge, MA: Harvard University Press, 1977), 167.

51. George H. Hitchings, Gertrude B. Elion, Elvira A. Falco, Peter B. Russell, and Henry Vander Werff, "Studies on analogs of purines and pyrimidines," in *Antimetabolites, Annals of the New York Academy of Sciences* 52 (July 7, 1950): 1197–1378, on 1318–1335; and George H. Hitchings, "A biochemical approach to chemotherapy," *Drug Intelligence and Clinical Pharmacy* 16 (1982): 843–848.

52. George H. Hitchings and Gertrude B. Elion, "The chemistry and biochemistry of purine analogs," in Roy Waldo Miner, editor, *6-Mercaptopurine, Annals of the New York Academy of Sciences* 60 (December 6, 1954): 183–508, on 195–199.

53. Y. SubbaRow et al., "Folic acid," *Annals of the New York Academy of Sciences* 48 (1946): 255–350; T.H. Jukes, A.L. Franklin, and E.L.R. Stockstad, "Pteroylglutamic acid antagonists," in *Antimetabolites* (note 51), 1336–1341; C. Chester Stock, John J. Biesele, Joseph H. Burchenal, David A. Karnovsky, Alice E. Moore, and Kanematsu Sugiura, "Folic acid analogs and experimental tumors," in *Antimetabolites* (note 51), 1369–1378. Woolley, *A Study of Antimetabolites* (note 42), 41–43, 77–78, 166, 179–181, 204–205; Sidney Farber et al., "Temporary remissions in acute leukemia in children produced by folic acid antagonist, 4-aminopteroylglutamic acid (aminopterin)," *NEJM* 238 (June 3, 1948): 787–793; and Cynthia P. Margolies and Kenneth B. McCredie, *Understanding Leukemia* (New York: Charles Scribner's Sons, 1983), 85.

54. C. Chester Stock et al., "Folic acid analogs and experimental tumors" (note 53), 1360; George Bosworth Brown, "The biosynthesis of nucleic acids as a basis for an approach to chemotherapy," in *6-Mercaptopurine* (note 52), 185–194; and R. Wayne Rundles and John A. Crago, "6-Mercaptopurine in neoplastic disease," in *6-Mercaptopurine* (note 52), 425–429. On the Sloan-Kettering program, see R.F. Bud, "Strategy in American cancer research after World War II: a case study," *Social Studies of Science* 8 (1978): 425–459.

55. George H. Hitchings and Gertrude B. Elion, "The chemistry and biochemistry of purine analogs" (note 52), 196–198; Rundles and Crago, "6-Mercaptopurine in neoplastic disease" (note 54), 425–429; and Joseph H. Burchenal, R.R. Ellison, M.L. Murphy, D.A. Karnovsky, M.P. Sykes, T.C. Tan, A.C. Mermann, M. Yuceoglu, W.P.L. Myers, I. Krakoff, and A. Alberstadt, "Clinical studies on 6-mercaptopurine," in *6-Mercaptopurine* (note 52), 359–368. For other early experimental and clinical reports on 6-mercaptopurine, see the same collection, Roy Waldo Miner, editor, *6-Mercaptopurine* (note 52). On the place of 6-mercaptopurine in the chemotherapy of leukemia, see, e.g., Margolies and McCredie, *Understanding Leukemia* (note 53), 86–87, 91.

56. S.R.M. Bushby and G.H. Hitchings, "Trimethoprim, a sulphonamide inhibitor," *British Journal of Pharmacology and Chemotherapy* 33 (1968): 72–90; James J. Burchall, "The development of the diaminopyrimidines," *Journal of Antimicrobial Chemotherapy* 5 (suppl. B, 1979): 3–14.

57. Bushby and Hitchings, "Trimethoprim" (note 56), 72–73, 86–88; Burchall, "The development of the diaminopyrimidines" (note 56), 6.

58. Adrian J. Salter, "Trimethoprim-sulfamethoxazole: an assessment of more than 12 years of use," *Reviews of Infectious Diseases* 4 (1982): 196–236, on 197.

59. Bushby and Hitchings, "Trimethoprim" (note 56), 87 (quote); Burchall, "The development of the diaminopyrimidines" (note 56), 7–8, 11.

Chapter 12

1. Lionel Whitby, "Chemotherapy of bacterial infections," *Lancet* (November 12, 1938): 1095–1103, on 1095; Eli Kennerly Marshall, Jr., "Medical research: the story of sulfanilamide," *North Carolina Medical Journal* 1 (1940): 125–129; C.R. Addinall, "Fifty years' progress in medicinal chemistry," *MR* 50(1) (January 1941): 13–16; Ronald D.

Mann, *Modern Drug Use: An Enquiry on Historical Principles* (Lancaster: MTP Press Ltd., 1984): 556; Lewis Thomas, *The Youngest Science: Notes of a Medicine-Watcher* (New York: Viking Press, 1983): 35. For a compact description of treatment of lobar pneumonia before type-specific serum and the sulfa drugs—"a therapeutic skirmish with fate"—see M.R. Dinkelspiel, "Fifty years of medical progress: some historic bequests to the patient," *MR* 50(1) (January 1941): 8–11. On the impact of the sulfa drugs and antibiotics on morbidity and death from serious bacteremic infections at Boston City Hospital, see also Maxwell Finland, "Changing patterns of susceptibility of common bacterial pathogens to antimicrobial agents," *AIM* 76 (1972): 1009–1036, on 1019.

2. Nicholas Wells, *Medicines: 50 Years of Progress 1930–1980* (London: Office of Health Economics, 1980), 5–11 (quote on 10); Mann, *Modern Drug Use* (note 1), 556. For a similar view, see also M.A.F. Lake, "25 years of sulphapyridine," *Chemist and Druggist* (October 26, 1963). My copy is an unpaginated reprint of 4 pp.

3. Harry F. Dowling, *Fighting Infection: Conquests of the Twentieth Century* (Cambridge, MA: Harvard University Press, 1977). 228–249. On the numerous factors affecting overall mortality rates, see also Irene B. Taeubner and Conrad Taeubner, *People of the United States in the 20th Century* (U.S. Bureau of the Census Monograph, Washington, DC: U.S. Government Printing Office, 1971), 495–579, esp. 517–518. On the difficulties involved in interpreting the causes behind the epidemiological transition, see also Gerald N. Grob, *The Deadly Truth: A History of Disease in America* (Cambridge, MA: Harvard University Press, 2002), 200–216.

4. Andrea F. Balis, *Miracle Medicine: The Impact of Sulfa Drugs on Medicine, the Pharmaceutical Industry and Government Regulation in the U.S. in the 1930s* (Ph.D. dissertation, New York: City University of New York, 2000), 7–15, 107; Irvine Loudon, *Death in Childbirth: An International Study of Maternal Care and Maternal Mortality, 1800–1950* (New York: Oxford University Press, 1992), 254–273; and Loudon, *The Tragedy of Childbed Fever* (New York: Oxford University Press, 2000), 169–188. Loudon concludes that the introduction of the sulfa drugs began a trend that "transformed the process of childbirth" (*Death in Childbirth*, 271–272).

5. Merck & Co. Inc., "Backgrounder 3. Drug Research" (December, 1959), MA, box R7-4.8.1, p. 4.

6. Harry F. Dowling, "Frustration and foundation: management of pneumonia before antibiotics," *JAMA* 220 (June 5, 1972): 1341–1345; Dowling, *Fighting Infection* (note 3), 192. On the transition from serotherapy to chemotherapy, see Scott H. Podolsky, *Pneumonia Before Antibiotics: Therapeutic Evolution and Evaluation in Twentieth-Century America* (Baltimore, MD: Johns Hopkins University Press, forthcoming).

7. W. Michael Scheld and Gerald L. Mandell, "Sulfonamides and meningitis," *JAMA* 251 (February 10, 1984): 791–794.

8. Percy Stokes, "Vital statistics of 1942," *Lancet* (May 29, 1943): 672–675. On the sulfa drugs in the U.S. military during World War II, see pages 225–250.

9. James Harvey Young, "The 'Elixir Sulfanilamide' Disaster," *Emery University Quarterly* 14 (1958): 230–237; Thomas, *The Youngest Science* (note 1), 26–35, on 28.

10. Balis, *Miracle Medicine* (note 4), 76–123; Podolsky, *Pneumonia before Antibiotics* (note 6).

11. G.M. Maxwell, "Sulphanilamide and the doctor," *JAMA* 112 (March 27, 1939): 28. I have omitted ten lines in this quotation.

12. Dowling, *Fighting Infection* (note 3), 113–114; Balis, *Miracle Medicine* (note 4), 7–15, 107–114, 237–239; Rosemary Stevens, *In Sickness and in Wealth: American Hospitals in the Twentieth Century* (Baltimore, MD: Johns Hopkins University Press, 1989), 177–178, 206; John C. Burnham, "American medicine's golden age: what happened to it?"

Science 215 (March 19, 1982): 1474–1479. On the U.S. reception of sulfanilamide and sulfapyridine, see chapters 6 and 7.

13. Walsh McDermott, with David E. Rogers, "Social ramifications of control of microbial disease," *Johns Hopkins Medical Journal* 151 (1982): 302–312. McDermott gives a vivid description of the typical distribution of cases on the male medical ward at Bellevue Hospital in New York City in the early 1930s, on 305–306.

14. Balis, *Miracle Medicine* (note 4), 241–242.

15. McDermott and Rogers, "Social ramifications" (note 13), 308–309.

16. John P. Swann, *Academic Scientists and the Pharmaceutical Industry: Cooperative Research in Twentieth Century America* (Baltimore, MD: Johns Hopkins University Press, 1988); Swann, "The evolution of the American pharmaceutical industry," *PH* 37 (1995): 76–86; Balis, *Miracle Medicine* (note 4), 27–75; 160–164; David L. Cowen, "The on-going pharmaceutical revolution: the role of the industry," in *Farmacia e industrializacion: libro homenaje al Doctor Guillermo Folch Jou* (Madrid: Sociedad Española de Historia de la Farmacia, 1985), 95–104, on 98; Wells, *Medicines* (note 2), 10–11; Louis Lasagna, "1938–1968: the FDA, the drug industry, the medical profession, and the public," in John B. Blake, editor, *Safeguarding the Public: Historical Aspects of Medicinal Drug Control* (Baltimore, MD: Johns Hopkins University Press, 1970), 171–179, on 171; Jordan Goodman, "Pharmaceutical industry," in Roger Cooter and John Pickstone, editors, *Companion to Medicine in the Twentieth Century* (London: Routledge, 2000), 141–154; and chapter 8.

17. Louis Galambos with Jane Eliot Sewell, *Networks of Innovation: Vaccine Development at Merck, Sharp & Dohme, and Mulford, 1895–1995* (Cambridge: Cambridge University Press, 1995), 35–38; Wesley W. Spink, *Infectious Diseases: Prevention and Treatment in the Nineteenth and Twentieth Centuries* (Minneapolis: University of Minnesota Press, 1978), 65. On the example of meningococcal vaccines, see, e.g., Martha L. Lepow and Ronald Gold, "Further conquest of the meningococcus," *NEJM* 297 (1977): 721–722.

18. Cowen, "The on-going pharmaceutical revolution" (note 16), 95–97; Lasagna, "1938–1968" (note 16), 171; Peter Temin, *Taking Your Medicine: Drug Regulation in the United States* (Cambridge, MA: Harvard University Press, 1980), 5–6; Galambos and Sewell, *Networks of Innovation* (note 17); and Elizabeth Siegel Watkins, *On the Pill: A Social History of Oral Contraceptives 1950–1970* (Baltimore, MD: Johns Hopkins University Press, 1998), 23–24.

19. See chapters 8 and 9, and Lasagna, "1938–1968" (note 16), 171.

20. Wells, *Medicines* (note 2), 10–11; Dowling, "Frustration and foundation" (note 6), 1341–1345; Dowling, *Fighting Infection* (note 3), 113–114.

21. Iago Galdston, *Behind the Sulfa Drugs: A Short History of Chemotherapy* (New York: D. Appleton-Century Co., 1943), viii–ix, xv–xvi. On early American and British press coverage, see chapters 6 and 8.

22. "Freedom from disease in fifty years' time?" *Birmingham Gazette*, July 4, 1938; Henry E. Sigerist, "Foreword," in F. Sherwood Taylor, *The Conquest of Bacteria: From Salvarsan to Sulphapyridine* (New York: Philosophical Library, 1942); Dowling, "Frustration and foundation" (note 6), 1343; Wells, *Medicines* (note 2), 11–12; Marcel H. Bickel, "The development of sulfonamides (1932–1938) as a focal point in the history of chemotherapy," *Gesnerus* 45 (1988): 67–86, on 79.

23. Boris Sokoloff, *The Miracle Drugs* (Chicago: Ziff-Davis Publishing Co., 1949), 247. See also Samuel Epstein and Beryl Williams, *Miracles from Microbes: The Road to Streptomycin* (New Brunswick, NJ: Rutgers University Press, 1946). On the popular reception of penicillin in the United States, see David P. Adams, "The penicillin mystique and the popular press (1935–1950)," *PH* 26 (1984): 134–142.

24. Richard O. Roblin, Jr., "Chemotherapy," in David E. Green and W. Eugene Knox, editors, *Research in Medical Science* (New York: Macmillan Co., 1950), 154–165 (quotes on 154). The mood of optimism generated by the success of the sulfa drugs and penicillin also helped to motivate the search for and acceptance of contraceptives in pill form. See Watkins, *On the Pill* (note 18), 19–20.

25. See chapter 7, and Harry M. Marks, *The Progress of Experiment: Science and Therapeutic Reform in the United States, 1900–1990* (Cambridge: Cambridge University Press, 1997), 71–97, 138, 149–150; J. Rosser Matthews, *Quantification and the Quest for Medical Certainty* (Princeton, NJ: Princeton University Press, 1995), 131–140, 145; James Harvey Young, *The Medical Messiahs: A Social History of Health Quackery in Twentieth-Century America* (Princeton, NJ: Princeton University Press, 1992), 408–422; Lasagna, "1938–1968" (note 16); and Morton Mintz, *The Therapeutic Nightmare* (Boston, MA: Houghton-Mifflin Co., 1965), 50–53.

26. Dale E. Cooper, "Adequate controls for new drugs: good manufacturing practice and the 1938 Federal Food, Drug, and Cosmetic Act," *PH* 44 (2002): 12–23. On the sulfathiazole episode, see also John P. Swann, "The 1941 sulfathiazole disaster and the birth of good manufacturing practices," *PH* 40 (1999): 16–25.

27. "Sulfanilamide—a warning" (editorial), *JAMA* 109 (October 2, 1937): 1128; Thomas Parran, "Sulfanilamide—a responsibility of the pharmacist," *MR* 49 (1) (January 1940): 12–13.

28. Robert H. Moser, editor, *Diseases of Medical Progress: A Contemporary Analysis of Illness Produced by Drugs and Other Therapeutic Procedures*, 2nd ed. (Springfield, IL: Charles C. Thomas, 1964; 1st ed. 1959), xi, xviii.

29. Dowling, *Fighting Infection* (note 3), 241–244; Allan M. Brandt, *No Magic Bullet: A Social History of Venereal Disease in the United States Since 1880*, expanded ed. (New York: Oxford University Press, 1987), 161–182. One disorder that owed part of its increasing visibility to control of infectious diseases first by sulfa drugs, then by antibiotics, was sickle cell anemia. See Keith Wailoo, *Dying in the City of the Blues: Sickle Cell Anemia and the Politics of Race and Health* (Chapel Hill, NC: University of North Carolina Press, 2001), 9, 103–104, 115–116.

30. See chapter 10, and Walter T. Goodale and Louis Schwab, "Factors in the resistance of gonorrhea to sulfonamides," *Journal of Clinical Investigation* 23 (1944): 217–223; Maxwell Finland, "Emergence of antibiotic-resistant bacteria," *NEJM* 253 (1955): 909–922, 967–979, 1019–1028; Finland, "Changing patterns of susceptibility" (note 1); and Wesley W. Spink, *Infectious Diseases* (note 17), 86–87, 442–443.

31. Finland, "Emergence of antibiotic-resistant bacteria" (note 30).

32. Finland, "Changing patterns of susceptibility" (note 1), 1009–1010, 1021; Theodore C. Eickhoff and Maxwell Finland, "Changing susceptibility of meningococci to antimicrobial agents," *NEJM* 272 (1965): 395–398; Lepow and Gold, "Further conquest of the meningococcus" (note 17), 721–722.

33. Finland, "Changing patterns of susceptibility" (note 1), 1033. On misuse and overuse of antibiotics, see also James C. Whorton, " 'Antibiotic abandon': the resurgence of therapeutic rationalism," in John Parascandola, editor, *The History of Antibiotics: A Symposium* (Madison, WI: American Institute of the History of Pharmacy, 1980), 125–136.

34. Ronald Hare, *Pomp and Pestilence: Infectious Disease, Its Origins and Conquest* (New York: Philosophical Library Inc., 1955), 9–10.

35. René Dubos, *The Dreams of Reason: Science and Utopias* (New York: Columbia University Press, 1961), esp. 1–39 (quotes on 38–39), 63–98. On Dubos, see Carol L. Moberg and Zanvil A. Cohen, editors, *Launching the Antibiotic Era: Personal Accounts of*

the *Discovery and Use of the First Antibiotics* (New York: Rockefeller University Press, 1990), esp. 1–18, 69–97 (contributions by Rollin D. Hotchkiss, Bernard D. Davis, and Carol L. Moberg). Dubos's views on the persistence of disease have been seconded by Gerald N. Grob—see *The Deadly Truth* (note 3), 271–275.

36. Dubos, *The Dreams of Reason* (note 35), 69–97 (quote on 84).

37. Thomas P. Hughes, "The industrial revolution that never came," *American Heritage of Invention and Technology* 3(3) (1988): 58–64; and Hughes, *American Genesis: A Century of Invention and Technological Enthusiasm 1870–1970* (New York: Penguin Books, 1989).

38. Hughes, *American Genesis* (note 37), 443–472.

39. Walter Modell, "Hazards of new drugs," *Science* 139 (March 22, 1963): 1180–1185 (quotes on 1185).

40. Colin Dollery, *The End of an Age of Optimism: Medical Science in Retrospect and Prospect* (London: Nuffield Provincial Hospitals Trust, 1978), esp. 1–5, 87–92 (quotes on 1, 2, 87). John C. Burnham identifies a reaction to inflated expectations of medicine and physicians as a contributor to rising criticism of the U.S. medical profession. See Burnham, "American medicine's golden age: what happened to it?" (note 12).

41. Richard M. Weinshilboum, "The therapeutic revolution," *Clinical Pharmacology and Therapeutics* 42 (1987): 481–484.

42. Charles E. Rosenberg, "Holism in twentieth-century medicine," in Christopher Lawrence and George Weisz, editors, *Greater Than the Parts: Holism in Biomedicine, 1920–1950* (New York: Oxford University Press, 1998), 335–355, esp. 346–348.

43. Weinshilboum, "The therapeutic revolution" (note 38), 482. For more general discussions of the relationships of pharmaceuticals and the pharmaceutical industry to biomedical knowledge, see Alfred Goodman, "The contribution of pharmacodynamics and pharmacology to basic physiological thought," in Chandler M. Brooks and Paul Cranefield, editors, *The Historical Development of Physiological Thought* (New York: Hafner Pub. Co., 1959), 335–349; Ernst Chain, "Academic and industrial contributions to drug research," *Nature* 200 (1963): 441–451; and Jordan Goodman, "Can it ever be pure science? Pharmaceuticals, the pharmaceutical industry and biomedical research in the twentieth century," in Jean-Paul Gaudillière and Ilana Löwy, editors, *The Invisible Industrialist: Manufactures and the Production of Scientific Knowledge* (New York: St. Martins Press, Inc., 1998), 143–165.

44. Marcel H. Bickel, "Eli K. Marshall, Jr. (1889–1966): from biochemistry and physiology to pharmacology and pharmaco-kinetics," *Drug Metabolism Reviews* 28(3) (1996): 311–344, on 320–321. On sulfaguanidine in World War II, see chapter 10.

45. Weinshilboum, "The therapeutic revolution" (note 41), 483; Bickel, "Eli K. Marshall, Jr." (note 44), 324–325, 336; and A. McGehee Harvey, "The story of chemotherapy at Johns Hopkins: Perrin H. Long, Eleanor A. Bliss, and E. Kennerly Marshall, Jr.," *The Johns Hopkins Medical Journal* 138 (1976): 54–60, on 59.

46. Bickel, "The development of sulfonamides" (note 20), 80; and Bernard D. Davis, "New biologic concepts derived from research on sulfonamide drugs," *NEJM* 230 (1944): 734–739.

47. Dowling, *Fighting Infection* (note 3), 159–160.

48. On antimetabolite theory and its extensions, see chapter 11; Weinshilboum, "The therapeutic revolution" (note 38), 482–483; Bickel, "The development of sulfonamides" (note 22), 76, 80–81; and George H. Hitchings, "A biochemical approach to chemotherapy," *Drug Intelligence and Clinical Pharmacy* 16 (1982): 843–848.

49. Roblin, "Chemotherapy" (note 24), 154. See also Roy Waldo Miner, editor, *"6-Mercaptopurine," Annals of the New York Academy of Sciences* 60 (December 6, 1954): 183–508 (on 251, 298).

50. On links between cancer chemotherapy research programs and earlier antimicrobial chemotherapy, see chapter 11, and R.F. Bud, "Strategy in American cancer research after World War II: a case study," *Social Studies of Science* 8 (1978): 425–459, esp. 439–447; John Laszlo, *The Cure of Childhood Leukemia: Into the Age of Miracles* (New Brunswick, NJ: Rutgers University Press, 1995), 47–48, 60, 65–66, 97–98; and Peter Keating and Alberto Cambrosio, "From screening to clinical research: the cure of leukemia and the early development of the cooperative oncology groups, 1955–1966," *BHM* 76 (2002): 299–334.

51. For general discussion and overview of these developments, see Max Tishler, "Molecular modification in drug research," paper presented at the Symposium on Influence of Molecular Modification in Drug Design, Division of Medical Chemistry, American Chemical Society, September 9, 1963, MA, box R4-1.8.5; Tishler, "Perspectives in pharmaceutical research," *TVF* 36 (1965): 37–47 (my copy is from MA, box R4-1.8.5); and Robert G. Denkewalter and Max Tishler, "Drug research—whence and whither," *Fortschritte der Arzeimittelforschung* (*Progress in Drug Research, Progrès des recherches pharmaceutiques*) 10 (1966): 11–31, esp. 16–19.

52. Walsh McDermott, "The story of INH," *Journal of Infectious Diseases* 119 (1969): 678–685; H. Corwin Hinshaw and Walsh McDermott, "Thiosemicarbazone therapy of tuberculosis in humans," *American Review of Tuberculosis* 61 (1950): 145–157; Dowling, *Fighting Infection* (note 3), 167–171. For a more detailed discussion of the chemistry involved, see R. Slack and A.W. Nineham, *Medical and Veterinary Chemicals* (Oxford: Pergamon Press, 1968), 68–80, esp. 71–75.

53. John Parascandola, "Miracle at Carville: the introduction of the sulfones for the treatment of leprosy," *PH* 40 (1998): 59–66; Tishler, "Molecular modification in drug research" (note 47), 9–10.

54. C.G. Mackenzie and Julia B. Mackenzie, "Effect of sulfonamides and thioureas on the thyroid gland and basal metabolism," *Endocrinology* 32 (1943): 185–209; Davis, "New biologic concepts derived from research on sulfonamide drugs" (note 46), 738; Roblin, "Chemotherapy" (note 24), 161–162; and Harold N. Wright and Mildred Montag, *A Textbook of Pharmacology and Therapeutics*, 7th ed. (Philadelphia, PA: W.B. Saunders Co., 1959), 391–392.

55. Auguste Loubatières, "The discovery of hypoglycemic sulfonamides and particularly of their action mechanism," *Acta Diabetologica Latina* 6 (suppl. 1, 1969), 20–56, on 21–22.

56. Ibid., 24–32.

57. Ibid., 41–45.

58. Ibid., 45–46; Tishler, "Molecular modification in modern drug research" (note 51), 13–14; Tishler, "Perspectives in pharmaceutical chemistry," lecture given April 29, 1964, MA, box R4-1.8.5, 32-pp. typescript, on pp. 14–16; Tishler, "Perspectives in pharmaceutical research" (note 51), 40–41; Wright and Montag, *A Textbook of Pharmacology and Therapeutics* (note 50), 387; and Mann, *Modern Drug Use* (note 1), 557. In the 1960s, tolbutamide was the subject of a major clinical study, the University Group Diabetes Program, funded by the National Institutes of Health, and concerns about its safety emerging from this study occasioned a protracted controversy about the merits of oral hypoglycemic drugs and the methods of clinical evaluation. See Marks, *The Progress of Experiment* (note 25), 197–228.

59. "Backgrounder 4. Merck Research" (n.d., but probably 1958 or 1959), MA, box R7-4.8.1; Karl H. Beyer, Jr., "The renal program: some lessons in research," Gairdner Foundation Award lecture, December 5, 1964, MA, box R4-1.6.2, pp. 2–3; Beyer, "A career or two," MA, box R4-1.6.1, pp. 12–13.

60. Beyer, "The renal program: some lessons in research" (note 59), 2–4; Beyer, "A career or two" (note 59), 13–15.

61. "Backgrounder 4. Merck Research" (note 59); Beyer, "The renal program: some lessons in research" (note 59), 4–8; Beyer; "A career or two" (note 59), 15–16; Tishler, "Molecular modification in modern drug research" (note 51), 11–12; and Tishler, "Perspectives in pharmaceutical research" (note 51), 39.

62. Robert M. Kaiser, "The introduction of the thiazides: a case study in twentieth-century therapeutics," in Gregory J. Higby and Elaine C. Stroud, editors, *The Inside Story of Medicines: A Symposium* (Madison, WI: American Institute of the History of Pharmacy, 1997), 121–137, on 124–126; Tishler, "Perspectives in pharmaceutical research" (note 51), 39–40; Karl H. Beyer, Jr., interview conducted by Leon Gortler and Jeffrey Sturchio, April 16, 1988, MA, box 2-6.9.2, p. 34; and James M. Sprague, interview conducted by Leon Gortler, May 23, 1990, MA, box R2-5.1.1, pp. 25–26.

63. Beyer interview (note 62), 34; Sprague interview (note 62), 26–27.

64. Kaiser, "The introduction of the thiazides" (note 62), 125–126; Tishler, "Perspectives in pharmaceutical research" (note 51), 40; Beyer interview (note 62), 34; Sprague interview (note 62), 28–31; and John E. Baer, Karl H. Beyer, Jr., Frederick C. Novello, and James M. Sprague, "The thiazide story: where biology and chemistry meet," 19-pp. typescript and bibliography dated November 14, 1975, MA, box R4-1.6.2, pp. 13–15.

65. Kaiser, "The introduction of the thiazides" (note 62), 126–133; Tishler, "Perspectives in pharmaceutical research" (note 51), 40; and Peter W. Feit, "Bumetanide," in Jasjit S. Bindra and Daniel Lednicer, editors, *Chronicles of Drug Discovery*, vol. 1 (New York: John Wiley & Sons, 1982), 133–148, on 133–136. On the introduction of Diuril, see also Jeremy A. Greene, "Releasing the flood waters: Diuril and the reshaping of hypertension," *BHM* 79 (2005): 749–794.

66. Max Tishler, interview conducted by Leon Gortler, July 13, 1988, MA, box R2-5.2.1; and "Today's theory for tomorrow's therapy," *Medical World News* 6(22) (June 11, 1965): 37–48, 84–86, on 46.

67. "Asulox herbicide (active ingredient Asulam)," product description (May & Baker, June 1980), p. 2; R.W.E. Ball, Helen J. Cottrell, and B.J. Heywood, "Benzene-sulphonylcarbamate herbicides," in *2me symposium sur les nouveaux herbicides* (Organisé par le European Weed Research Council en liaison avec le Comité francais de Lutte contre les Mauvaises Herbes, Paris: Éditions Essor, 1965), 55–68, on 55–56; J.F. Hodgson, personal communication, February 11, 1994; E.W. Parnell, personal communication, June 24, 1994.

68. Tishler, "Perspectives in pharmaceutical research" (note 51), 38–39; Tishler, "Molecular modification in modern drug research" (note 51), 8.

69. Thomas P. Hughes, "The evolution of large technological systems," in Wiebe E. Bijker, Thomas P. Hughes, and Trevor Pinch, editors, *The Social Construction of Technological Systems* (Cambridge, MA: MIT Press, 1987), 51–82, on 57–62; and Ulrich Marsch, "Transferring strategy and structure: the German chemical industry as an exemplar for Great Britain," in John E. Lesch, editor, *The German Chemical Industry in the Twentieth Century* (Dordrecht: Kluwer Academic Publishers, 2000), 217–241, on 238.

70. Gerhard Domagk to Direktion der I.G. Farbenindustrie A.G. Wuppertal-Elberfeld, December 21, 1945; Domagk to Dr. Brüggemann, June 19, 1946; memo of discussion between Professor Domagk, Dr. Haberland, and Dr. Brüggemann, July 16, 1946; and Domagk to Direktion der I.G. Farbenindustrie, September 20, 1946; all in BA, file GD. For Mietzsch, see Fritz Mietzsch to Gerhard Domagk, July 13, 1953, BA, file GD; Fritz Mietzsch, "Neuere Entwicklung der synthetischen Chemotherapeutika," *Österreichische*

Chemiker-Zeitung 53 (1952): 178–187; Mietzsch, "Entwicklungslinien der Chemotherapie (Vom chemischen Standpunkt gesehen)," *KW* 29 (1951): 125–134; Mietzsch, "Chemie und wirtschaftliche Bedeutung der Sulfonamide," *Arbeitsgemeinschaft für Forschung des Landes Nordrhein-Westfalen* 31 (1954): 7–32; and Mietzsch, "Beiträge zur Entwicklung der Chemotherapie aus den Laboratorien der Farbenfabriken Bayer," *Arzneimittel-Forschung* (September 1956): 503–508.

71. Paul György, affidavit dated July 9, 1947, submitted as testimonial evidence for the Nuremberg trials, BA, Personalia, H. Hörlein, 271/2.

72. On Merck, and on cycles in pharmaceutical research and development, see Galambos and Sewell, *Networks of Innovation* (note 17), esp. 29–32, 35–39, 41–43, 120–126, and 241–249.

73. On Prontosil, see chapter 3. On sulfapyridine, see chapter 7. On the characteristics and virtues of the screening method, see also Roblin, "Chemotherapy" (note 24), 162–163.

74. Roblin, "Chemotherapy" (note 22), 163. On the antimetabolite concept, see chapter 11.

75. Alfred Gilman, "The contribution of pharmacodynamics and pharmacology to basic physiological thought," in Chandler M. Brooks and Paul F. Cranefield, editors, *The Historical Development of Physiological Thought* (New York: Hafner Publishing Co., 1959), 335–349; Denkewalter and Tishler, "Drug research-whence and whither" (note 47), 17–19; "Preface," in Jasjit S. Bindra and Daniel Lednicer, editors, *Chronicles of Drug Discovery*, vol. 1 (New York: John Wiley & Sons, 1982), vii–viii; and M.A. McKinlay and M.G. Rossmann, "Rational design of antiviral agents," *Annual Review of Pharmacology and Toxicology* 29 (1989): 111–122.

76. On Fourneau and Dale, see chapter 6. On May & Baker, see chapter 7. On Young, see chapter 1.

77. See chapter 8.

78. On the United States, see Balis, *Miracle Medicine* (note 4), 27–75. On Britain, see Judy Slinn, "Research and development in the UK pharmaceutical industry from the nineteenth century to the 1960s," in Roy Porter and Mikulás Teich, editors, *Drugs and Narcotics in History* (Cambridge: Cambridge University Press, 1995), 168–186. On France, see chapter 6. On Hörlein and I.G. Farben pharmaceutical research during the Third Reich, see chapters 4 and 5. On the international pharmaceutical industry, see "The nature of the pharmaceutical industry," in Slack and Nineham, *Medical and Veterinary Chemicals* (note 52), 3–29, esp. 9–10.

79. Slack and Nineham, *Medical and Veterinary Chemicals* (note 52), 10.

80. Ibid., 49. In 1952, sales of sulfonamides ranked fifth after antibiotics, vitamins, endocrines, and botanicals and represented a dollar equivalent of sixteen percent of antibiotic sales. John F. Bohmfalk, "Markets for pharmaceuticals," *Chemical and Engineering News* (November 30, 1953): 5006–5012.

Index